TEACHING MEDICAL PROFESSIONALISM

Until recently, professionalism was transmitted by respected role models, a method that depended heavily on the presence of a homogeneous society sharing values. This is no longer true, and medical schools and postgraduate training programs in the developed world are now actively teaching professionalism. In addition, licensing and certifying bodies are attempting to assess the professionalism of practicing physicians on an ongoing basis.

This is the only book available to provide guidance to those designing and implementing programs on teaching professionalism. It outlines the cognitive base of professionalism, provides a theoretical basis for teaching the subject, gives general principles for establishing programs at various levels (undergraduate, postgraduate, and continuing professional development), and documents the experience of institutions that are leaders in the field. Teaching aids that have been used successfully by contributors are included as an appendix.

Richard L. Cruess, M.D., is Professor of Orthopedic Surgery and a Member of the Centre for Medical Education at McGill University. He served as Chair of Orthopedics (1976–1981) and was Dean of the Faculty of Medicine at McGill University from 1981 to 1995. He was President of the Canadian Orthopedic Association (1977–1978), the American Orthopedic Research Society (1975–1976), and the Association of Canadian Medical Colleges (1992–1994). He is an Officer of The Order of Canada and of L'Ordre National du Québec.

Sylvia R. Cruess, M.D., is Professor of Medicine and a Member of the Centre for Medical Education at McGill University. She previously served as Director of the Metabolic Day Centre (1968–1978) and as Director of Professional Services (Medical Director) of the Royal Victoria Hospital (1978–1995) in Montreal.

Since 1995, Drs. Richard and Sylvia Cruess have taught and carried out independent research on professionalism in medicine. They have published widely on the subject and have been invited to speak at universities, hospitals, and professional organizations throughout the world.

Yvonne Steinert, Ph.D., a clinical psychologist, is a Professor of Family Medicine, Associate Dean for Faculty Development, and the Director of the Centre for Medical Education at McGill University. Dr. Steinert is actively involved in curriculum development at the undergraduate and postgraduate levels, the design and delivery of faculty development programs and activities, and research in medical education. A past President of the Canadian Association for Medical Education (2006–2008), she has published extensively in the area of faculty development and medical education and is frequently invited to present at national and international meetings.

Teaching Medical Professionalism

Edited by

Richard L. Cruess
McGill University
Montreal, Quebec

Sylvia R. Cruess
McGill University
Montreal, Quebec

Yvonne Steinert
McGill University
Montreal, Quebec

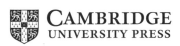
CAMBRIDGE
UNIVERSITY PRESS

CAMBRIDGE UNIVERSITY PRESS
Cambridge, New York, Melbourne, Madrid, Cape Town, Singapore, São Paulo, Delhi

Cambridge University Press
32 Avenue of the Americas, New York, NY 10013-2473, USA

www.cambridge.org
Information on this title: www.cambridge.org/9780521707428

First published 2009

Printed in the United States of America

A catalog record for this publication is available from the British Library.

Library of Congress Cataloging in Publication Data

Teaching medical professionalism / edited by Richard L. Cruess, Sylvia R. Cruess, Yvonne Steinert.
    p. ; cm.
    Includes bibliographical references and index.
    ISBN 978-0-521-88104-3 (hardback) – ISBN 978-0-521-70742-8 (paperback)
    1. Medical education. 2. Physicians–Professional ethics–Study and teaching. I. Cruess, Richard L. II.
Cruess, Sylvia R. (Sylvia Robinson). III. Steinert, Yvonne. IV. Title.
    [DNLM: 1. Professional Competence. 2. Education, Medical. 3. Physician's Role. W 21 T253 2008]
    R737.T38 2008
    610–dc22   2008025429

ISBN 978-0-521-88104-3 hardback
ISBN 978-0-521-70742-8 paperback

Contents

List of Contributors

Louise Arnold, Ph.D.
Professor and Associate Dean for Medical
 Education
University of Missouri–Kansas City School of
 Medicine, Kansas City, Missouri

Linda L. Blank
Vice President, The Culliton Group
 Washington, DC
Robert G. Petersdorf Scholar (2005–2007)
Association of American Medical Colleges
Washington, DC

Jordan J. Cohen, M.D.
President Emeritus
Association of American Medical Colleges
Professor of Medicine and Public Health
George Washington University
Washington, DC

Ann H. Cottingham, M.A.R.
Director of Special Programs
Medical Education and Curricular Affairs
Indiana University School of Medicine
Indianapolis, Indiana

Richard L. Cruess, M.D.
Professor of Surgery
Member, Center for Medical Education
Former Dean of Medicine
McGill University, Montreal, Quebec

Sylvia R. Cruess, M.D.
Professor of Medicine
Member, Center for Medical Education
 McGill University

Former Director of Professional Services
Royal Victoria Hospital, Montreal, Quebec

**Dave Davis, M.D., C.C.F.P., F.C.F.P.,
 F.R.C.P.C. (hon.)**
Vice President, Continuing Health Care
 Education and Improvement
Association of American Medical Colleges
Washington, DC
Adjunct Professor, Family and Community
 Medicine, and Health Policy, Management
 and Evaluation
University of Toronto, Toronto, Ontario

Richard M. Frankel, Ph.D.
Professor of Medicine and Geriatrics
Senior Research Scientist
Regenstrief Institute
Indiana University School of Medicine
Research Sociologist
Center on Implementing Evidence Based
 Practice
Richard L. Roudebush Veteran's
 Administration Medical Center
Indianapolis, Indiana

Erika Goldstein, M.D., M.P.H.
Professor, Internal Medicine
Director UWSOM Colleges Program
University of Washington School of Medicine
Seattle, Washington

Frederic William Hafferty, Ph.D.
Professor, Department of Behavioral Sciences
University of Minnesota Medical School
Duluth, Minnesota

Thomas S. Inui, Sc.M., M.D.
President and CEO, Regenstrief Institute
Sam Regenstrief Professor of Health Services
  Research
Associate Dean for Health Care Research, and
  Professor of Medicine
Indiana University School of Medicine
Indianapolis, Indiana

**Sir Donald Irvine, C.B.E., M.D., F.R.C.G.P.,
  F.Med.Sci.**
Chairman, Picker Institute Europe
Former President, UK General Medical Council

**Sharon Johnston, B.A. (gov.), B.A. (law),
  L.L.M., M.D.**
Assistant Professor
Department of Family Medicine
University of Ottawa
CT Lamont Primary Health Care Research
  Centre, Élisabeth Bruyère Research Institute
Ottawa, Ontario

David C. Leach, M.D.
CEO (retired), Accreditation Council for
  Graduate Medical Education
Chicago, Illinois

Debra K. Litzelman, M.A., M.D.
Associate Dean for Medical Education and
  Curricular Affairs
Richard Powell Professor of Medicine
Indiana University School of Medicine
Indianapolis, Indiana

**Gillian Maudsley, M.B.Ch.B., M.P.H. (dist.),
  Med. (dist.), M.D.**
Clinical Senior Lecturer in Public Health
  Medicine
Division of Public Health, School of
  Population, Community, and Behavioural
  Sciences, The University of Liverpool
Liverpool, UK

Mark A. Peacock, M.Ed.
Learning Solutions d'Apprentissage
Chelsea, Quebec

Linda Snell, M.D.
Professor of Medicine
McGill University

Associate Physician in Chief
McGill University Health Center
Member, Center for Medical Education
McGill University
Montreal, Quebec

Yvonne Steinert, Ph.D.
Professor of Family Medicine
Associate Dean for Faculty Development
Director, Center for Medical Education
McGill University
Montreal, Quebec

Anthony L. Suchman, M.D., M.A.
Senior Consultant
Relationship Centered Health Care
Clinical Professor of Medicine and Psychiatry
University of Rochester School of Medicine
  and Dentistry
Rochester, New York

Christine Sullivan, M.D., F.A.C.E.P.
Assistant Professor
Residency Program Director
Department of Emergency Medicine
University of Missouri–Kansas City School of
  Medicine, Truman Medical Center
Kansas City, Missouri

William M. Sullivan, Ph.D.
Senior Scholar
Carnegie Foundation for the Advancement of
  Teaching
Palo Alto, California

**The Reverend David C.M. Taylor, B.Sc., Med.,
  Ph.D.**
Deputy Director of Medical Studies (Quality,
  Assessment, and Research)
School of Medical Education
The University of Liverpool
Liverpool, UK

Penelope R. Williamson, Sc.D.
Senior Consultant
Relationship Centered Health Care
Associate Professor of Medicine
The Johns Hopkins University School of
  Medicine
Baltimore, Maryland

Teaching Medical Professionalism

William M. Sullivan, Ph.D.

This is a pioneering book. It brings together leading figures in both the theory and the practice of teaching professionalism in medicine. The volume's chapters provide a thorough and useful guide to one of the most important topics in medical education today: how to ensure that future physicians can meet the increased expectations the public now places on medicine. The key to securing medicine's future, the authors of the volume argue, lies in understanding, transmitting, and enhancing medical professionalism.

The public wants both better medical care and a profession more responsive to its needs. But most of all, people want competent and caring physicians who are committed to the healing of their patients. Nearly all of us will be patients. We will be vulnerable and in need of medical expertise. We will want the best prepared and most knowledgeable doctors we can find. But more than that, we will need to be able to trust that our physicians will be dedicated above all else to care for us with all their ability.

ADDRESSING THREATS TO THE INTEGRITY OF THE PRACTICE OF MEDICINE

Medicine as a profession is defined by its blending of expertise in healing with responsibility for patient care. Teaching professionalism, as the authors present it, directly addresses the formation of physicians who manifest this needed integration of expertise with dedication to the care of patients. They write this in full knowledge that medicine's integrity has for some time been under threat. Those threats to the integrity of medical practice are two. One stems from the success of the new technological medicine itself. Advances in biological science and technology are steadily transforming medical care for the better. However, they have also strengthened the false idea that medicine is simply an application of scientific knowledge rather than a complex and artful sociobiological practice. The other threat is embodied in the largely well-intentioned efforts to make medicine safer, more predictable, and more efficient through applying techniques of financial and organizational management.

Both these developments, the misunderstanding of medicine as either applied technology, on the one hand, or as the delivery of standardized services, on the other, reduce medicine to a too limited perspective. Each fails to recognize that medicine is a complex practice defined by its own goals and internal values of competence and dedication. Indeed, the idea of professionalism has come to stand for recovery of the full dimensions of the practice of medicine. Medicine's purpose is to maintain and develop medical art in the service of patient care. Achieving these aims depends upon physicians' orientation and commitment to these purposes in their daily work. And the individual physician's understanding and dedication themselves depend importantly upon the vitality and intensity with which the community of practitioners supports practices with these ends.

Biomedical research and managerial technique can be valuable assets in society's quest for better health care, but they can contribute most by enriching and extending the forms of medical practice. They cannot by themselves substitute for the expertise and orientation to service cultivated within the professional community. Medical practice, in other words, has an integrity, even a wisdom, that needs to be understood, assessed, and enhanced, not supplanted.

PROFESSIONALISM AS A FRAMEWORK
FOR PREPARING PHYSICIANS

In their practice, physicians employ their expertise in the service of patients' healing and society's health. Within their relationships with patients, physicians can find a unique fulfillment through employing their capacities in resourceful, caring, and creative ways. This is the promise of medicine as a vocation. But to practice medicine means joining a professional community as well as deploying the art of healing. The fulfillment of medicine's promise depends upon sustaining the confidence of individual patients and also the trust of the larger society the profession is pledged to serve.

As the editors, Sylvia and Richard Cruess and Yvonne Steinert emphasize, there is an implicit but vital contract between medicine and the larger society, a compact according to which the profession is granted discretion and self-regulation in exchange for service and high standards of care. For both patients and physicians, however, the promise can only be redeemed when it is well understood and shapes the whole orientation of physicians in their development as professionals. Ensuring that this happens is the task of teaching medical professionalism.

As the authors in this volume demonstrate, teaching professionalism is not so much a particular segment of the medical curriculum as a defining dimension of medical education as a whole. Professionalism provides an angle of approach to the whole trajectory of formation in the practice of medicine, from beginning student through continuing professional development. The peculiar intensity of medical education ensures that it is deeply formative. As Frederic Hafferty shows in his contribution, the implications of the formative intensity of medical education are still not fully understood by all medical educators. This is an important issue, Hafferty argues, because effective educational interventions to strengthen professionalism will not succeed until the inconsistencies in existing practice are more clearly understood and addressed.

The positive aspect of recognizing the formative nature of medical preparation is the opportunity it presents to medical educators to become more self-aware and intentional about how future physicians actually develop. A formative perspective further suggests ways in which medical students and residents might be enabled to become more self-aware in developing their own expertise and dedication at each stage in their professional training. A professionalism curriculum is intended to place the values of medical practice at the center of all phases of medical training so that the defining aims and shaping experiences of the profession become a primary focus of attention and standard of assessment in the student's progress toward taking up the life of a physician.

PROFESSIONALISM ACROSS THE CONTINUUM OF MEDICAL EDUCATION

The great challenge confronting medical education is to provide a sense of overall direction and continuity across a long trajectory of preparation. The arc of development from the beginning of medical school to advanced residency spans a very long and exceptionally complicated educational process. Future physicians begin their training in school-like settings in which they are often encouraged to continue the role and thinking of students. There, they are mostly concerned with solving well-structured problems by learning and applying routine techniques. As their education progresses, however, they must gradually replace that familiar stance by learning to think and act in clinical settings as a novice and then a more experienced practitioner. As clinicians, future physicians must learn to configure their knowledge to define problems in context in order to meet novel challenges, becoming ever more authentically engaged with the practice of medicine in its multiple dimensions.

This path of development is not a one-directional movement from simple to complex but a series of iterations, a growing sophistication in understanding the overall sense and goal of the medical arts. Professionalism provides a continuing thread by which to remind students of the basic continuity of aim that unites the disparate domains of theory, practice, setting, and forms of teaching and learning they encounter. A number of authors in this volume draw upon the rich literature of learning theory in order to address ways of ensuring progress in fostering an integrated and integrating professional stance throughout the movement from student to advanced resident and beyond. In different ways, the authors develop recent insights into the cultivation of expertise in order to form a professional identity as a physician.

Learning theorists argue that expertise is best developed through learning by doing. Learning by doing is always to some degree formative, but it is not necessarily self-consciously so. This requires that the instructor communicate as clearly as possible the aims as well as the content that is taught. Effective learning requires practice, response to feedback on that practice, and recurrent attention to the goals as well as the actions and understandings that constitute the practice being learned. Assessment is critical to this process since what is assessed communicates to learners what is important about the subject and how it is to be engaged.

Such pedagogy shapes the perception, imagination, and deportment of anyone who undergoes it. However, unless it also contains a reflexive dimension, unless it is intentionally aimed at affecting the learner (or is so appropriated by the learner) – as in encouraging learning to learn, or taking responsibility for one's own development – it can remain less than fully effective. Formative teaching, however, enables students to grow in a very concrete sense: they acquire abilities but also sensibilities that expand their repertoire beyond what that had been previously. Such education thereby influences individuals' sense of what is possible and worth doing and of who they are and might become. This is perhaps especially so with regard to learning something as complex and integrative as professionalism.

The principles and examples presented in *Teaching Medical Professionalism* develop these themes for the variety of stages and settings of preparing doctors. Gillian Maudsley and David Taylor explain how professionalism fits into a problem-based curriculum, while Erika Goldstein shows how it can be integrated with an organ system–based approach. Both approaches emphasize explicit goal setting, early involvement of students in basic elements of clinical practice, and effective assessment. Continuing that theme, Christine

Sullivan and Louise Arnold provide an overview of how to make assessment effective in the professionalism curriculum. Addressing the other end of the educational trajectory, David Leach presents principles that motivate the ACGME's performance-based standards for professionalism. Thomas Inui and his colleagues extend these concerns beyond the curriculum into an analysis of how the institutional settings must be structured, or restructured, in order to support the development of professionalism considered as an essential element of medical expertise.

PUTTING THE PRACTICE AT THE CENTER

A striking feature of *Teaching Medical Professionalism* is that it reveals how teaching professionalism reflects and maps onto the challenge of initiating students into the practice of medicine itself. The heart of medical practice – and training – is a distinctive way of thinking that focuses upon the unfolding of patient's experience with health and illness. Medicine makes sense of disease by understanding patients' experience against the background of biomedical science and clinical procedures. This is conveyed through the device of the case narrative.

The case narrative, as Kathryn Montgomery has argued, "is the principal means of thinking and remembering – of *knowing* – in medicine." The case narrative, that is, represents nothing less than "clinical judgment . . . in all its situated and circumstantial uncertainty."[1] It enables practitioners to make sense of the contingent unfolding of the disease or medical situation by setting up a kind of conversation, a back-and-forth, between the patient's particular story with various general, analytical accounts derived from scientific pathophysiology. The crucial point is that case reasoning is not a hold-over from the prescientific past but a representation of clinical judgment itself. This is the foundation of all medical skill. Thus, Montgomery concludes that it is important to recognize – and we might add, to teach – that medicine is more than a science. It is rather a complex practice of healing in which "diagnosis and treatment are intensively science-using activities," though not "in and of themselves, science."[2]

Case-based reasoning is also the focal point of medical training. It is neither classical deduction of particulars from general laws nor the induction of principles from particulars. Instead, case reasoning is a kind of circular or iterative process. In it, doctors form hypotheses about the possible causes of

---

[1] Kathryn Montgomery, *How Doctors Think: Clinical Judgment and the Practice of Medicine* (New York: Oxford University Press, 2006). p. 46.

[2] Ibid. pp. 46 and 52.

a particular patient's situation and then test those possibilities against details revealed by closer examination of the patient. Medical judgment employs analytical, scientific knowledge as well as clinical experience in the service of the interpretive work of isolating probable causes of illness by eliminating alternative possibilities to arrive at a "differential diagnosis."

This procedure moves between generalities of disease, on the one hand, and unfolding of a particular patient's situation. It initiates a back-and-forth dialogue between these two modes of thinking until a judgment is reached as to what is happening to the patient and how to respond to it. It enables practitioners to make sense of the contingent unfolding of a disease or medical situation in its particular context. Clinical medical education works by bringing learners into this conversation, guiding them by modeling, questioning, and mentored practice into the back-and-forth of clinical reasoning, as it moves between the patient's particular story and general analytical knowledge and standard procedures.

If one understands medical practice as case reasoning in this way, the core medical practice and teaching appear well suited to incorporate the themes of medical professionalism. Teaching ways of explicitly attending to the patient's experience and to the social or organizational as well as biological context of the case represent natural developments of the back-and-forth between formal knowledge and developing situation that are the basic features of medical art. Seen in the perspective of case reasoning, the themes of professionalism represent an expansion and deepening of the physician's perception, reasoning, and judgment that are already the center of medical practice and learning. It is to recover the full dimensions of medical practice.

PROFESSIONALISM AS THE INTEGRATION OF APPRENTICESHIP

The expansion of knowledge about learning has put new life into the old metaphor of education as apprenticeship. The key idea, derived from the study of a variety of domains of thought and action, has been the discovery that all learning resembles the development of expertise. When medical educators make key features of expert practice visible and available to novices for appropriation, they are providing students with access to the practices that constitute the profession. By giving learners opportunities to practice approximations to expert performance, and giving these students feedback to help them improve their own performance, educators are providing an apprentice-like experience of the mind, a "cognitive apprenticeship."

Clinical teaching, when well done, already models and promotes the blending of analytical and practical habits of mind that medical practice demands. The contributors to this volume show why and how that complex educational achievement must be carefully nurtured within a growing understanding of self as physician and member of the profession. To hold these several dimensions together in one view – to see medical formation steadily and to see it whole – I want to propose the metaphor of professional education as a three-fold "apprenticeship." This three-fold apprenticeship addresses the key dimensions of understanding, judgment, and responsibility.[3]

The first apprenticeship could be called academic or intellectual, with a focus on the scientific analytical mode of thinking. Its chief focus is understanding and concerns the academic knowledge base of the domain of medicine, including the habits of mind that the faculty judge most important to the profession. The setting is the classroom and the pedagogies employed reinforce the familiar student role, assessing formal knowledge and reasoning through formal testing. Despite its evident removal from the settings of professional practice, this apprenticeship always has high prestige since it links the faculty and the school, and implicitly the whole profession, to those intellectual values that confer legitimacy in the modern university and beyond.

The students' second apprenticeship emphasizes the cultivation of judgment. Here, the student "apprentices" to the often tacit body of skills shared by competent practitioners. Students encounter this skills-based kind of learning through quite different pedagogies, and often from different faculty members, from those through which they are introduced to the first intellectual apprenticeship. One of the distinctive aspects of the second apprenticeship in medicine is the extensive use of near-peers, resident physicians, who play an important role as teachers of students and transmitters of professional values as well as practices. Here, the learner must take up the stance of an apprentice to the practice, gradually growing into taking responsibility for the outcomes of their interventions with patients.

The third apprenticeship introduces students to the values and dispositions shared by the professional community. It is in this dimension of professional education that the acceptance of responsibility presents the chief formative challenge. It is this dimension of medical education that brings professionalism to the explicit awareness of students and educators alike. Like the second, this apprenticeship is also often taught through dramatic

---

[3] In this, I am drawing upon work in which I have been engaged at the Carnegie Foundation for the Advancement of Teaching, a comparative study of professional preparation across five fields: law, engineering, the clergy, nursing, and medicine. I have sketched an overview of the approach in William M. Sullivan, *Work and Integrity: The Crisis and Promise of Professionalism in America*, 2nd edition (San Francisco: Jossey-Bass Publisher, 2005).

pedagogies of participation. Traditional apprenticeship emphasizes the transmission of expert knowledge through face-to-face contact. When it is employed in today's professional training, especially in situations in which practitioners rather than pure academics do the teaching, apprenticeship often reveals these ancient roots. In a famous study of surgical residency in a high-technology medical center, Charles Bosk reported that students were rarely washed out for errors of skill alone. They were dismissed when their mentors judged that they lacked the proper character for surgery, especially qualities of dedication, interest, and thoroughness.[4]

To be a professional in the full sense is to understand oneself as claimed by a practice that derives its integrity from service to others. Precisely because that purpose is a public one, today's physicians need more than a haphazard understanding of the organizational contexts of medical practice. Understanding alone, however, is not enough. Medical education needs to develop physicians who are not only experts but also citizens, both as contributors to their professional communities and as participants and leaders in addressing the health concerns of the larger society. These are the dimensions of professionalism that need most development. In their contributions to the volume, Donald Irvine and Jordan Cohen with Linda Blank speak from experience of struggling with these issues in the United Kingdom and the United States, respectively. Their chapters propose ways of using professionalism as a focus for strengthening links between the preparation of physicians and accrediting bodies as well as the broad public.

Taken together, the contributors articulate an understanding of formative education that is more than "socialization" seen as molding human clay from without. Rather, their focus on medical professionalism helps us see that the key lies in enabling students to become self-reflective about and self-directing in their own development. Seen from the perspective of professionalism, medical education can provide the richest context possible for students to explore and make their own profession's possibilities for a socially useful and personally fulfilling life.

---

[4] Charles Bosk, *Forgive and Remember: Managing Medical Failure* (Chicago: University of Chicago Press, 1979).

Introduction

Richard L. Cruess, M.D., Sylvia R. Cruess, M.D., and Yvonne Steinert, Ph.D.

The practice of medicine is an art, not a trade; a calling, not a business; a calling in which your heart will be exercised equally with your head.[1]

This book is about education. While the subject is about teaching and learning professionalism, the authors discuss how best to educate the physicians of the future who will be responsible for much of the health and well-being of their fellow citizens. While medical education often appears to have developed in isolation from the formal world of pedagogy, medical students are adult learners and the science of cognition applies to them as it does to other learners. Through the centuries, we have come to understand a great deal about education, but there is still much that we do not know and probably will never fully comprehend. For a period of time, both general and medical education placed great emphasis on the acquisition of knowledge and skills. In our knowledge-based world, this is certainly appropriate, as one cannot function without a minimal level of knowledge. However, recent times have seen a return to an earlier belief that education represents more than facts and figures. It has been said that education is what remains after what has been learned has been forgotten. Michael Polanyi, that wonderful combination of chemist and philosopher, coined the term "tacit knowledge" to help us understand this phenomenon. He stated that "one knows things which one cannot tell."[2] Tacit knowledge is acquired through experiencing a broad spectrum of life's challenges.

The authors who have contributed such rich material to this book have addressed the challenge of teaching and learning professionalism. They and others have uniformly concluded that knowledge and skills remain important but that something much more intangible and difficult to impart is necessary to produce a true professional and that it can no longer remain tacit. Physicians must be able to both "know" professionalism and "tell" what it is.

In recent decades, medicine has lost public trust through a combination of its own failings as a profession and health care systems which often discourage professional behavior. Medicine's fundamental role as healer depends upon patient trust, and its loss must be addressed, as without it healing is impaired. As the profession has attempted to respond and take corrective action in the domain over which it exerts control, two linked areas for action have emerged. It has been concluded that the profession must respond to societal concerns about its own performance, particularly the perception that it is less altruistic than it once was, that it self-regulates poorly, and that it has abused its privileged position in society for financial gain. Individual physicians and medicine's associations and regulatory bodies must react to this reality. Of equal importance, it has been concluded that professionalism as a subject must be addressed directly and explicitly at all levels of medical education. For over 2,000 years, it was not thought necessary to actively teach professionalism. The ideals and values of the profession were transmitted by mentors and role models and were important components of the tacit knowledge base of physicians. This method sufficed because times were simpler and both the profession and the society that it served were relatively homogeneous in most countries, sharing common values. This is no longer true. Medicine and society are wonderfully diverse and health care systems are now part of a global network. The professionalism of yesteryear has difficulty in coping with contemporary funding and regulatory mechanisms and with a society that has also changed profoundly. It is now believed that a professionalism appropriate to the times must be taught explicitly and that this requires decisive action on the part of medicine's educational institutions. We must also pay attention to the environment in which we educate future generations of physicians and remember that, while role models remain central to the process, the role models themselves must understand the professionalism that they are modeling.

It is hoped that this book will be of assistance to those responsible for designing and implementing programs of instruction on professionalism. It should also be of interest to both teachers and learners. While being aimed specifically at the medical community, it should be noted that the terms profession, professional, and professionalism are generic and applicable to other occupations both within and outside the health care field. The authors hope that the chapters in this book will also be of assistance to those responsible for training other members of the health care team with whom future physicians will most certainly interact.

The book discusses many aspects of becoming a professional, including an understanding of the process of socialization that is essential to transmitting the values, attitudes, and behaviors of the profession. An overview of the cognitive base underlying professionalism is provided, as well as a discussion of educational theories and strategies that can underpin our work in this area. A number of chapters examine the special needs of programs at the undergraduate, postgraduate, and continuing professional development levels, as well as the environment in which we teach. The importance of evaluation to teaching and learning professionalism is stressed, as is the necessary link between remediation and evaluation. Faculty development, essential to the success of any program in professionalism, is described in detail, and a template for its implementation is presented. Generational differences, which lead to particular approaches for the teaching and learning of diverse age-groups are examined, together with strategies for bridging generational gaps. The relationship of professionalism with the regulatory and licensing bodies and the importance of enlisting the public in support of medical professionalism, along with methods that might be used, is discussed. This discourse on professionalism ends with a series of chapters illustrating how programs have been and can be established in different curricular designs (organ-based or problem-based) in undergraduate, postgraduate, and continuing professional development settings. The appendix is designed to provide educational resource materials that the authors have found to be helpful in their programs.

It has been an extraordinary experience for the editors to work with such a group of scholarly, creative, and enthusiastic authors known for their individual contributions to the field of medical professionalism. Those who read the book from cover to cover can obtain a comprehensive background for program development and teaching in the field of medical professionalism. However, each chapter can stand alone and be used by readers with specific areas of interest.

The editors would like to thank each and every author for their support, diligence, and commitment to the project as well as for the true excellence of their chapters. We are also grateful to the students and residents of McGill University for teaching us so much about professionalism and to our colleagues at the Centre for Medical Education and in the Faculty of Medicine for their intellectual engagement, honest feedback, and creative suggestions as we have tested our concepts and beliefs.

Finally, we would like to acknowledge the contribution of the McConnell Family Foundation whose generous support both validated the project and made much of the work possible. As well, we would like to thank Cambridge University Press for their patient assistance and especially Beth Barry, without whose enthusiasm and support this book would not have been written.

Elliot Freidson, a distinguished sociologist, believed that professionalism was the "soul" of the practice of medicine.[3] We are sure that each author who has contributed to this book hopes that their efforts help to preserve this soul.

REFERENCES

1. Osler, W. The master word in medicine. In *Aequanimitas, with Other Addresses to Medical Students, Nurses and Practitioners of Medicine*. 3rd ed. Philadelphia, PA: P. Blakiston; 1932.
2. Polanyi, M. *Personal Knowledge: Towards a Post-critical Philosophy*. Chicago: University of Chicago Press; 1958.
3. Freidson, E. *Professionalism: The Third Logic*. Chicago: University of Chicago Press; 2001.

PART ONE

What Is to Be Taught

1 The Cognitive Base of Professionalism

Sylvia R. Cruess, M.D., and Richard L. Cruess, M.D.

As physicians, patients, and members of the general public have come to believe that medicine's professionalism is under threat, virtually all have concluded that any action to address the issue must include a major educational initiative aimed at ensuring that physicians both understand the nature of contemporary medical professionalism and live according to its precepts.[1–6] As a result, there is now a substantial literature containing a variety of opinions as to how this can be best accomplished. One of the common themes that has emerged is that the approaches of the past are no longer sufficient.

For centuries, professionalism as a subject was not addressed directly. There were no courses on professionalism and it was not included in the standard medical curriculum. This is not because it was deemed unimportant. The Hippocratic Oath, subsequent codes of ethics, and a host of writers including Osler addressed the values and beliefs of the medical profession, often linking them to the word professionalism. However, it was assumed that these values and beliefs, which are the foundation of the profession, would be acquired during the process of socialization of students as they "acquire the complex ensemble of analytic thinking, skillful practice, and wise judgment."[5] The learning of professionalism depended heavily upon role models where students, residents, and indeed practicing physicians patterned their behavior on "individuals admired for their ways of being and acting as professionals."[7] While this method remains essential and powerful, by itself it is no longer felt to be adequate.[2,4,6,8–10] There appears to be general agreement among educators that professionalism must be taught and evaluated as a specific topic. Indeed, certifying and accrediting bodies now require it.[11–14] What in the past was largely implicit in medical education must now be made explicit.

For this to occur, it is necessary to define professionalism, not only so that it can be taught but also so that the professionalism of students, residents,

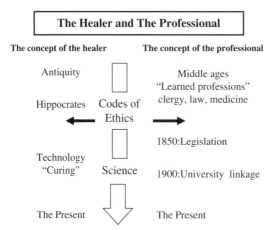

Figure 1.1. The healer and the professional have different origins and have evolved in parallel but separately. As shown on the left, all societies have required the services of healers. The Western tradition of healing began in Hellenic Greece and is the part of the self-image of the medical profession. Curing became possible only with the advent of scientific medicine. The modern professions arose in the guilds and universities of medieval Europe and England. They acquired their present form in the middle of the nineteenth century when licensing laws granted a monopoly over practice to allopathic medicine. When science caused medicine to be more knowledge based, the profession moved closer to universities. Codes of ethics have always guided the behavior of both the healer and the professional, and science empowers both.

and practicing physicians can be evaluated. This chapter will outline the origins and evolution of the modern medical profession, will provide definitions of professionalism and a list of its attributes, and will relate professionalism to medicine's social contract. The objective is to provide information drawn from the literature on professionalism to form a cognitive base for those designing and implementing teaching programs.

HISTORICAL ROOTS

The concept of professionalism has a long history and the word has been in use for at least 2,000 years (Figure 1.1). Its first appearance in connection with medicine has been ascribed to a Roman physician, Scribonius,[15] who defined professionalism as "a commitment to compassion or clemency in the relief of suffering."[16(p29)] He linked it to the act and the tradition of professing inherent in the Hippocratic Oath. This meaning carried forward to the Middle Ages when the learned professions of medicine, law, and the clergy emerged. They arose in their new form from the guilds and universities of Europe and England.[17–20] The professions were given status in society and a considerable degree of autonomy. Medicine, which served a small elite and had minimal curative powers, exerted little impact on the average citizen. In the nineteenth century, science began to transform medicine, making it more effective and therefore worth purchasing, at the same time as the industrial revolution provided sufficient wealth so that patients could pay for health care. Some form of organization of the delivery of medical services was required, and society turned to the pre-existing profession to accomplish this.[1,17,19] Essentially, public policy in health care was built around the concept of the professions. The medical profession was enthusiastically complicit in this endeavor. By the middle of the nineteenth century, in most developed countries physicians had come together to form national professional medical associations and developed codes of ethics governing the behavior of their members. These bodies successfully lobbied governments to establish medical licensure that granted a monopoly over practice to allopathic medicine.[17,19] At this point, the foundations of the present day professions were laid.[17] Contemporary interpretation of these events indicates that the granting of professional status to medicine served then, and continues to serve, as the basis of a social contract between medicine and society.[5,21,22] Under the terms of this contract, medicine is given a monopoly over the use of its knowledge base, considerable autonomy in practice, prestige and status, the privilege of self-regulation, and financial rewards. In return, physicians and the profession are expected to be altruistic, demonstrate honesty and integrity, assure the competence of practitioners, and be devoted to the public good. While the operational details of both professionalism and the social contract have changed as both medicine and society have evolved,[1,3,18–20] the basic "bargain" has not.

THE CHALLENGE OF DEFINING PROFESSIONALISM

Although there is general agreement on the salient features of professionalism,[4,23] it has proven difficult to actually develop definitions of "profession" and the words "professional" and "professionalism" that are derived from it. In part, this stems from the use of the words as if they are interchangeable, which they are not. However, another cause is the difference in the background and approach of those studying all professions, including medicine.[23,24] The largest independent body of literature referring to the professions is found in the social sciences. Sociologists have been studying and writing about the professions for over a century and medicine has figured prominently in this literature. While there are certainly different approaches within the field of sociology, the primary interest is in the organization of society (and of work within society) and the role of the professions in this organization.[23] While sociologists recognize the importance of the doctor-patient relationship, they are much more interested in the interface between the medical profession and the society it serves. The analysis of the medical profession and the accompanying definitions drawn from the sociology literature offer a series of snapshots of this interface over the past 100 years.

To members of the medical profession, the definition must convey something more than the organization of society, important as this may be. Physicians require something that can assist in defining their own identity, establishing the ideology of the profession,[3,5,20,23] and helping to establish the ideals to which they can aspire. Many physicians studying professionalism feel that the emphasis should be on medicine's base in morality and the nature of the doctor-patient relationship is stressed.[25–27] For others, the definition, while in no way diminishing the importance of medicine's moral base, must be broader to include the relationship between medicine and society and the very fundamental obligations derived from this aspect of professionalism.[1,9,28–30]

Those responsible for teaching professionalism must address aspects relating to the relationship of physicians with both patients and society as there are clearly expressed concerns about the performance of individual practitioners and of the profession in both areas.[3,5,25,31,32] These concerns relate to issues of morality, conflicts of interest, the state of the doctor-patient relationship, and self-regulation and to the impact of the health care system on the practice of medicine. For this reason, we believe that any definition of medical professionalism must encompass the approaches found in both the medical and the sociological literature.

There are individuals and organizations that prefer short and succinct definitions including three or four major points.[17,23,33,34] These have the obvious advantage of being simpler and easier to commit to memory. Others feel that the definition must be all inclusive and therefore embrace definitions that are more comprehensive, often including a list of traits or attributes, and are consequently longer.[1,28–30] Either approach is acceptable and can be effective. When short definitions are used, they must subsequently be expanded during the course of teaching as all elements of professionalism must be taught and learned. To leave anything out is to imply that it is not important. Longer definitions are more difficult to remember but can be helpful to guide teaching, having the advantage of including everything.

DEFINITIONS

The literature contains many definitions of profession, professionalism, and medical professionalism. Most are similar and present common concepts because they generally begin with the assumption that the physician is a virtuous person and that the practice of medicine is a moral en-deavor.[4,23,25,26] These concepts can serve as the cognitive base of teaching programs if placed in a proper perspective. Profession, derived from the word "profess," is the etymological root of the frequently used terms professional and professionalism.[35] Profession, professional, and professionalism are generic and their definitions are therefore applicable to the other "status professions" such as law and engineering. For that reason, the word "medical professionalism" has been developed and is frequently used to allow for a definition that is specific to the practice of medicine.

It seems to us preferable to start with a definition of the root word "profession." In recognition of the two different approaches – short and long – we will provide two definitions, either of which can easily serve as the basis of a program to teach and evaluate professionalism in medicine.

Those preferring a short definition that stresses broad categories generally include descriptions of professions as containing common elements; work based on command of a complex body of knowledge, autonomy (sometimes linked to self-regulation), and a service orientation. We would suggest the following, which was developed by Starr in his seminal book, *The Social Transformation of American Medicine*.[17]

> **Profession:** *An occupation that regulates itself through systematic, required training and collegial discipline; that has a base in technical specialized knowledge; and that has a service rather than profit orientation, enshrined in its code of ethics.*[17(p15)]

It must be stressed that if this definition is to be used as the cognitive base for teaching professionalism, the attributes of the profession that are outlined below must also be taught and should be linked to one of the broad principles covered in the definition.

For those who prefer a more complete definition, the following is offered. It is based on that of the *Oxford English Dictionary*[35] to which have been added elements drawn from the medical and social sciences literature that are felt to be fundamental parts of contemporary professionalism. Its disadvantage is its length and complexity but it does contain the major elements that the literature indicates should be included. In addition, it indicates that professional status is granted by society, with the important implication that society can alter the terms should it wish to do so.

> **Profession:** *An occupation whose core element is work based upon the mastery of a complex body of knowledge and skills. It is a vocation in which knowledge of some department of science or learning or the practice of an art founded upon it is used in the service of others. Its members are governed*

by codes of ethics and profess a commitment to competence, integrity and morality, altruism, and the promotion of the public good within their domain. These commitments form the basis of a social contract between a profession and society, which in return grants the profession a monopoly over the use of its knowledge base, the right to considerable autonomy in practice and the privilege of self-regulation. Professions and their members are accountable to those served, to the profession, and to the society.[36]

It should be pointed out that there are other examples of long and short definitions of profession, professionalism, and medical professionalism that are both acceptable and operationally useful (see Appendix A). In particular, the "International Charter on Medical Professionalism" explicitly outlines the nature of professionalism, stressing the obligations of a medical professional in contemporary society[30] as does Swick's "Towards a Normative Definition of Medical Professionalism."[28] Both are comprehensive and can serve effectively as the basis of a program on teaching and learning professionalism.

It is important to stress that the medical profession does not define professionalism, society does by delegating powers and responsibilities to the profession.[1,17–20] There is a tendency among medical educators to attempt to promote buy-in by asking focus groups to define the word. This can be effective but one must use the method with caution as there are two potential difficulties. First, it can transmit the impression that the medical profession itself can determine the nature of professionalism. Second, if the group leader is not familiar with the literature on the subject, there can be important omissions or an unbalanced definition can emerge.

THE ATTRIBUTES

As society uses the concept and structures of the professions to organize the services of the healer, any consideration of the attributes expected of a physician must recognize this by either separating the two roles (healer and professional) or including the attributes of both when discussing professionalism. In our teaching, we have preferred to separate the roles, stating that physicians in their day-to-day activities must simultaneously fulfill the roles of healer and professional.

The Faculty of Medicine of McGill University has established a longitudinal four-year undergraduate program of instruction on physicianship.[37–41] There are two separate but interlocking and complementary blocks of teaching, one on the role of the healer[39] and the other devoted to the role of the professional.[37–38] This approach can be justified in historical terms because the origin and evolution of the two roles, while parallel, have been different (Figure 1.1). The healer has been found in all societies throughout recorded history. The evolution of the concept in Western society can be traced through Hellenic Greece to the present, with the Hippocratic and Aesculapian traditions being part of the foundation of Western medicine.[1,42,43] Other cultures and religions have their own traditions, but the role of the healer seems to be remarkably constant, almost certainly because it responds to a basic and universal human need.

The professions have different origins and have evolved independently throughout history. The modern professions arose in the guilds and universities of medieval Europe and England.[3,5,17–19] They acquired their present form in the middle of the nineteenth century when most Western societies granted them a monopoly over the practice of medicine by establishing licensure. As stated earlier, society used the professions as a means of organizing the delivery of the complex services it came to require,[1,5] in this case, those of the healer. Although the division is obviously somewhat arbitrary, one can postulate that those qualities traditionally associated with the relationship between a doctor and a patient are derived from the role of the healer, while medicine's relationship with society as a whole owes more to the development of the modern profession.[1]

An equally valid and widely used method is to use the term "medical professionalism" to cover the combined roles of the healer and the professional. If this is the approach chosen, great care must be taken to include all aspects

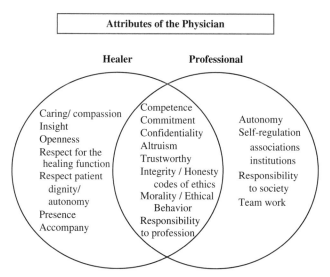

Figure 1.2. The attributes traditionally associated with the healer are shown in the left-hand circle and those with the professional on the right. As can be seen, there are attributes unique to each role. Those shared by both are found in the large area of overlap of the circles. This list of attributes is drawn from the literature on healing and professionalism.

of both roles as the definition dictates not only what is taught but also what will be evaluated.

Figure 1.2 is a diagram of the attributes of the physician/medical professional that have been derived from the literature on healing and professionalism. As can be seen, there are attributes, such as caring and compassion, which have been long recognized as fundamental to the healing function.[42–44] In contrast, there are others associated with being a contemporary professional that historically have not been linked with the traditional healing role, such as responsibility to society or teamwork. In the middle are a group of important shared attributes, each of which is fundamental to the practice of medicine.

The nature of these attributes is so well known to the medical profession that it does not seem necessary to give a detailed description of each. Table 1.1 lists them with operational definitions that can be used for teaching purposes.

However, it is important to discuss the evolution of medical professionalism because some attributes have changed greatly in their meaning, while others are relatively new to the list. Castellani and Hafferty have warned that we must not practice or teach "nostalgic professionalism," an idealized version that is rooted in the past and does not recognize the emergence of a professionalism that must cope with the presence of health care systems, some of which encourage "entrepreneurial professionalism."[24] Others have concurred in this opinion, calling for a "reborn professionalism,"[45] "civic professionalism,"[5] or redefining the term, stating that many of the traditional aspects are no longer appropriate.[46] In addition, as many have pointed out, students and young physicians are emerging from a society that places great emphasis on lifestyle for whom nostalgic professionalism, with an approach to altruism, which they regard as being open ended, is not acceptable.[24] This is covered in Chapter 9.

The professionalism that is taught must recognize these forces and be capable of providing a moral base for the physicians of the future whose task is to ensure that both the role and the values of the healer survive. It is the services of the healer that society needs, and if this need is properly met, it seems likely that a form of professionalism acceptable to both society and medicine will evolve.

Changes in the Attributes

Those attributes whose operational definitions have changed significantly require some discussion because there is a danger that the "idealized" version drawn from nostalgic professionalism will be taught.

Table 1.1. The attributes of the medical professional or the dual roles (healer and professional) of the physician

Attributes of the healer

Caring and compassion: a sympathetic consciousness of another's distress together with a desire to alleviate it.

Insight: self-awareness; the ability to recognize and understand the patient's and one's actions, motivations, and emotions.

Openness: willingness to hear, accept, and deal with the views of others without reserve or pretense.

Respect for the healing function: the ability to recognize, elicit, and foster the power to heal inherent in each patient.

Respect for patient dignity and autonomy: the commitment to respect and ensure subjective well-being and sense of worth in others and recognize the patient's personal freedom of choice and right to participate fully in his/her care.

Presence: to be fully present for a patient without distraction and to fully support and accompany the patient throughout care.

Attributes of both the healer and the professional

Competence: to master and keep current the knowledge and skills relevant to medical practice.

Commitment: being obligated or emotionally impelled to act in the best interest of the patient; a pledge given by way of the Hippocratic Oath or its modern equivalent.

Confidentiality: to not divulge patient information without just cause.

Autonomy: the physician's freedom to make independent decisions in the best interest of the patients and for the good of society.

Altruism: the unselfish regard for, or devotion to, the welfare of others; placing the needs of the patient before one's self-interest.

Integrity and honesty: firm adherence to a code of moral values; incorruptibility.

Morality and ethical conduct: to act for the public good; conformity to the ideals of right human conduct in dealings with patients, colleagues, and society.

Trustworthiness: worthy of trust, reliable.

Attributes of the professional

Responsibility to the profession: the commitment to maintain the integrity of the moral and collegial nature of the profession and to be accountable for one's conduct to the profession.

Self-regulation: the privilege of setting standards; being accountable for one's actions and conduct in medical practice and for the conduct of one's colleagues.

Responsibility to society: the obligation to use one's expertise for, and to be accountable to, society for those actions, both personal and of the profession, which relate to the public good.

Teamwork: the ability to recognize and respect the expertise of others and work with them in the patient's best interest.

Changes in the Attributes of the Healer

The role of the healer appears to have been relatively constant throughout the ages. Consequently, its attributes appear to have changed little. Caring and compassion, openness, and presence, the need for the physician to be there for the patient, are timeless and cross both national and cultural boundaries.[42–44] The concept of respecting patient autonomy is the attribute that has undergone the greatest transformation. The doctor-patient relationship of the past was paternalistic in nature and this is no longer acceptable. It is widely recognized that patients must control the direction and details of their own care, with the physician offering expert advice.[47,48] This is a fundamental aspect of patient-centered care and it is now a societal expectation.[49]

Changes in the Attributes of the Professional

Some attributes ascribed to the professional either are new or have changed significantly. Physician autonomy has been limited in part because of the growth of patient autonomy. However, the most severe intrusions into physician autonomy have resulted from the new levels of accountability expected of contemporary physicians who are now accountable not only to their patients but also to third-party payers, be they government or corporate, and to society for the health of populations.[50–52] Essentially, physician autonomy and physician accountability are reciprocal. The more that physicians and the medical profession are held accountable, the less autonomous they become and society is quite properly demanding new levels of accountability. This dimension of medical professionalism, which now represents an important societal expectation, must be taught and learned in order that it may be met.

Medicine's responsibility to society is not in the Hippocratic tradition but is now a major expectation.[53,54] The importance of modern scientific health care to society, in the presence of apparently infinite demand for health care services, makes responsiveness to societal needs imperative. Contemporary physicians must balance their fiduciary duty to place their patient's interests first with the knowledge that resources devoted to health care are limited and must benefit the largest possible number of individuals. This has been described as representing a conflict between the "social purposes" of medicine and a physician's fiduciary duty to an individual patient.[53,54] This ongoing conflict leads to considerable tension in the practice of medicine, which must be addressed in teaching programs on professionalism.

Self-regulation is a privilege granted to the medical profession, not because it is good for medicine, but because it was assumed that only the profession was competent to make judgments in an area of great complexity.[3,5,17–19] Well-publicized failures in self-regulation on the part of the medical profession have cast doubt upon this assumption[31,55,56] and medicine's regulatory powers are being diminished or altered by actions of the state, the courts, or the corporate sector.[57-59] For this reason, teaching the details of self-regulation and the role of medicine's associations and regulatory bodies becomes an important part of the cognitive base of professionalism. This is addressed in Chapter 10.

Finally, a new requirement is the necessity to practice in teams of health care professionals.[49,60,61] The historical image of the solo practitioner serving a single patient has not represented reality for some time. Because of the complexity of contemporary health care, a major expectation of current society is that physicians will function as members of a health care team. This often conflicts with a student's, resident's, or practitioner's image of themselves as independent and autonomous practitioners. This image must be challenged and, if present, altered in teaching programs. Establishing programs where clinical activities and professionalism may be learned in an interprofessional setting should be considered.

Changes in the Attributes Shared by the Healer and the Professional

Perhaps the greatest changes, and consequently the greatest challenges, between nostalgic and contemporary professionalism are found in this category.

Historically, physicians were licensed and certified as being competent in their chosen field of medicine and it was assumed that they would remain so for the rest of their professional lives. As outlined in Chapter 10, it has been amply demonstrated that this is not true and the graduates of the future will be required to demonstrate that they remain competent throughout their careers.[62-64] Furthermore, as long as the profession retains the right to self-regulate, it will remain a professional obligation to accept responsibility for one's own competence as well as for the competence of one's colleagues.[6,19,20,62] This concept must be introduced at a very early stage of medical education and be reinforced throughout the continuum.

The subject of altruism must also be addressed as it remains a fundamental societal expectation.[25,26,49,65-68] Simply put, it is expected that physicians will place the patient's interests above their own, something that is essential if a patient is to trust a physician.[4,8,16,20,65-70] One traditionally important aspect of altruism has been the expectation that a patient's physicians will be available when needed. The current generation of graduates comes from a society in which lifestyle is of primary importance, resulting in a questioning of the concept of altruism.[71-74] It is of note that there appears to be very little objection to other aspects that are closely linked to altruism such as commitment, caring, and compassion. The balance between altruism and lifestyle must be addressed in programs aimed at teaching professionalism. Denial of the obligation to be altruistic could mean that it is acceptable for a physician to place his or her own interests above that of their patient. Students and residents must understand that altruism is fundamental to patient trust and that in the absence of trust, healing will be severely impaired. However, with proper planning and with the organization of practice so that someone competent and informed is always available, it should be possible to meet patient's legitimate expectations while maintaining a satisfactory balance between work and personal life. Establishing this system is the responsibility of the physician caring for the patient. Students and residents should be encouraged to consider possible methods of balancing the needs of patients with their own desired lifestyle before they actually enter practice, remembering that they must both place and be seen to place the meeting of their patient's needs above their own.

The final group of attributes that must be stressed because they are under threat at the present time is the constellation of honesty, integrity, morality, and ethical behavior. The threats come from a variety of sources including health care systems that rely on market forces, competition,[32,66,75] the presence of a powerful and well-funded pharmaceutical, medical device, and hospital industry.[32,76] They endanger "the ethical foundations of medicine, including the commitment of physicians to put the needs of patients ahead of personal gain, to deal with patients honestly, competently, and compassionately, and to avoid conflicts of interest that could undermine public trust in the altruism of medicine."[32(p2668)] Students, residents, and practicing physicians must understand that conflicts of interest, which are more present than they have ever been in history, are not going to disappear and that their professionalism requires that they manage these conflicts in a way that does not diminish their trustworthiness.[77] These issues must be discussed openly in the context of professional behavior and individuals must be encouraged to reflect on them in a safe environment before they must actually deal with them in practice.

MEDICINE'S SOCIAL CONTRACT WITH SOCIETY

The services of the healer require an organizational framework within which they can be delivered and there is wide agreement that Western society has relied heavily upon the concept of the independent and self-regulating profession as the most appropriate means of accomplishing this.[17–19,77] It helps to explain why professionalism has been said to be the basis of medicine's relationship with society. This relationship was not analyzed in great detail when both medicine and society appeared to be satisfied with the state of affairs. This is no longer true. One observer has noted that "a better informed community is asking for accountability, transparency, and sound professional standards," whereas the profession feels that its "autonomy is severely restricted by budgets, bureaucracy, guidelines, and peer review."[78] Because of the evident discontent on both sides, the interface between medicine and society has come under scrutiny during recent years. Most observers conclude that the most accurate and useful descriptor of the relationship is the historical concept of the "social contract."[1,5,24,29,79–83] Originally elaborated over two centuries ago, it has always been based upon the presence of reciprocal rights and obligations on the part of the parties to the contract. An advantage of using this term is that it has been a part of the discourse on the organization of society for so long and is therefore widely understood.

Because professionalism serves as the basis of this contract and because a change in the contract must of necessity lead to a change in the nature of professionalism, the social contract is an important part of the cognitive base of professionalism that must be taught and learned. It is also useful in setting the context as the idea of a contract does imply a series of obligations on both sides that lead to expectations. If reasonable expectations are not met, one can anticipate changes in the contract.

A useful definition of social contract is, "The rights and duties of the state and its citizens are reciprocal and the recognition of this reciprocity constitutes a relationship which by analogy can be called a social contract."[84]

Medicine's social contract with society is not an identifiable legal document to which one can refer, although important parts of it are written. The written parts of the contract are found in a variety of sources: the laws and rules governing the regulatory framework of medicine, including education, licensure, certification, and revalidation; the legislation establishing the health care system of any given country; and legal judgments found in jurisprudence. There are also documents produced by the profession itself such as the Hippocratic Oath and contemporary codes of ethics, the "International Charter on Medical Professionalism,"[30] and "Good Medical Practice."[13] However, there are also extremely important aspects of the contract relating to the moral basis of the practice of medicine that are unwritten. Altruism and commitment are fundamental to the social contract, representing almost existential expectations on the part of individual patients and society. They cannot be legislated and must arise from within individual physicians.[4,5,16,20,25,26,65,67]

As shown in Figure 1.3, medicine's social contract is complex, beginning with the relationship between individual physicians and medicine's institutions on one side. The profession rarely enjoys unanimity of opinion on many issues that are basic to the contract. There are differences between the desires of generalists and specialists and among specialists,[80] among generations,[71–74] and between the national and the specialty associations.[81] Individual

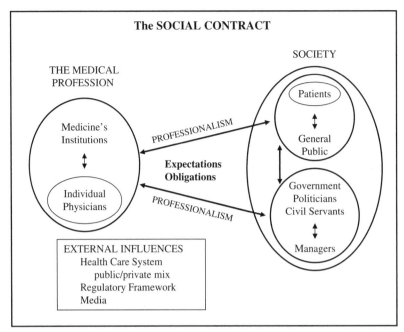

Figure 1.3. This figure represents a schematic representation of medicine's social contract with society. The medical profession consists of individual physicians and the profession's organizations and institutions. There is a dynamic interplay between them that results in medicine's stance on important issues. Society consists of patients and the general public, between whom there is a dynamic interplay, and government, which is made up of politicians, civil servants, and managers. The external influences that can have a profound impact on the nature of the contract are the national health care system specific to each country, the regulatory framework, and the media. Professionalism serves as the basis of medicine's relationship with society as a whole, the patients/public component, and government.

physicians frequently profoundly disagree with the actions of their own associations.[3,17] Nevertheless, the stance of the medical profession on matters that affect it must eventually emerge from the interplay between and among individual practitioners and their organizations. In teaching professionalism, this dynamic and the role of the various organizations are important to teach if present and future physicians are to understand the "system," how they relate to it, and how they may effect change should they so desire. Only in this way can they become involved as professionals in the communities they serve, something that most observers believe to be obligations important to the future of professionalism.[3,5,20,68,81]

Society, the other party to the social contract, is also complex.[5,17,85–88] In a democratic society, it can be said to consist of citizens and those selected to govern them. Individual patients and patient's groups as well as the general public have a legitimate interest in health care. In addition, important groupings in society such as other health care professions (many of whom have their own social contract with society) and the pharmaceutical, medical device, and insurance industries have a vested interest in health care. Public opinion, often expressed in voting patterns, is the result of the interplay between these individuals and groups. In recent years, the relationship of citizens with government has become of great importance as it is government action that ultimately determines the structure as well as the method and level of financing of the health care system.

Finally, government itself is not monolithic, consisting of elected politicians, civil servants, and managers of the health care system, a category which is more important in countries with national health care systems.[85–88] Each of these groups has its own vested interests and opinions. Public policy is the end result of their deliberations, with the political process having a great influence on the resulting health care system and hence the social contract.

As indicated in Figure 1.3, there are external influences that have a significant impact on the nature of the social contract.[85,86] The most important is the nature of the health care system itself, including the presence or absence of a national health plan and the involvement of the private sector. The changes required for the professionalism of medicine, including some perceived to be threats to its fundamental nature, are very different in the United States, which does not have a comprehensive system, than those found in United Kingdom or Canada which do.[17–19] In the United States, physicians are forced to function as entrepreneurs in a competitive marketplace.[17,24,32] It is difficult to merge the values of the healer with those of the marketplace. In countries with national health plans, tensions arise between medicine's fiduciary duty to individual patients and the wider population.[18,19,88]

The nature of the regulatory framework also affects the social contract and hence professionalism. The changes in self-regulation occurring in the United Kingdom following highly publicized failures of medicine's internal regulatory processes highlight the importance of medicine meeting its obligations, in this case to assure the competence of its members.[31,56]

Finally, the media can have a profound effect upon the social contract. While it certainly expresses public opinion, it is also capable of leading it as has been shown in many instances, including in the United Kingdom following medicine's regulatory failures.

Implications of the Use of the Term "Social Contract"

Because professionalism is the basis of medicine's relationship to society,[1,5,9,82] the nature of society's expectations of individual physicians and the medical profession is determined by what it means to be a professional.

An important consequence of using this concept is that it highlights the reciprocal nature of the "bargain" and the rights and obligations associated with it. Medicine's obligations have been recognized for some time. However, individual physicians and the profession can claim that they have legitimate expectations of society.[5,22,81,82] As was stated earlier in this chapter, physicians are granted a monopoly over practice, considerable autonomy, prestige and status, the privilege of self-regulation, and financial rewards on the expectation that they will be altruistic, demonstrate honesty and integrity, ensure the competence of their colleagues, and be devoted to the public good. If individual practitioners or the profession fail to meet society's expectations, the contract will be changed. In contrast, if society does not meet the legitimate expectations of the profession, it can be expected that the profession will desire change. The predominance of the corporate sector in the American health care system has altered aspects of the professionalism of some members of the medical profession, causing them to embrace "entrepreneurial professionalism," something that has changed the social contract.[24,32]

There are other advantages to the use of the term social contract.[81] It identifies the parties to the relationship, something that is essential if the complexities of contemporary health care are to be fully understood. It allows the discussion to be focused on areas of disagreement as well as consensus. Finally, as contracts are subject to negotiation, using this approach can logically lead both individuals and the profession to negotiate with society in an attempt to create a health care system that actually supports professional values.[68,81]

There is also a pedagogic advantage. Presenting professionalism as the basis of a social contract emphasizes its relevance to the practice of medicine and makes the profession's obligations and the reasons for their existence more understandable. Emphasizing the reciprocal nature of medicine's relationship to society can logically lead to an understanding of the consequences of a failure of medicine or society to meet the reasonable and legitimate expectations of the other.

SUMMARY

Fundamental to any teaching program on professionalism is a cognitive base whose objective is transmitting knowledge about the subject and providing a rationale for the behaviors expected of physicians as healers and professionals. This must start with a faculty-wide agreement on a definition of medical professionalism that recognizes medicine's obligations to individual patients and society. It also includes the attributes of a physician that are the basis of society's expectations and hence of medicine's obligations. Finally, the concept that the relationship with society constitutes a social contract based on professionalism provides a rationale for the existence of both rights and obligations on the part of the profession and society, an approach that can facilitate the teaching of professionalism.

It has been stated that "Entry into the profession is a voluntary act, and most people who perform it are disposed to learn its ways and take its ideology seriously. They only need to be told how."[89(p336)] We believe that twenty-first-century learners require more. They need to be told "why?" Using the concept of the social contract to emphasize the fundamental importance of professionalism to medicine's relationship with both individual patients and society helps to provide an answer to that question.

REFERENCES

1. Cruess, RL, Cruess, SR. Teaching medicine as a profession in the service of healing. *Acad Med*. 1997; 72: 941–952.

2. Cruess, SR, Cruess, RL. Professionalism must be taught. *BMJ*. 1997; 315: 1674–1677.

3. Freidson, E. *Professionalism: The Third Logic*. Chicago, IL: University of Chicago Press; 2001.

4. Inui, TS. *A Flag in the Wind: Educating for Professionalism in Medicine*. Association of American Medical Colleges. Washington, DC: Association of American Medical Colleges; 2003.

5. Sullivan, W. *Work and Integrity: The Crisis and Promise of Professionalism in North America*. 2nd ed. San Francisco, CA: Jossey-Bass; 2005.

6. Cohen, JJ. Professionalism in medical education, an American perspective: from evidence to accountability. *Med Educ*. 2006; 40: 607–617.

7. Cote, L, Leclere, H. How clinical teachers perceive the doctor-patient relationship and themselves as role models. *Acad Med*. 2000; 75: 1117–1124.

8. Hensel, WA, Dickey, NW. Teaching professionalism: passing the torch. *Acad Med*. 1998; 73: 865–870.

9. Ludmerer, KM. Instilling professionalism in medical education. *JAMA*. 1999; 282: 881–882.

10. Gordon, J. Fostering students' personal and professional development in medicine: a new framework for PPD. *Med Educ*. 2003; 37: 341–349.

11. Bataldan, P, Leach, D, Swing, S, Dreyfus, H, Dreyfus, S. General competencies and accreditation in graduate medical education. *Health Aff*. 2002; 21: 103–110.

12. Royal College of Physicians and Surgeons of Canada. *The CanMEDS Roles Framework*. 2005. http://rcpsc.medil.org.canmeds/index.php. Accessed February 5, 2007.

13. General Medical Council. *Good Medical Practice*. London; 2006.

14. Liaison Committee on Medical Education. Functions and Structure of a Medical School: Standards for Accreditation of Medical Education Programs Leading to the M.D. Degree. Washington, DC: Liaison Committee on Medical Education; 2007.

15. Hamilton, JS. Scribonius Largus on the medical profession. *Bull Hist Med.* 1986; 60: 209–216.

16. DeRosa, P. Professionalism and virtues. *Clin Orthop Relat Res.* 2006; 44: 28–33.

17. Starr, P. *The Social Transformation of American Medicine.* New York: Basic Books; 1982.

18. Hafferty, FW, McKinley, JB. *The Changing Medical Profession: An International Perspective.* Oxford: Oxford University Press; 1993.

19. Krause, E. *Death of the Guilds: Professions, States and the Advance of Capitalism, 1930 to the Present.* New Haven, CT: Yale University Press; 1996.

20. Sox, HC. The ethical foundations of professionalism: a sociologic history. *Chest.* 2007; 131: 1532–1540.

21. Cruess, RL, Cruess, SR, Johnston, SE. Professionalism and medicine's social contract. *J Bone Joint Surg.* 2000; 82A: 1189–1194.

22. Cruess, SR. Professionalism and medicine's social contract with society. *Clinical Orthop Relat Res.* 2006; 449: 170–176.

23. Hafferty, FW. Definitions of professionalism: a search for meaning and identity. *Clin Orthop Relat Res.* 2006; 449: 193–2043.

24. Castellani, B, Hafferty, FW. The complexities of medical professionalism: a preliminary investigation. In Wear, D, Aultman, JM (eds.) *Professionalism in Medicine: Critical Perspectives.* New York: Springer; 2006, 3–25.

25. Pellegrino, ED. Medical morality and medical economics. *Hastings Cent Rep.* 1978; 4: 8–11.

26. Coulehan, J. Today's professionalism: engaging the mind but not the heart. *Acad Med.* 2005; 80: 892–898.

27. Huddle, TS. Teaching professionalism: is medical morality a competency? *Acad Med.* 2005; 80: 885–891.

28. Swick, HM. Towards a normative definition of professionalism. *Acad Med.* 2000; 75: 612–616.

29. ABIM (American Board of Internal Medicine) Foundation; ACP (American College of Physicians) Foundation; European Federation of Internal Medicine. Medical professionalism in the new millennium: a physician charter. *Ann Intern Med.* 2002; 136: 243–246. *Lancet.* 359: 520–523.

30. Barondess, JA. Medicine and professionalism. *Arch Int Med.* 2003: 163; 145–149.

31. Smith, R. All changed, changed utterly. British medicine will be transformed by the Bristol case. *BMJ.* 1998; 316: 1917–1918.

32. Relman, AS. Medical professionalism in a commercialized health care market. *JAMA.* 2007; 298: 2668–2670.

33. American Board of Internal Medicine(ABIM). *Project Professionalism* (revised). Philadelphia, PA. 1999. www.abimfoundation.org/mppprof.html. Publisher ABIM Foundation. Accessed April 28, 2008.

34. Stern, DT. A framework for measuring professionalism. In Stern, DT (ed.) *Measuring Medical Professionalism.* New York: Oxford University Press; 2005, 3–15.

35. *Oxford English Dictionary*, 2nd ed. Oxford, UK: Clarendon Press; 1989.

36. Cruess, SR, Johnston, S, Cruess, RL. Profession: a working definition for medical educators. *Teach Learn Med.* 2004; 16: 74–76.

37. Cruess, R. Teaching professionalism. *Clinical Orthop Relat Res.* 2006; 449: 177–185.

38. Cruess, R, Cruess, S. Teaching professionalism: general principles. *Med Teacher.* 2006; 28: 205–208.

39. Boudreau, JD, Cassell, EJ, Fuks, A. A healing curriculum. *Med Educ.* 2007; 41: 1193–1201.

40. Steinert, Y, Cruess, SR, Cruess, RL, Snell, L. Faculty development for teaching and evaluating professionalism: from programme design to curricular change. *Med Educ.* 2005; 39: 127–136.

41. Steinert, Y, Cruess, RL, Cruess, SR, Boudreau, JD, Fuks, A. Faculty development as an instrument of change: a case study on teaching professionalism. *Acad Med.* 2007; 82: 1057–1064.

42. Dixon, DM, Sweeney, KG, Pereira Gray, DJ. The physician healer: ancient magic or modern science? *Brit J Gen Pract* 1998; 49: 309–312.

43. Novak, DH, Epstein, RM, Paulsen, RH. Toward creating physician-healers: fostering medical students' self-awareness, personal growth, and well-being. *Acad Med.* 1999; 74: 516–520.

44. Kearney, M. *A Place of Healing: Working with Suffering in Living and Dying.* Oxford: Oxford University Press; 2000.

45. Freidson, E. *Professionalism Reborn: Theory, Prophecy, and Policy.* Cambridge, UK: Polity Press; 1994.

46. Royal College of Physicians of London. *Doctors in Society: Medical Professionalism in a Changing World.* London: Royal college of Physicians of London; 2005.

47. Emanuel, EJ, Emanuel, LL. Four models of the patient-physician relationship. *JAMA.* 1992; 267: 1221–1226.

48. Chisholm, A, Cairncross, L, Askham, J. *Setting Standards: The Views of Members of the Public and Doctors on the Standards of Care and Practice that They Expect of Doctors.* Oxford, UK:Picker Institute Europe; 2006.

49. Coulter, A. Patient's views of the good doctor. *BMJ.* 2002; 325: 668–669.

50. Emanuel, EJ, Emanuel, LL. What is accountability in health care? *Ann Intern Med.* 1996; 124: 229–239.

51. Moran, M, Wood, B. *States, Regulation and the Medical Profession.* Buckingham, UK: Open University Press; 1993.

52. Broadbent, J, Laughlin, R. "Accounting logic" and controlling professionals. In Broadbent, J, Dietrich, M, Roberts, J (eds.) *The End of Professions? The Restructuring of Professional Work.* London: Routlegde; 1997, 34–49.

53. Bloche, MG. Clinical loyalties and the social purposes of medicine. *JAMA.* 1999; 268: 274–281.

54. Gruen, RL, Campbell, EG, Blumenthal, D. Public roles of US physicians: community participation, political involvement, and collective advocacy. *JAMA.* 2006; 296: 2467–2475.

55. Institute of Medicine. *To Err Is Human: Building a Safer Health System.* Washington, DC: National Academy Press; 1999.

56. Irvine, D. *The Doctor's Tale: Professionalism and Public Trust.* Abington, UK. Radcliffe Medical Press; 2003.

57. Vogel, D. *National Styles of Self-regulation*. Ithaca, NY: Cornell University Press; 1986.

58. Rosenbaum, S. The impact of United States law on medicine as a profession. *JAMA*. 2003; 289: 1546–1566.

59. Secretary of State for Health. Trust, Assurance, and Safety—The Regulation of Health Professionals in the 21st Century. London: Stationary Office; 2007.

60. Neufeld, VR, Maudsley, RF, Pickering RJ Turnbull, JM, Weston, WW, Brown, MG, Simpson, JC. Educating future physicians for Ontario. *Acad Med*. 1998; 73: 1133–1148.

61. Coulter, A. What do patients and the public want from primary care? *BMJ*. 2005; 331: 1199–1201.

62. Irvine, D. Patients, professionalism, and revalidation. *BMJ*. 2005; 330: 1265–1268.

63. Dauphinee, WD. Revalidation of doctors in Canada. *BMJ*. 1999; 319: 1188–1190.

64. Norcini, JJ. Recertification in the United States. *BMJ*. 1999; 319: 1183–1185.

65. Pellegrino, ED. The medical profession as a moral community. *Bulletin N.Y. Acad Med*. 1990; 66: 221–232.

66. Mechanic, D, Schlesinger, M. The impact of managed care on patient's trust in medical care and their physicians. *JAMA*. 1996; 275: 1693–1697.

67. May, WF. Money and the medical profession. *Kennedy Inst Ethics J*. 1997; 7: 1–13.

68. Wynia, MK, Latham, SR, Kao, AC, Berg, JW, Emanuel, LL. Medical professionalism in society. *NEJM*. 1999; 341: 1612–1616.

69. McGaghie, WM, Mytco, JJ, Brown, N, Cameron, JR. Altruism and compassion in the health professions: a search for clarity and precision. *Med Teacher*. 2002; 24: 374–378.

70. Hall, MA. The importance of trust for ethics, law, and public policy. *Camb Q Healthc Ethics*. 2005; 14: 156–167.

71. Levinson, W, Lurie, N. When most doctors are women: what lies ahead? *Ann Int Med*. 2004; 141: 471–479.

72. Borges, NJ, Stephen, MR, Elam, C, Jones, BJ. Comparing millennial and generation X medical students at one medical school. *Acad Med*. 2006; 81: 571–576.

73. Watson, DE, Slade, S, Buske, L, Tepper, J. Intergenerational differences in workloads: a ten year population-based study. *Health Aff*. 2006; 25: 1620–1628.

74. Johnston, S. See one, do one, teach one: developing professionalism across the generations. *Clin Orthop Relat Res*. 2006; 449: 186–192.

75. Sullivan, W. What is left of professionalism after managed care. *Hastings Cent Rep*. 1999; 29: 7–13.

76. Brennan, TA, Rothman, DJ, Blank, L, Blumenthal, D, Chimonas, SC, Cohen, J, Goldman, J, Kassirer, JP, Kimball, H, Naughton, J, Smelser, N. Health industry practices that create conflicts of interest. *JAMA*. 2006; 295: 429–433.

77. Cohen, JJ, Cruess, SR, Davidson, C. Alliance between society and medicine: the public's stake in medical professionalism. *JAMA*. 2007; 298: 670–673.

78. Dunning, AJ. Status of the doctor—present and future. *Lancet*. 1999; 354(suppl.): SIV 18.

79. Rosenblatt, RE, Shaw, S, Rosenbaum, S. *Law and the American Health Care System*. New York: Foundation Press; 1997.

80. Ludmerer, KM. *Time to Heal.* Oxford: Oxford University Press; 1999.

81. Stevens, R. Public roles for the medical profession in the United States: beyond theories of decline and fall. *Milbank Q.* 2001; 79: 327–353.

82. Kurlander, JK, Morin, K, Wynia, MK. The social-contract model of professionalism: baby or bathwater? *Am J Bioethics.* 2004; 4: 33–36.

83. Iglehart, JK. The emergence of physician-owned specialty hospitals. *NEJM.* 2005; 352: 78–84.

84. Gough, JW. *The Social Contract: A Critical Study of Its Development.* Oxford: The Clarendon Press; 1957.

85. Ham, C, Alberti, KJ. The medical profession, the public, and the government. *BMJ.* 2002; 324: 838–842.

86. Rosen, R, Dewar, S. *On Being a Good Doctor: Redefining Medical Professionalism for Better Patient Care.* London, UK: King's Fund; 2004.

87. Salter, B. Patients and doctors: reformulating the UK health policy community? *Soc Sci Med.* 2003; 57: 927–936.

88. Tuohy, C. Agency, contract, and governance: shifting shapes of accountability in the health care arena. *J Health Pol Policy Law.* 2003; 29: 195–215.

89. Kultgen, JH. *Ethics and Professionalism.* Philadelphia, PA: University of Pennsylvania Press; 1998.

PART TWO

Theory

2 Educational Theory and Strategies for Teaching and Learning Professionalism

Yvonne Steinert, Ph.D.

There is nothing so practical as a good theory.[1]

As the chapters in this book demonstrate, professionalism is taught and learned in diverse and complex ways. Indeed, the past decade has witnessed a significant increase in the teaching and learning of professionalism in undergraduate and postgraduate medical education.[2–4] However, despite this rapid growth, few authors have described the educational frameworks that underpin their work in this area,[5] even though we all hold different assumptions about *what* we teach and *how* we try to achieve our goals.

For example, one contemporary school of thought has emphasized that professionalism needs to be taught explicitly, either by defining core content or outlining professionalism as a list of traits or characteristics.[6–8] From this perspective, the goal is to ensure that every physician understands the nature of professionalism, its basis in morality, the reasons for its existence, its characteristics, and the obligations necessary to sustain it. Others have stated that the teaching of professionalism should be approached primarily as a moral endeavor, emphasizing altruism and service, the importance of role modeling, self-awareness, community service, and other methods of acquiring experiential knowledge.[9,10] In this school of thought, explicit teaching receives less attention, and learning is embedded in an authentic activity. Although both approaches are needed to promote the teaching and learning of professionalism,[11] as teachers and educators we must clarify the assumptions that we hold and try to answer the following question: *What is our guiding theory or educational framework?*

The goal of this chapter is to situate the teaching and learning of professionalism in a theoretical context, to review the key features of instructional design, and to describe a number of educational strategies that can guide our work in this area. The teaching and learning of professionalism often occur in a spontaneous, unplanned fashion. By describing several educationally relevant frameworks, this chapter will hopefully facilitate a more systematic approach.

WHY THEORY?

Theory has been defined as "a conception or mental scheme of something to be done; a systematic statement of rules or principles to be followed."[12] In diverse ways, theories represent various aspects of reality in an understandable way.[13] That is, they simplify reality by ignoring a large number of variables (like a map) and they often stress the importance of certain variables by giving them special names or stressing their importance in words, figures, or formulas. However, theory is not simply a summary of the data; rather, it is a specification of loosely construed mechanisms that give rise to observed effects.[14]

The particular theory we subscribe to, whether consciously or not, is likely to dictate how we work.[15] Thus, an awareness of different theoretical frameworks will allow us to make informed choices about how we approach teaching and learning; it will also enable us to share what we do in a scholarly manner. Without theoretical frameworks to guide our practice, there is a danger that there will be too much reliance on intuition or common sense. Theory can help to ensure that interactions are intentional.

In summary, theory can influence practice, provide a structure for interactions that move toward identifiable outcomes, and create the shared understanding and terminology that is a necessary prerequisite for discussion and debate. "New" theories can also pave the way for progress and innovation when "old" theories are found wanting.[16]

A THEORETICAL FRAMEWORK TO GUIDE THE TEACHING AND LEARNING OF PROFESSIONALISM

Although many educational theories can be applied to the teaching and learning of professionalism (e.g., constructivism,[17] social learning,[18] and self-efficacy[19]), we have chosen to carefully examine situated learning[20,21] as an overarching framework. Principles of adult learning and experiential learning, which are also pertinent, will be described in the following section as they primarily influence the design and delivery of instructional programs.

Why Situated Learning?

Situated learning is based upon the notion that knowledge is *contextually situated* and fundamentally influenced by the *activity, context,* and *culture* in which it is used.[20] This view of knowledge as *situated* in *authentic contexts*

Table 2.1. Key Components of Situated Learning[21]

Cognitive apprenticeship
Collaborative learning
Reflection
Practice
Articulation of learning skills

has important implications for our understanding of teaching and learning professionalism as well as the design and delivery of instructional programs and activities in this area.

We have chosen to describe situated learning theory for a number of reasons. Although only two articles in the literature have specifically addressed educational theory and the teaching and learning of professionalism, they have both referred to the concepts and principles of situated learning.[11,22] As Maudsley and Strivens[22] have remarked, "Of the educational theories available, situated learning theory best describes the most effective design model to transform students from members of the lay public to expert members of a profession possessing skills and a commitment to a common set of values." It has also been said that situated learning is particularly appropriate to educating the professions that are communities or cultures joined by "intricate, socially constructed webs of belief."[20] This description is particularly relevant to medicine.

Situated learning theory brings together the cognitive base and experiential learning that is needed to facilitate the acquisition of professionalism. That is, it bridges the gap between the "know what" and the "know how" of teaching and learning by embedding learning in authentic activities. It also helps to transform knowledge from the abstract and theoretical to the useable and useful.[11] The proponents of situated learning suggest that there should be a balance between the explicit teaching of a subject and the activities in which the knowledge learned is used in an authentic context – both essential principles in the teaching and learning of professionalism.

The Situated Learning Model

As mentioned previously, situated learning is based upon the notion that knowledge is contextually situated and fundamentally influenced by the activity, context, and culture in which it is used.[20] Some of the key components of situated learning (outlined in Table 2.1) include cognitive apprenticeship, collaborative learning, reflection, practice, and articulation of learning skills.[21]

Cognitive apprenticeship, a fundamental element of situated learning, has particular relevance to clinical teaching and learning, and therefore to professionalism. Apprenticeship is a familiar and pervasive method of learning in medicine.[23] Cognitive apprenticeship builds on this traditional form of learning and consists of four distinct phases: modeling, scaffolding, fading, and coaching (all of which will be detailed below).

In traditional apprenticeship, the expert shows the apprentice how to do a task, watches as the apprentice practices portions of the task, and then turns over more and more responsibility until the apprentice is proficient enough to accomplish the task independently.[24] Cognitive apprenticeship differs from a more traditional approach in that the process of carrying out the task that is to be learned is not always observable; learning is not always situated in the workplace (and the value of the final product is not always evident); and transfer of skills to new situations is required. Thus, in order to translate the model of traditional apprenticeship to cognitive apprenticeship, teachers need to *identify the processes* of the task and make them visible, or explicit, to the student; *situate* abstract tasks in authentic contexts, so that students understand the relevance of their work; *vary* the diversity of learning situations; and *articulate* common aspects so that students can transfer their new knowledge and learning to new situations.[21]

In **modeling**, the learner observes and then mimics the teacher in the performance of a task. Modeling is most effective when teachers make the target processes visible, often by explicitly showing the learner, or apprentice, what to do. Through modeling, students observe normally invisible processes and begin to integrate *what* occurs with *why* it happens.[25]

Scaffolding refers to the support teachers give the learner in carrying out a task. This can range from almost doing the entire task to giving occasional hints as to what to do next. Scaffolding supports and simplifies a task as much as necessary to enable learners to manage their learning, allowing them to accomplish otherwise difficult tasks with optimal challenge. Too little challenge will prove boring; too much challenge will foster frustration.[26] By supporting the integration of established understanding and know-how, scaffolding facilitates the transfer of what students already know to the task at hand.[27]

Fading is the notion of slowly removing support, giving the learner more and more responsibility. It is a critical step in the trajectory of becoming an independent practitioner.

Coaching is the thread that runs through the entire apprenticeship experience and involves helping individuals while they attempt to learn or perform a task. It includes directing learner attention, providing hints and feedback, challenging and structuring tasks, and providing additional challenges or problems. Coaches explain activities in terms of the learners' understanding and background knowledge, and provide additional directions about how, when, and why to proceed; they also identify errors, misconceptions, or faulty reasoning in learners' thinking and help to correct them. In situated learning environments, advice and guidance help students to maximize use of their own cognitive resources and knowledge, as in many ways these strategies are nondirective.[25]

Collaborative learning is another important feature of situated learning and cognitive apprenticeship. Brown *et al.*[20] have identified the following strategies to promote collaborative learning: collective problem solving, displaying and identifying multiple roles, confronting ineffective strategies and misconceptions, and developing collaborative work skills. Small group work, peer teaching, and group projects can also facilitate the acquisition of collaborative skills. As interprofessional teamwork is an essential component of professionalism, collaborative learning should be incorporated into a variety of teaching and learning situations.

Reflection, an essential ingredient of situated learning, has received increasing attention in the medical literature[28]; it is also viewed as a core skill in professional competence.[29] In practice, there are three kinds of reflective activity. Schön[28] describes a spontaneous reaction (i.e., thinking on your feet) as "reflection *in* action." This type of reflection, which is frequently described as a subliminal process of which the participant is only partially aware, most likely involves pattern recognition; as well, it is usually triggered by recognition that "something doesn't seem right."[28,30] Thinking of a situation after it has happened and initiating the ability to re-evaluate the situation is referred to as "reflection *on* action." This type of reflection, in which the participant is fully aware of what has occurred, allows the participant to mentally reconstruct the experience, paying particular attention to context. Reflection on action also forms a bridge between the relived situation and knowledge retrieved from internal memory or other external sources.[31] While the development of the capacity to reflect "in" and "on" action has become an important feature of medical practice, "reflection *for* action"[32] forms an additional avenue for professional training and improvement of practice. As Lachman and Pawlina[32] have observed, "The benefits of reflective practice, whilst meeting the objectives of new and revised curricula, extend beyond the construct of a medical curriculum. The process of reflection and its basis of critical thinking allows for the integration of theoretical concepts into practice; increased learning through experience; enhanced critical thinking and judgment in complex situations; and the encouragement of student-centred learning".

Clearly, all these benefits are of vital importance in the promotion of professionalism.

Boud et al.[33] describe three elements critical to the reflective process. All these can help to promote the teaching and learning of professionalism.

- Returning to experience – which refers to the recollection of salient events, the replaying of the initial experience in the mind of the learner, or the recounting to others of the key features of the experience.
- Attending to feelings – which includes utilizing positive feelings and removing negative feelings, both of which are needed for learning to occur.
- Re-evaluating experience – which is clearly the most important and is often not completed if the other two phases are ignored. Re-evaluation involves a re-examination of the original experience in light of the learner's goals, associating new knowledge with that which is already processed, and integrating new knowledge into the learner's conceptual framework.

According to Roth,[34] a true reflective process requires that the educational process provide the opportunity to keep an open mind about "what," "how," and "why" things are being done. From this perspective, learning of professionalism can be achieved through questioning, investigating, evaluating, analyzing, theorizing, seeking feedback, and incorporating the ideas and viewpoints of team members.

Practice is another central component of situated learning. Repeated practice serves to test, refine, and extend skills into a web of increasing expertise in a social context of collaboration and reflection.[21] It also enables skills to become deeply rooted and "automatically" mobilized as needed. The notion of *experiential learning* (outlined in Chapter 4) is closely tied to the concept of practice.

Articulation includes two aspects.[21] First, it refers to the concept of articulating or separating out different component skills in order to learn them more effectively. An example of this is effective communication with patients. Second, articulation refers to the goal of getting students to articulate their knowledge, reasoning, or problem-solving processes in a specific domain. By articulating problem-solving processes, students come to a better understanding of their thinking processes, and they are better able to explain things to themselves and to others. Articulation also helps to make learning – and reflection – visible.

In summary, situated learning is based upon the idea that knowledge is contextually situated and fundamentally influenced by the activity, context, and culture in which it is used. Adherence to a situated learning model also leads to different perceptions of the teacher's role. That is, teachers must assume the role of *coach* in addition to that of pedagogue, and they must act as *models* for performing learner tasks to students.[35] At the same time, students become *experts* and engage in reciprocal teaching,[36] and the role of *apprentice* and *master* are shared. In many ways, situated learning (and its key components of apprenticeship, collaboration, reflection, practice, and articulation of skills) provides a useful framework by which to understand how professionalism can be taught and learned. An understanding of this model can also help to guide the design and delivery of diverse educational programs and activities.

Closely tied to the notion of situated learning is the concept of "legitimate peripheral participation."[37] This social practice, which combines "learning by doing" (also known as experiential learning) and apprenticeship into a single theoretical perspective, is the process by which a novice becomes an expert. That is, from a situated learning perspective, learners build new knowledge and understanding through gradual participation in the community of which they are becoming a part. As learners, they begin at the edge – or periphery – of the community, where because of their status as learners, they have what is called "legitimate peripheral participation."[31] Mann[23] provides a useful example. As students in a clinical rotation, or residents at the beginning of their training, gain experiences, they slowly become involved in a community of physicians. They gradually participate in more of the community's work, and they move from the periphery toward the centre. They also take on increasing responsibility for the work of the community, namely the care of patients. In the process, they learn to "talk the talk" and "walk the walk." A key element of participation in the community is the opportunity to see and participate in the framing of problems and understand how knowledge is structured. According to Wenger,[38] social participation within the community is the key to informal learning. It is embedded in the practices and relationships of the workplace and helps to create identity and meaning. It also complements, and can substitute for, formal learning mechanisms. Informal learning is often not acknowledged as learning within organizations; rather, it is typically regarded as being "part of the job" or a mechanism for "doing the job properly." However, "learning at work" is a key component of medical education, and there is value in rendering this learning as visible as possible so that it can be valued as an important curricular component.

Research by Boud and Middleton[39] has further identified a range of informal learning that occurs in workplaces and illustrates the complexities of

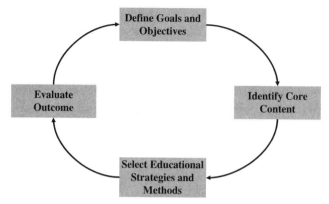

Figure 2.1. The instructional design cycle.

learning. For example, there is a diverse range of people that we learn from at work, very few of whom are recognized by the organization as individuals with a role in promoting learning. In a large organization, the range and diversity of communities of practice in which we may legitimately participate increases with seniority; as a result, the range of opportunities for informal learning also increases. Some learning networks manifest features of communities of practice, but others do not – and do not build identity and meaning. Awareness of these networks, often labeled part of the informal or hidden curriculum, is fundamental to our understanding of where teaching and learning of professionalism takes place.

THE CYCLE OF INSTRUCTIONAL DESIGN

Figure 2.1. summarizes the key steps in designing an instructional unit, be it an entire curriculum, a specific course, or one teaching and learning activity. The main components include defining educational goals and objectives, identifying core content, selecting educational strategies and methods, and evaluating outcome. Each of these steps will be explained below. However, two additional theoretical frameworks will influence the design of any activity structured to promote the teaching and learning of professionalism and they will be addressed first: principles of adult learning and experiential learning.

Some have argued that the principles of instructional design are not compatible with situated learning because instructional design refers to a systematic process that follows a step-wise progression – and this is not always the case in work-based learning. As well, the theoretical framework of instructional design assumes that what people learn is relatively stable across situations and that people apply what is learned in a logical, planned way.[40]

However, the two perspectives are not incompatible; teachers and educators need to plan for student "apprenticeships" and create learning experiences that are situated in the real world. At the same time, the basic premises of instructional design *can* be maintained in a situated learning model.[40] For example, teaching strategies must still be based on what is known about the students and what they have to master; they must also be chosen rationally and modified as needed. Most importantly, thinking about instructional design forces us to think about how we can facilitate learning in authentic contexts.

Principles of Adult Learning

Although some have argued that adult learning is not a theory[41] and merely a description of the adult learner, others believe that principles of adult learning (also referred to as andragogy) form an important theoretical construct.[42] In either case, andragogy captures essential characteristics of adult learners and offers important guidelines for planning instruction.

Knowles[43,44] first introduced the concept of andragogy, defining it as "the art and science of helping adults learn." Key principles include the following:

- Adults are independent.
- Adults come to learning situations with a variety of motivations and definite expectations about particular learning goals and teaching methods.
- Adults demonstrate different learning styles.
- Much of adult learning is "relearning" rather than new learning.
- Adult learning often involves changes in attitudes as well as skills.
- Most adults prefer to learn through experience.
- Incentives for adult learning usually come from within the individual.
- Feedback is usually more important than tests and evaluations.

Clearly, the incorporation of these principles into the design of any educational program, with medical students, residents, or practicing physicians, will enhance receptivity, relevance, and engagement. An understanding of these principles can also influence pacing, meaning, and motivation. Kaufman *et al.*[45] have outlined a number of recommendations for program planning based on principles of adult learning that are equally relevant in the context of teaching and learning professionalism. To paraphrase these authors, teachers, and educators should try to

- establish an effective learning climate, so that learners will feel "safe" and be able to express themselves without judgment or ridicule;

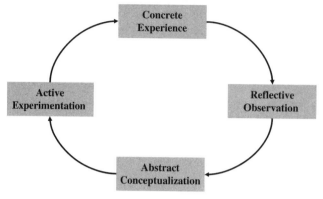

Figure 2.2. The experiential learning cycle.[46]

- involve learners in the planning of curricular content and methods, to enhance "buy in," collaboration, and relevance;
- enable learners to diagnose their own needs and formulate their own learning objectives, to ensure motivation and meaningful learning;
- encourage learners to identify available resources and devise strategies to achieve their objectives;
- help learners to carry out their learning plans and try to ensure successful completion of necessary tasks;
- involve learners in the evaluation of learning, an essential step in self-directed learning.

In many ways, adult learning theory "offers us a means of thinking about student learners in a way that is consistent with what is known about learning and development."[45] Interestingly, the criteria of self-directedness, relevance, learning from experience, and self-assessment, which are important in promoting effective learning, are also essential aspects of the practice of medicine.

The Experiential Learning Cycle

Kolb and Fry[46] have provided a description of the learning cycle that highlights the role of experience in the learning process. More specifically, they describe how experience is translated into concepts, which in turn guide the choice of new experiences.[33] In this model, which should be considered in the design of all instructional events, learning is viewed as a four-stage cycle (outlined in Figure 2.2.). Immediate concrete experience is the basis for observation and reflection; observations are then assimilated into a personal theory, from which new implications for action can be deduced; and all these steps eventually lead to new experiences. According to Kolb and Fry,[46] learners need opportunities to experience each step of the learning cycle. That is, they need the ability to experience diverse situations (in both the classroom and the clinical setting), observe and reflect on what they have learned (often in a large group session), develop their own theory and understanding of the world, and experiment new ways of being in order for learning to occur. Attention to the experiential learning cycle will facilitate both the teaching *and* learning of professionalism and ensure that different learning styles are respected and nurtured.

Steps to Instructional Design

Defining Goals and Objectives

The goals (and objectives) for the teaching and learning of professionalism must be carefully determined, in collaboration with students, their teachers, and other members of the health care team. Often, a formal (or an informal) analysis of needs will guide the articulation of goals and objectives; at other times, the requirements of licensing or accrediting bodies will determine the learning outcomes. Chapter 15 outlines a series of needs assessment methods that can be used in this context as well.

Identifying Core Content

The needs of the students, their teachers, and other members of the health care team will help to define the core content to be taught – and learned. Core content includes the competencies underlying professionalism and addresses knowledge, attitudes, and skills. Chapter 1 provides an overview of the cognitive base of professionalism; other chapters in this book address the attitudes and skills needed to behave in a professional manner. What is key to remember is that the core content must be chosen in line with the learners' needs, the institutional context, the available time, and accessible resources. Moreover, clearly determining content is a critical step in the design process, as this will determine educational strategies and methods.

Selecting Educational Strategies and Methods

Once the core content has been identified, teachers must select the strategies they wish to use in light of their goals and objectives as well as students' capabilities, prior knowledge, and skills. For example, interactive lectures and large group sessions can be used to convey the cognitive base of professionalism. Case vignettes and small group discussions allow for an exploration of personal beliefs, values, and assumptions. Clinical and simulated teaching environments enable skill acquisition, practice, and feedback. As outlined in Chapter 8, strategy selection should also be influenced by generational preferences.

It has been said that professional identity arises "from a long term combination of experience and reflection on experience."[47] The choice of educational strategies should therefore ensure stage-appropriate opportunities for gaining experience and reflecting upon them; these methods should also provide students, residents, and practitioners with structured occasions to discuss, reflect, and internalize professional issues in a safe environment.[22,48,49] In addition, the choice of methods should be influenced by the view that multiple instructional modes are considered to be more effective than a single method[50] and that active learning methods are more effective than passive ones.[51,52] With this in mind, educators should consider a variety of strategies to meet diverse objectives.

Evaluating Outcome

Evaluating outcome includes both the assessment of learning (and thereby the evaluation of students) as well as program evaluation (and whether the goals and objectives have been met). Student learning can be measured in a number of ways that include written assessments (e.g., essays, multiple choice questions), clinical assessments (e.g., global rating scales, oral examinations), clinical simulations (e.g., standardized patients), and multisource assessments (e.g., peer assessments, self-assessments, portfolios). It is beyond the scope of this chapter to describe diverse methods of student assessment. However, a review by Epstein[53] can be a very useful resource. Chapter 7 also provides a rich description of how to assess professionalism among students and residents. These methods should be incorporated into the design of any instructional program on professionalism.

To evaluate the educational activity, be it a one-time event or a curricular unit, teachers should consider available data sources (e.g., students, peers, patients), common methods of evaluation (e.g., questionnaires, focus groups, observations), resources to support assessment, and models of program evaluation (e.g., goal attainment, decision facilitation).[54,55] Kirkpatrick's levels of evaluation are also helpful in conceptualizing and framing the evaluation of effectiveness.[56] They include the following:

- Reaction – participants' views on the learning experience.
- Learning – change in participants' attitudes, knowledge, or skills.
- Behavior – change in participants' behavior.
- Results – changes in the organizational system, the patient, or the learner.

At a minimum, a practical and feasible evaluation should include an assessment of utility and relevance, content, and educational methods. Moreover, as evaluation is an integral part of the educational cycle, it should be conceptualized at the beginning of any program and whenever possible should include qualitative and quantitative assessments of learning and behavior change, using a variety of methods and data sources.

STRATEGIES TO PROMOTE TEACHING AND LEARNING

As noted in the different chapters of this book, strategies for teaching and learning professionalism span the spectrum from large group didactic lectures to small group discussions,[57] role plays and simulations,[58] narrative medicine,[59] and independent learning. In this section, we will highlight role modeling, an oft-neglected teaching strategy as well as several methods that have particular appeal in teaching and learning professionalism (e.g., the use of case vignettes, art and video, narrative medicine, and portfolios) and that tie in closely with principles of situated learning. For a more comprehensive review of teaching and learning methods in general, work by Dent and Harden[60] as well as Newble and Cannon[61] should be consulted.

Role Modeling

Coulehan[9] has said that the "first requirement for a sea change in professionalism is to increase dramatically the number of physicians who are able to role-model professional virtue at every stage of medical education." Role modeling has been described as one of the most important educational methods for instilling the attitudes, behaviors, ethics, and professional values of medicine to students and residents.[62–66] However, although role modeling is at the heart of "character formation,"[67] medical students and residents have observed that many of us are poor role models. As teachers, we also frequently undermine this powerful method of teaching and learning.

The characteristics of effective role models are described in Chapter 4. As previously stated, these include *clinical competence*, which encompasses knowledge and skills, communication with patients and staff, and sound clinical reasoning and decision making; *teaching skills*, which comprise effective communication, feedback, and opportunities for reflection that promote student-centered learning; and *personal qualities* such as compassion, honesty, and integrity as well as effective interpersonal relationships, enthusiasm for practice and teaching, and an uncompromising quest for excellence. All these characteristics are essential to effective role modeling. The challenge is to articulate the process and make the implicit explicit.

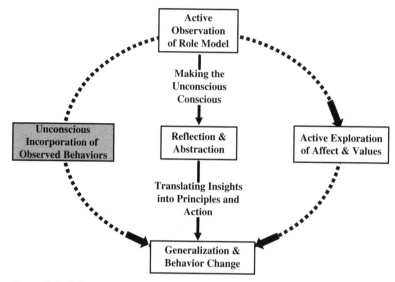

Figure 2.3. Schematic representation of the process of role modeling.[68] The process of incorporating the attributes of a role model can proceed through two different mechanisms.[69] The first, shown on the right, involves an active thought process, which leads to change. Related to this, but somewhat different, is a change brought about by active reflection, often expressing ideas in abstract terms. This can convert an unconscious feeling into one which is conscious and can be actively translated into principles and action. There is also an equally powerful process, shown on the left, in which observed behaviors are unconsciously incorporated into the belief patterns and behaviors of the student. Role models should be aware of these components of observational learning.

Learning from role models occurs through observation and reflection. Figure 2.3. provides a schematic representation of the process of role modeling, a complex mix of conscious and unconscious activities.[68,69] While we are all aware of the conscious observation of observed behaviors, understanding the power of the unconscious component is essential to effective role modeling. More importantly, as Swick[2] has cautioned, we must pay attention to the professionalism manifested by practicing physicians, not only for what it means to the patients they care for but also for the impact it has on students who observe them providing care.

The Use of Case Vignettes and Case Presentations

The use of case vignettes and/or case presentations can be particularly powerful in the teaching and learning of professionalism. For example, case studies that involve clinical concepts allow students to critically evaluate specific problems by integrating and applying basic knowledge.[32] Vignettes that integrate context and conflict in medical professionalism can also be useful tools.[70] However, application to other situations may be limited. For example, Goldie *et al.*[71] used vignettes describing a dilemma concerning professionalism to study knowledge of professional norms. More specifically, their vignettes addressed situations in which clinical clerks were confronted with suboptimal practice as well as value clashes and personal emotions. The results of this educational intervention indicated a positive effect; however, students did not generalize their knowledge to new vignettes or clinical scenarios. At the same time, Kon[72] observed that educators should consider using both student-generated and instructor-generated cases, as the former facilitate relevance and personal interest. Irrespective of the origin, case vignettes allow for an exploration of understanding, attitudes, and beliefs; case presentations offer the same value, with the added benefit of authenticity and relevance.

The Use of Art and Video

The use of art and video clips (from movies and television) can also be useful adjuncts to teaching and learning professionalism, especially as these media engage the residents emotionally and can evoke their own professional ideals that initially led them to choose a career in medicine. Winter and Birnberg[73] have described a seminar in which residents are asked to read a selection on "Virtues and Ideals in Professional Life," view two paintings depicting different but complementary aspects of the medical profession, and discuss three video clips, to explore whether or not physicians have legitimate self-interests. As the author stated, it was clear that "the paintings and video clips touched the residents on an emotional level and had a much greater impact than would otherwise have been experienced from didactic lectures and isolated clinical vignettes." This multimedia approach also enabled the residents to discuss their professional beliefs without feeling that their personal integrity was being threatened and fostered a deeper and more sophisticated understanding of professionalism and the work-related expectations that they have for one another.

Narrative Medicine

Stories are an essential part of situated learning and the social *construction* of knowledge.[21] Stories help people to keep track of their discoveries and provide a meaningful structure for remembering what has been learned. Stories have also been described as a type of "expert system" for storing, linking, and readily accessing information,[21] and there appears to be an increasing emphasis on stories as a tool for learning, understanding, and remembering. For this and other reasons, the use of narrative medicine[74] becomes a compelling strategy in the teaching and learning of professionalism.

Narrative competence can be understood as "the ability to acknowledge, absorb, interpret, and act on the stories and plights of others."[59] The narrative medicine movement provides a way of reframing the knowledge, skills, and attitudes of good doctoring under the aegis of language, symbol, story, and the cultural construction of illness.[75] It draws upon the centrality of clinical empathy in establishing and maintaining therapeutic relationships and builds upon the broader, more imaginative empathy that allows observers to "connect with" the experience of persons not immediately known to them.[76] Coulehan[9] has proposed a narrative-based approach to learning professionalism to help students address the tension between self-interest and altruism. In doing so, he states that "one of the prerequisites for developing narrative-based professionalism is to provide, throughout medical school and residency, a safe venue for students and residents to share their experiences and enhance their personal awareness." Physicians in training need to understand their own beliefs, feelings, attitudes, and response patterns, and narrative competence is one way to achieve this objective.

As previously stated, the student's own life experience, molded by positive role modeling and reflective practice, can serve as the basic material from which narrative competence may develop.[9,59] However, students may enhance their repertoires of life experience by exposure to the written, filmed, and oral narratives of real and fictional physicians,[75–78] and they may increase awareness of their own developing professional identities by writing personal and professional narratives consistently and with discipline.

Portfolio Learning

Portfolio learning is closely tied to reflection and a narrative-based approach to learning professionalism. Portfolios have been defined as "a purposeful collection of student work that demonstrates the student's efforts and progress in selected domains."[79] In medicine, portfolios can encourage self-directed learning, foster reflection, and demonstrate progress toward identifiable outcomes.[80] Portfolios also have the added advantage of respecting individuality and diversity while developing life-long learning skills.

Portfolios were originally introduced in medicine to assess performance in authentic contexts and stimulate learners to reflect on their own functioning.[81,82] Their use has been extended beyond this original intent and much has been written about the role and value of portfolios, both electronic and paper based, in medical training.[83,84] For more details about the use and structure of portfolios, the work of Driessen *et al.*[83] and Wilkinson *et al.*[84] should be consulted. In this context, it is important to appreciate how portfolios can support the teaching and learning of professionalism, as they promote reflection in authentic contexts.

The Culture of Medicine

No discussion of educational theory, design, or strategies for teaching and learning professionalism can neglect the environment in which teaching and learning take place. As highlighted by Inui,[48] Wear and Kuczewski,[85] and Brainard and Brislen,[86] the environment in which our students and residents learn is sometimes "toxic" and can negate the impact of what we are trying to achieve. The academic environment may also impede the students' learning and professional development.

As a number of authors have stated, professionalism is an important construct, though the movement to teach and evaluate professionalism presents a conundrum to medical educators.[85] Its intent is laudable: to produce humanistic and virtuous physicians who will be better able to cope with and overcome the dehumanizing features of health care systems. However, its impact on medical education is likely to be small and misleading if professionalism curricula continue to focus on lists of rules and behaviors.[9] As a result, educators are proposing a more comprehensive approach to changing the culture of medical education to favor an approach that facilitates organizational change and development.

As many of the authors in this book have highlighted, there is general agreement that the institutional culture can support – or subvert – professional behaviors. Medical education is carried out in an environment heavily influenced by economic, cultural, and organizational forces,[48] and many of these institutional factors can negate the impact of our "formal" educational programs.[87,88] There is also an extremely powerful informal curriculum, consisting of unscripted, unplanned, and highly interpersonal forms of teaching and learning that take place among and between faculty and students, and attention must be paid to both the informal and the hidden curriculum, whose influence can be extremely positive or negative.[89] Accordingly, all teachers and educators must work together to change the institutional culture and try to influence the informal and hidden curriculum, while structuring formal teaching and learning programs.[90] Brainard and Brislen,[86] two medical students, propose that the main barrier to the teaching and learning of professionalism is unprofessional conduct by their teachers. They also maintain that deficiencies in the learning environment, combined with the subjective nature of many evaluations, often leave students feeling persecuted and/or confused. They therefore recommend that teachers and administrators, and students and residents, show a personal commitment to the explicit professionalism curriculum and address the hidden curriculum openly and proactively. It would be wise to heed their recommendations.

CONCLUSIONS

Educational programs to promote the teaching and learning of professionalism clearly need to pay attention to the academic environment in which students learn. However, knowledge of a theoretical framework for teaching and learning, as well as an understanding of principles of adult learning, experiential learning, and instructional design, will strengthen the educational program and promote pedagogical excellence and coherence.

Cruess and Cruess[11] have stated that professionalism is a fundamental aspect of the process of socialization, during which individuals acquire the values, attitudes, interests, skills, and knowledge of the groups they seek to join. Situated learning, with its emphasis on cognitive apprenticeship, collaboration, reflection, practice, and articulation of skills within an authentic context, provides a useful framework for the teaching and learning of professionalism.

REFERENCES

1. Lewin, K. *Field Theory in Social Science: Selected Theoretical Papers.* New York: Harper & Row; 1951.
2. Swick, HM. Veiwpoint: professionalism and humanism beyond the academic health center. *Acad Med.* 2007;82(11):1022–8.
3. Ludmerer, KM. Instilling professionalism in medical education. *JAMA.* 1999; 282(9):881–2.
4. Wear, D, Bickel, J. *Educating for Professionalism: Creating a Culture of Humanism in Medical Education.* Iowa City (IA): University of Iowa Press; 2000.
5. Gordon, J. Fostering students' personal and professional development in medicine: a new framework for PPD. *Med Educ.* 2003;37(4):341–9.
6. Cruess, RL, Cruess, SR. Teaching medicine as a profession in the service of healing. *Acad Med.* 1997;72(11):941–52.
7. Cruess, SR, Cruess, RL. Professionalism must be taught. *BMJ.* 1997;315(7123): 1674–7.
8. Swick, HM. Towards a normative definition of professionalism. *Acad Med.* 2000;75(6):612–6.
9. Coulehan, J. Today's professionalism: engaging the mind but not the heart. *Acad Med.* 2005;80(10):892–8.

10. Huddle, TS. Viewpoint: teaching professionalism: is medical morality a competency? *Acad Med.* 2005;80(10):885–91.

11. Cruess, RL, Cruess, SR. Teaching professionalism: general principles. *Med Teach.* 2006;28(3):205–8.

12. *Oxford English Dictionary.* 2nd ed. Oxford: Oxford University Press; 1989 [cited November 27, 2007]. Available from: http://dictionary.oed.com/cgi/entry/50250688.

13. Krumboltz, JD, Nichols, CW. Integrating the social learning theory of career decision making. In Walsh, WB, Osipow, SH, editors. *Career Counseling: Contemporary Topics in Vocational Psychology.* Hillsdale (NJ): Lawrence Erlbaum Associates; 1990,159–92.

14. Adger, D. *Why Theory Is Essential: The Relationship between Theory, Analysis and Data.* Southampton (UK): The Higher Education Academy, University of Southampton; 2002 [cited November 27, 2007]. Available from: http://www.llas.ac.uk/resources/goodpractice.aspx?resourceid=405.

15. Bailey, KD. *Sociology and the New Systems Theory: Toward a Theoretical Synthesis.* New York: State of New York Press; 1994.

16. Marris, L. *A Practitioner's Perspective* [monograph on the internet]. Coventry (UK): National Guidance Research Forum; 2003[cited November 27, 2007]. Available from: http://www.guidance-research.org/EG/impprac/ImpP2/ImpP2ii/ImpP2iia.

17. Steffe L, Gale J, editors. *Constructivism in Education.* Hillsdale (NJ): Lawrence Erlbaum; 1995.

18. Bandura, A. *Social Learning Theory.* Englewood Cliff (NJ): Prentice Hall; 1977.

19. Bandura, A. *Self-efficacy: The Exercise of Control.* New York: W.H. Freeman; 1997.

20. Brown, JS, Collins, A, Duguid, S. Situated cognition and the culture of learning. *Educ Res.* 1989;18(1):32–42.

21. McLellan, H. *Situated Learning Perspectives.* Englewood Cliffs (NJ): Educational Technology Publications; 1996.

22. Maudsley, G, Strivens, J. Promoting professional knowledge, experiential learning, and critical thinking for medical students. *Med Educ.* 2000;34(7):535–44.

23. Mann, K. Learning and teaching in professional character development. In Kenney, N, editor. *Lost Virtue: Professional Character Development in Medical Education.* New York: Elsevier; 2006.

24. Collins, A, Brown, JS, Holum, A. Cognitive apprenticeship: making thinking visible. *Am Educ.* 1991;15(3):6–11,38–46.

25. Choi, JI, Hannafin, M. Situated cognition and learning environments: roles, structures, and implications for design. *Educ Technol Res Dev.* 1995;43(2):53–69.

26. Brandt, BL, Farmer, JA, Buckmaster, A. Cognitive apprenticeship approach to helping adults learn. *New Dir Adult Contin Educ.* 1993;59:69–78.

27. Harley, S. Situated learning and classroom instruction. *Educ Technol.* 1993;33(3):46–51.

28. Schön, DA. *The Reflective Practitioner: How Professionals Think in Action.* New York: Basic Books; 1983.

29. Epstein, RM, Hundert, EM. Defining and assessing professional competence. *JAMA*. 2002;287(2):226–35.

30. Hewson, MG. Reflection in clinical teaching: an analysis of reflection-on-action and its implications for staffing residents. *Med Teach*. 1991;13(3):227–31.

31. Robertson, K. Reflection in professional practice and education. *Aust Fam Physician*. 2005;34(9):781–3.

32. Lachman, N, Pawlina, W. Integrating professionalism in early medical education: the theory and application of reflective practice in the anatomy curriculum. *Clin Anat*. 2006;19(5):456–60.

33. Boud, D, Keogh, R, Walker, D. *Reflection: Turning Experience into Learning*. London: Kogan Page; 1985.

34. Roth, RA. Preparing the reflective practitioner: transforming the apprentice through the dialectic. *J Teach Educ*. 1989;40(2):31–5.

35. Brown, AL, Palincsar, AS. Guided, cooperative learning and individual knowledge acquisition. In Resnick, LB, editor. *Knowing, Learning, and Instruction: Essays in Honor of Robert Glaser*. Hillsdale (NJ): Erlbaum; 1989, 393–444.

36. Palincsar, AS, Ransom, K, Derber, S. Collaborative research and development of reciprocal teaching. *Educ Leadersh*. 1988;46(4):37–40.

37. Lave, J, Wenger, E. *Situated Learning: Legitimate Peripheral Participation*. Cambridge (UK): Cambridge University Press; 1991.

38. Wenger, E. *Communities of Practice: Learning, Meaning and Identity*. New York: Cambridge University Press; 1998.

39. Boud, D, Middleton, H. Learning from others at work: communities of practice and informal learning. *J Workplace Learn*. 2003;15(5):194–202.

40. Winn, W. Some implications of cognitive theory for instructional design. *Instr Sci*. 1990;19(1):53–69.

41. Norman, GR. The adult learner: a mythical species. *Acad Med*. 1999;74(8):886–9.

42. Merriam, SB. Updating our knowledge of adult learning. *J Contin Educ Health Prof*. 1996;16:136–43.

43. Knowles, MS. *Andragogy in Action*. San Francisco (CA): Jossey-Bass; 1985.

44. Knowles, MS. *The Modern Practice of Adult Education: From Pedagogy to Andragogy*. New York: Cambridge Books; 1988.

45. Kaufman, DM, Mann, KV, Jennett, PA. *Teaching and Learning in Medical Education: How Theory Can Inform Practice*. Edinburgh (UK): Association for the Study of Medical Education; 2000.

46. Kolb, DA, Fry, R. Towards an applied theory of experiential learning. In Cooper, CL, editor. *Theories of Group Processes*. London: John Wiley; 1975, 33–58.

47. Hilton, SR, Slotnick, HB. Proto-professionalism: how professionalisation occurs across the continuum of medical education. *Med Educ*. 2005;39(1):58–65.

48. Inui, TS. *A Flag in the Wind: Educating for Professionalism*. Washington (DC): Association of American Medical Colleges; 2003.

49. Wear, DP, Castellani, BP. The development of professionalism: curriculum matters. *Acad Med*. 2000;75(6):602–1.

50. Evans, BJ, Stanley, RO, Mestrovic, R, Rose, L. Effects of communication skills training on students' diagnostic efficiency. *Med Educ*. 1991;25(6):517–26.

51. Novack, DH, Dube, C, Goldstein, MG. Teaching medical interviewing: a basic course on interviewing and the physician-patient relationship. *Arch Intern Med.* 1992;152(9):1814–20.

52. Burack, JH, Irby, DM, Carline, JD, Root, RK, Larson, EB. Teaching compassion and respect: attending physicians' responses to problematic behaviors. *J Gen Intern Med.* 1999;14(1):49–55.

53. Epstein, R. Assessment in medical education. *N Engl J Med.* 2007;356(4):387–96.

54. Popham, WJ. *Educational Evaluation.* Boston (MA): Allyn and Bacon; 1993.

55. Wholey, IS, Hatry, HP, Newcomer, KE. *Handbook of Practical Program Evaluation.* San Francisco (CA): Jossey-Bass; 1994.

56. Kirkpatrick, DL. *Evaluating Training Programs: The Four Levels.* San Francisco (CA): Berrett-Koehler Publishers; 1997.

57. Steinert, Y. Twelve tips for effective small-group teaching in the health professions. *Med Teach.* 1996;18(3):203–7.

58. Steinert, Y. Twelve tips for using role plays in clinical teaching. *Med Teach.* 1993;15(4):283–91.

59. Charon, R. Narrative medicine: a model for empathy, reflection, profession, and trust. *JAMA.* 2001;286(15):1897–902.

60. Dent, JA, Harden, R. *A Practical Guide for Medical Teachers.* Toronto (ON): Elsevier; 2005.

61. Newble, D, Cannon, R. *A Handbook for Medical Teachers.* Boston (MA): MTP Press Limited; 1987.

62. Wright, S. Examining what residents look for in their role models. *Acad Med.* 1996;71(3):290–2.

63. Ficklin, FL, Browne, VL, Powell, RC, Carter, JE. Faculty and house staff members as role models. *J Med. Educ.* 1988;63(5):392–6.

64. Shuval, JT, Adler, I. The role of models in professional socialization. *Soc Sci Med.* 1980;14A:5–14.

65. Wright, SM, Wong, A, Newill, C. The impact of role models on medical students. *J Gen Intern Med.* 1997;12:53–6.

66. Wright, SM, Carrese, JA. Which values do attending physicians try to pass on to house officers? *Med Educ.* 2001;35(10):941–5.

67. Kenney, NP, Mann, KV, MacLeod, HM. Role modeling in physicians' professional formation: reconsidering an essential but untapped educational strategy. *Acad Med.* 2003;78(12):1203–10.

68. Cruess, S, Cruess, R, Steinert, Y. Role modelling – making the most of a powerful teaching strategy. *BMJ.* 2008;336:718–721.

69. Epstein, RM, Cole, DR, Gawinski, BA, Piotrowski-Lee, S, Ruddy, NB. How students learn from community-based preceptors. *Arch Fam Med.* 1998;7:149–54.

70. Boenink, AD, de Jonge, P, Smal, K, Oderwald, A, van Tilburg, W. The effects of teaching medical professionalism by means of vignettes: an exploratory study. *Med Teach.* 2005;27(5):429–32.

71. Goldie, J, Schwartz, L, McConnachie, A, Morrison, J. The impact of three years' ethics teaching, in an integrated medical curriculum, on students' proposed behaviour on meeting ethical dilemmas. *Med Educ.* 2002;36(5):489–97.

72. Kon, AA. Resident-generated versus instructor-generated cases in ethics and professionalism training. *Philos Ethics Humanit Med.* 2006;1(1):E10.

73. Winter, RO, Birnberg, BA. Teaching professionalism artfully. *Fam Med.* 2006; 38(3):169–71.

74. Charon, R. Narrative and medicine. *N Engl J Med.* 2004;350(9):862–4.

75. Morris, DB. Narrative, ethics and thinking with stories. *Narrative.* 2001;9:55–77.

76. Coulehan, J, Clary, P. Healing the healer: poetry in palliative care. *J Palliat Med.* 2005;8(2):382–9.

77. Bolton, G. Stories at work: reflective writing for practitioners. *Lancet.* 1999;354(9174):243–5.

78. DasGupta, SM, Charon, RM. Personal illness narratives: using reflective writing to teach empathy. *Acad Med.* 2004;79(4):351–6.

79. Kalet, A, Sanger, J, Chase, J, Keller, A, Schwartz, M, Fishman, ML, Garfall, A, Kitay, A. Promoting professionalism through an online professionalism development portfolio: successes, joys and frustrations. *Acad Med.* 2007;82(11):1065–72.

80. Gordon, J. Assessing students' personal and professional development using portfolios and interviews. *Med Educ.* 2003;37(4):335–40.

81. Snadden, D, Thomas, M. The use of portfolio learning in medical education. *Med Teach.* 1998;20(3):192–9.

82. Davis, MH, Friedman Ben-David, M, Harden, RM, Howie, P, Ker, J, McGhee, C, Pippard, MJ, Snadden, D. Portfolio assessment in medical students' final examinations. *Med Teach.* 2001; 23(4):357–66.

83. Driessen, EW, van Tartwijk, J, Overeem, K, Vermunt, JD, van der Vleuten, CPM. Conditions for reflective use of portfolios in undergraduate education. *Med Educ.* 2005;39(12):1230–5.

84. Wilkinson, TJ, Challis, M, Hobma, SO, Newble, DI, Parboosingh, JT, Sibbald, RG, Wakeford, R. The use of portfolios for assessment of the competence and performance of doctors in practice. *Med Educ.* 2002:36(10);918–24.

85. Wear, D, Kuczewski, MG. The professionalism movement: can we pause? *Am J Bioeth.* 2004;4(2):1–10.

86. Brainard, AH, Brislen HC. Viewpoint: learning professionalism: a view from the trenches. *Acad Med.* 2007;82(11):1010–4.

87. Hafferty, FW. Beyond curriculum reform: confronting medicine's hidden curriculum. *Acad Med.* 1998;73(4):403–7.

88. Hafferty, FW, Franks, R. The hidden curriculum, ethics teaching, and the structure of medical education. *Acad Med.* 2006;69(11):861–71.

89. Suchman, AL, Williamson, PR, Litzelman, DK, Frankel, RM, Mossbarger, DL, Inui, TS. Relationship-Centered Care Initiative Discovery Team. Toward an informal curriculum that teaches professionalism: transforming the social environment of a medical school. *J Gen Intern Med.* 2004;19(5 Pt. 2):501–4.

90. Steinert, Y, Cruess, S, Cruess, R, Snell, L. Faculty development for teaching and evaluating professionalism: from programme design to curriculum change. *Med Educ.* 2005;39(2):127–36.

3 Professionalism and the Socialization of Medical Students

Frederic William Hafferty, Ph.D.

History is opaque. You see what comes out, not the script that produces events, the generator of history.[1]

INTRODUCTION

In this chapter, we will examine issues of professions and professionalism through a particular lens, socialization theory. The fundamental assumption driving this chapter is my belief that current discussions about professionalism contain a bevy of unexamined assumptions about what happens to trainees as they move from the social and social-psychological status of lay outsiders to full members in a particular occupational group, in this case, medicine. These tacit renderings, in turn, block or otherwise distort meaningful efforts by medical educators to link medical training with principles and practices of professionalism. Until these disconnects and contradictions are pinpointed and made more explicit, efforts to develop targeted and effective educational interventions will continue to be thwarted.

To facilitate this examination, I treat medicine's current professionalism movement as *discourse* and analyze "how the specialized language of academic medicine disciplines has defined, organized, contained, and made seemingly immutable a group of attitudes, values, and behaviors subsumed under the label of professionalism."[2] My principal focus will be on the discourse of professionalism that has emerged since the mid-1980s, a period I consider organized medicine's "modern day professionalism movement." For analytical reasons discussed below, I label this discourse "nostalgic professionalism."[3] This discourse is marked by calls for physicians to recommit themselves to an ethic of professionalism – an ethic grounded in selfless service (e.g., altruism) and an ethic calling for the transformation of practitioners at the level of core value and self-identity. This discourse also identifies medical education as the principle vehicle for change and often calls for change at the level of organizational culture, but with few if any details about how to link the structure, process, and content of education with these outcomes. Furthermore, this discourse is awash with often inconsistent and conflicting references to professionalism across a broad variety of social-cognitive entities such as behaviors, attitudes, values, motives, tendencies. In bringing these inconsistencies to the surface, I argue that approaching/defining professionalism at the level of values and self-identity calls for a fundamentally different educational enterprise than approaching professionalism at the level of attitudes or behavior. In short, *how* we conceptualize professionalism must be reflected in how we structure our pedagogical practices to arrive at that end.

In preparing this chapter, I sought to understand exactly how professionalism is being handled within the modern day professionalism literature. Thus, if a given article referred to "professional attitudes," I asked; "In what way is professionalism treated as an attitude?" Conversely, if a given article specifies "professional values," I wanted to understand how the author actually framed professionalism as a value. As the reader might anticipate, it is not unusual for authors to refer to professionalism as a value *and* as an attitude, and do so in ways that are largely tacit, implying that the entities listed (attitudes, values, etc.) are interchangeable. While values, attitudes, and other dimensions of social life certainly coexist in a complex web of mutualities, they are not synonyms. While there is nothing inherently wrong with approaching professionalism as behavior (Does it really matter what one *believes* as long as one *acts* professionally?), the fundamental uncertainties that underscore clinical decision making, and the ambiguities that permeate medical practice, require a professional presence that is best grounded in who one *is* rather than what one *does*.

I organize this chapter in four parts. First, I present a brief overview of the modern-day professionalism movement and its emergent discourse of nostalgic professionalism. I then subject this discourse to a critical review by highlighting its tacit assumptions and conceptual weaknesses. Second, and taking an "if-then" form of argument, I conclude that if professionalism is to be conceptualized as values, then this calls for a particular framing of medical education – in this case education-as-socialization. To this end, I briefly review some principles of socialization and apply them to the particular case of medical education as professional preparation. Third, I take a more explicit look at professionalization as a form of social control and the implications of such a framing for a socialization approach to medical education. I close with some thoughts on how better to frame medical education as socialization.

MEDICAL PROFESSIONALISM: A TRUNCATED HISTORY

> Professionalism can be defined for all time as the means by which individual doctors fulfill the medical profession's contract with society. The specific attributes that have long been understood to animate professionalism include altruism, respect, honesty, integrity, dutifulness, honour, excellence, and accountability.[4]

> This version of professionalism is now moribund.[5]

Background

For the purposes of this chapter, the rise of a modern professionalism literature within medicine can be traced to the 1980s and 1990s with the emergence of what has been termed "nostalgic professionalism."[3] This particular discourse emerged from a consensus among medical leaders that medicine had strayed from its "traditional commitments" to patient welfare and had violated its social contract with society. In response, organized medicine embarked on a collective "professionalism project." Across a broad number of initiatives, medicine began to develop definitions, assessment tools, standards/competencies, and curricula.[4,6–12] It also identified "market forces" and "market incentives" as *the* primary threat to professionalism.[13]

The Rise of Nostalgic Professionalism

The rise of a professionalism movement within organized medicine produced a deluge of materials within the medical literature calling for a "rediscovery" and subsequent "recommitment" to "traditional values" and "core professional principles." Across a bevy of publications,[6,14–27] "key attributes and qualities" began to shape medicine's professionalism discourse. At its core, professionalism was characterized as "the essence of the physician-patient relationship" with strong ties to social forces such as trust and altruism.

As a whole, this literature produced a decidedly "old school" or "nostalgic" view of professionalism.[3] In addition to being framed as something essential to the identity of both medicine and its practitioners, professionalism was cast as something "central to sustaining the public's trust in the medical profession" by emphasizing "the primacy of patient welfare and the subordination of self-interest."[4,14,25] Writers referred to "avowed standards" and listed "core characteristics" such as altruism, respect, and honesty. Physicians, meanwhile, were expected to "pledge[ing] fidelity to their professional ethic" and to "pursue their professional prerogatives in the public interest."[4]

Warnings about commercialism were a key element in this discourse. Medical leaders saw a rise in unprofessional behavior, with professionalism being marginalized by the "irreconcilable ethics of the marketplace."[4] The fear was that medicine would evolve into "just another business" as physicians became increasingly disillusioned, frustrated, and cynical.

In addition to creating definitions, codes, statements of standards, and tools for assessment, the discourse of nostalgic professionalism identified medical education as *the* principle agent of remediation. Organized medical education responded. The Accreditation Council for Graduate Medical Education, for example, identified professionalism as one of its six "core competencies" and tied residency accreditation to meeting these competencies. Formal coursework in professionalism became ubiquitous throughout undergraduate medical training in the United States, Canada, and the United Kingdom. Targets for change included admissions practices, an emphasis on small group and experiential learning, and a general "purging" of educational environments of unprofessional practices.[4] Even personality factors were identified as barriers. Former AAMC President Jordan Cohen, for example, insisted that physicians (like all humans) were "hard-wired for self-interest," leading to "self-serving decisions under the guise of respectability."[4] For these and similar reasons, he called for "substantial change in the culture and environment of medical education" and for medical educators to "assume greater responsibility and accountability for strengthening the resolve of future doctors to sustain their commitment to the ethics of professionalism."[4] Educators were encouraged to develop learning experiences that would enable trainees to "inculcate" and "internalize" those principles.

This movement, while impressive in its collective breadth, energy, and commitment was not without opposition. Some medical school faculty, for example, questioned whether "something like professionalism" could be taught to medical students and/or residents.[28-31] Students, in turn, complained that the sudden infusion of professionalism materials within the formal curriculum is "unnecessary," "too rule driven," or "just another way to keep us in line."[32,33] Furthermore, students appeared to embrace new definitions of professionalism by emphasizing issues of lifestyle and balance over traditional medical concerns with altruism and "selfless service to others."[3,34] Meanwhile, many older faculty found themselves bewildered by what they saw as a younger generation of physicians who "no longer want to work hard."[35]

Where, then, do things stand with respect to professionalism and organized medical education? On the one hand, we have today a genuinely broad-based movement with considerable progress in defining and assessing professionalism and in establishing curricula and standards. On the other hand, there appears to be some measure of student and faculty resistance to the ways in which professionalism is represented within the movement. Finally, there appear to be disconnects between the discourse of nostalgic professionalism and what we expect (and should expect) from our underlying medical educational system if, in fact, we are going to formally train physicians based upon what is called for within that discourse. For example, if commercialism is antithetical to professionalism and the nostalgic professionalism literature is quite specific on this point, then the pedagogical task is not how to be a professional *in principle* but rather how to be a professional within a den of industry iniquity. After all, pedagogy shorn of context is little more than rhetoric.

The problem is not so much a lack of definition(s) within the medical professionalism literature as it is an ongoing vagueness about the underlying *nature* of what it is we aspire to. In turn, confusions about this nature have direct implications for, and impact on, the integrity of the educational mission as we seek to translate our professionalism ideals into educational outcomes.

Deconstructing Nostalgia

What then are we to make of these calls to professionalism – particularly the calls for necessary and substantial changes in the culture of the educational enterprise and/or the internalization of core values by trainees?

First, we need to agree upon what it is we are dealing with – and thus what we seek to address. Are we talking about "professional values," "professional attitudes," "professional attributes," "character traits," or perhaps, more restrictively, "professional behaviors"? For example, Cohen (and he is by no means alone) references all five, oftentimes interchangeably, along with using professionalism as an adjective attached to a wide variety of entities. The implication is that all the above terms are equivalent entities, which, of course they are not.

Second, regardless of our target (e.g., professionalism) what are we asking medical educators to do? Teach? Instruct? Transmit? Inform? Model? Inculcate? Or perhaps we anticipate structuring student learning across multiple fronts and expect medical schools to stress one modality of learning at one time and others at different phases or stages of training? The use of the verb "inculcation," for example, posits change at the level of self-identity.[6] Inculcation, however, is a fundamentally different social act than calling upon students to "*learn the principles* of professionalism" (italics mine) or to *master* behavioral skills or competencies, or to have students *model* themselves upon exemplary faculty.

Third, and related, what do we expect from students? Do we expect them to *learn* about professionalism – *appreciate* key professionalism principles – *behave* in professionally appropriate ways? Or do we expect them to *identify* with the precepts of professionalism, *be* or *become* professionals, and make these precepts part of their core identity? Knowing, behaving, and identification are very different ends.

Fourth, what about professionalism's "core expectation" – namely to subordinate self-interest in deference to the interest of others? This call to altruism is a key element in virtually all statements of nostalgic professionalism; yet, there appear to be substantive shifts in how the newest cohorts of students and practitioners view what it means to practice medicine. Can one actually be professional without being altruistic? Is it possible – or perhaps preferable – to approach altruism as a behavior rather than as a core attribute of one's personality or character? Teaching students to *act* or behave in an altruistic fashion calls for a different set of pedagogical practices than a developing learning environment to promote altruism as a matter of being or identity.

Fifth, what about marketplace ethics and their threat as a "corrupting influence?" What exactly is being corrupted – and how? At what level does "corruption" operate? Does it function more as a surface phenomenon (e.g., it may change what you do but not who you are) or does it operate more at the level of character and identity, with a corresponding invisibleness to the social actor? The understanding that the framing of commercialism as antithetical to professionalism within the medical literature often is more a rallying cry than nuanced analytical distinction, but efforts by faculty and students to tease out the social-psychological nature of this alteration and alteration has important implications for how best to train students to counter its influences.

To summarize, the call within the nostalgic professionalism literature for trainees to *embrace* the principles and practices of professionalism, and for educators to "strengthen the resolve" of their trainees "to the ethics of professionalism"[4] have fundamental implications for how we structure our educational endeavors. To further raise the pedagogical stakes, this literature calls for this reaffirmation in the face of social forces (including commercialism, corporatization, and capitalism) deemed antiprofessional in nature, and to do so in the face of a human nature that is characterized as "hard-wired" for selfishness. Finally, all of this is to take place within an educational milieu populated with role models and mentors whom themselves (according to medicine itself) have wandered somewhat afield from medicine's core mission and work.

THE MEDICAL SCHOOL AS A SITE OF OCCUPATIONAL SOCIALIZATION

Professional schools are an institutional context in which the organized profession can exert significant control. They are perhaps the sole sites where the professions' standards of good work set the agenda for learning. Professional schools are not only where expert knowledge and judgment are communicated from advanced practitioner to beginner but are also the place where the profession puts its defining values and exemplars on display, where future practitioners can begin both to assume and to critically examine their future identities. This is a complex educational process, however, and its value depends, in large part, on how well the several aspects of professional training are understood and woven into a whole.[36]

Introduction

The notion of the medical school as a special place permeates the medical education and professions literatures. One hallmark of medicine's status as a profession is that it controls both the selection and the education of future physicians. As such, and as noted in Sullivan's quote, medical schools and residency training programs are formidable – and formative – settings that structure and shape how future physicians will think, act, and identify themselves with core occupational values.

Although neither uses the concept directly, both Sullivan and Cohen (as quoted directly above) consider medical training as a site of occupational socialization and the medical school as a setting of deep learning.[37] They and others also frame the learning process as multifaceted, and thus at least implicitly recognize that *becoming* a doctor requires educators to take explicit steps to coordinate the multiplicity of learning environments that make up medical education, and in doing so to produce a professionally infused tapestry of physicianhood.

If we heed Sullivan's call and if we frame the educational undertaking at the level of identity, and do so utilizing "defining values and exemplars," then we are talking about socialization. If we accept Cohen's framing and conceptualize the medical school as a site of occupational culture, we are talking about changes in the structure and process of occupational socialization. While there will always be room for educators to decide whether we wish to emphasize a professionalism of attitudes or behaviors versus a professionalism of values and identity, the fact remains that if we wish to frame the general issue at the level of identity and at the level of organizational culture, then we are dealing at a fundamental level more with norms and values than with attitudes and behaviors.

To date (at least within this chapter), we have seen professionalism cast as a little bit of everything (attitude, identity, value, norm, behavior, attributes, perception, etc.), sometimes in the same document and often interchangeably. While it certainly is reasonable, or even warranted, for educators to identify "professional attitudes" *and* "professional values" as dually important objects of pedagogy, attitudes, and values are different social-psychological creatures with different implications for how we transform neophyte outsiders into well-established insiders.

One approach – and only one, I might add – to this conceptual conundrum is to examine medical education from within the framework of socialization theory.

Socialization Theory

There is no one (singular) theory of socialization. Core meanings and foci have evolved over time and across academic disciplines.[38,39] Within the medical education literature, references to socialization have a moderate presence, but most often appear as an isolated term without explanation or explication. In some instances, the term is used in a throwaway fashion, often as a synonym for "medical education," which most certainly is not, or as a vague reference to an unspecified social process (see Fineberg *et al.*[40] as an exception). In this same way, one also encounters references to "professional socialization" but without understanding whether the author is referring to the training of a particular occupational group (e.g., professionals) or as a particular (or special) type of socialization (e.g., childhood or adult socialization). Recognizing this distinction – referring to a particular occupational group versus a particular type of socialization – is critical because it directs our attention either to the *product* of a social process (e.g., the socialization of professionals) or to the social process itself (e.g., socialization). As Wentworth notes in his detailed analysis of socialization theory, contemporary writings on socialization tend to stress product over process, thus narrowing our understanding – and appreciation – of the social dynamics that underscore this particular form of social learning.[39]

Differences in time and discipline notwithstanding, there are some basic principles of socialization theory we can draw upon in exploring issues of medical education and professionalism. First, while the socialization literatures address issues of behavior and attitudes, socialization fundamentally involves training for self-image and identity. One can behave in certain respects because of underlying beliefs and one can have attitudes about the objects involved in the process, but the underlying dimension of socialization is personal transformation. Furthermore, while any occupational training involves learning new knowledge and skills, it is the melding of knowledge and skills with an altered sense of self that differentiates "training" from "socialization."

Second, much of what takes place during socialization, whether that be as child or adult, takes place at a tacit level. The very object of socialization is to take that which is unusual, nonroutine, or discordant to an outsider and render it commonplace and taken for granted by those within the group one seeks to join. Socialization works best when it unfolds in a subtle and incremental fashion rather than under the scrutiny of reflection at the group or personal level (how this "nature of" socialization dovetails with the recent emphasis within the professionalism literature on reflection and mindfulness will not be explored in this chapter).

Third, the identification of medical education as a site of occupational culture links us directly to the concept of socialization.[41] Furthermore, while there is great value in attending to organizational ceremonies and rituals in the transmission of group values and norms, the role of the less dramatic, routine, and taken-for-granted nature of everyday social life in the transmission and reinforcement of group values and normative standards has been underappreciated within the occupational training literature.[42] Finally, distinctions between the recognized and taken for granted, the formal and tacit, or the espoused and underlying, echo properties of the formal, informal, and hidden curriculum. The informal curriculum, for example, is awash with usualness. In turn, the hidden curriculum is closely aligned with Schein's model of occupational culture, including the presence of artifacts, espoused values (often within the formal curriculum), and the presence of basic underlying assumptions.

Fourth, while references to medical education as transformation without explication are common within the medical education literature, explicit references to the nature of medicine as a moral community and the medical school as sites of moral acculturation are relatively rare.[43,44] In contrast to other arenas of professional/occupational training, such as the military[45–48] and ministry,[49,50] medicine appears relatively reluctant to formally identify itself as a locus of personal and moral transformation. The consequence, for medical students at least, is not an absence of normative messages within the educational process, but rather a deluge of them – often at the individual (e.g., "this is how I do things around here") rather than group (e.g., "this is what we do") level. The consequence is a learning experience that is more disjointed and chaotic than unifying and directive. None of this is to imply that physicians should think like soldiers or profess like ministers, but it is to challenge the notion that medicine is best practiced at the level of knowledge and/or skills.

Finally, the experience of medical education is hardly a benign process. Some consider it "challenging," others "stressful," and still others rife with "bullying"[51] and "abuse."[52] Moreover, and independent of such environmental pressures, medical students are a tense, anxious, and highly goal-directed lot. They are high achievers, placed within settings of considerable tension and ambiguity, where all intensely want to become in-group members (e.g., physicians). As such, and to invoke the imagery of a "perfect storm" with intentional analogies to massive turbulence and kinetic energy, medical students are the "perfect objects" for socialization. This "fitness for socialization" is heightened by a medical culture that at least until recently devalues introspection and reflection.

To sum, if the object of our pedagogical attention is socialization as opposed to other types of learning, then we are committing ourselves to working with a pedagogical sandbox of values and personal/group identity rather than some other focus of learning. This framing, in turn, has appreciable implications for how we structure the medical learning process.

PROFESSIONALISM AS A FORM OF SOCIAL CONTROL

There are other reasons to place the concept of socialization at the forefront of any discussion of professionalism and medical education. Whether our referent literature is sociology or medicine, the concept of professionalism is linked indelibly to the notion of social control. While the specifics of medicine's rise as a profession have been detailed elsewhere,[53–55] medicine's ascendancy as a profession, its acquisition of occupational autonomy, and its promise to act as a fiduciary rests on two promises about, and related forms of, social control. The first is the widely cited (within the medical professionalism literature) promise by medicine to police itself in the public's interest. This is the concept – and promise – of peer review. This is social control at a collective level. An ineffective, dysfunctional, or otherwise corrupt process of peer review significantly weakens medicine's claim to professional status.

The second form of social control – taking place at the level of the self (e.g., self-review) is more foundational, yet only recently has it become the object of analytic attention within the medical professions literature.[6,56–59] This form of social control involves both the ability (with skill sets involved) and willingness of individuals to regulate their own selves and do so in the public's interest. The nature of this "willingness" is a core issue in this chapter.

Self-regulation (review/reflection) is a precursor for, and condition of, peer review. Peer review sans self-review is ritualized social action. It is the promise without the product. At a fundamental and definitional level, professionals are professionals because they *self*-regulate. Moreover, they do not so because of external rules or the threat of sanctions but rather because this is who they are. In short, self-review functions, or should function, as a core value within the overall normative framework of what it means to be a professional. In these respects, the notion of the physician – as professional revolves around the internalization of core occupational values that include a work ethic linked to a committed, concerned, and continuous self-monitoring on the public's behalf. Professionals, by definition – at least as represented within the nostalgic professionalism literature) – do not require the same types of external controls afforded, for example, by bureaucratic structures. Once again, we have core theoretical reasons within both sociology and the medical professionalism literature, for treating professionalism as the product of deep learning and internalization, something that functions at the level of personality and self-identity. Professionals regulate themselves because this is who they are and because of the special nature of their work – in that they work on behalf of "the other" (the patient).

Considerable work still needs to be done to better link self to peer review, self and peer review to the social contract, the social contract to broader issues of professionalism, and broader issues of professionalism to the nature of social control – particularly the control of work,[53] but this does not detract from the core argument linking self-regulation to socialization.

Medical Education as Resocialization

As noted above, socialization is hardly a monolithic entity. There are many different types of socialization, along with dimensions to this process. Some are widely referenced in the literature (primary/secondary, child/adult, political, gender, religious), while others are less visible (e.g., anticipatory,[60] emotional,[61] and resocialization[62]).

On a general level, professional socialization is a type of adult, and therefore secondary, socialization. Nonetheless, because of its structure (hierarchical, extended), it's setting (something often linked to Erving Goffman's concept of the "total institution"[63]), and because of its cognitive and emotional demands (intensive, stressful, etc.), it is reasonable to frame medical education as special or particular type of socialization.[64] The image of medical education as stressful and self-altering is a ubiquitous part of the medical education literature as well as a prominent message within autobiographical accounts of physician training[65–67] – even if the term itself never appears on the printed page.

Framing medical education as resocialization moves us away from an image of training as an additive process in which adult experiences are "simply" layered onto that which has been formulated via primary socialization – oftentimes in a passive and incidental fashion. Instead, postulating medical training as resocialization allows us to view medical training as more active, more purposeful social process where certain aspects of one's prior self are *replaced* by new ways of thinking, acting, and valuing. In other words, the concept of resocialization allows us to view certain types of occupational preparation as involving a dual process of moving into new and moving away from the old. This symbiotic interface of entering/embracing versus exiting/rejecting has been observed in studies of medical education, including educational experiences as early as the first few months of training.[68,69]

Of additional relevance in this linking of resocialization and medical training is the long-standing association of resocialization with brainwashing, including intentional efforts to reshape the identities and ideologies of "deviants" such as political prisoners or the "reprogramming" of "rescued" religious cult members. Although rarely used within the medical education literature, the concept is considered germane to the study of certain types of occupational training including professions (law and medicine), along with certain occupations (soldiers, firefighters, police officers) where the training itself is considered mentally and/or physically arduous, where the work is considered dangerous or even life threatening, and where that danger to self is accompanied by some kind of service ethic. By its very nature, then, resocialization involves some degree of intentionality as well as a reorientation or restructuring of self-identity.

The concept of resocialization also raises – once again – the role of environmental stresses, which are often purposefully manipulated in the case of resocialization, and the corresponding and often causally linked anxieties experienced by the trainee/socializee. Resocialization is most effective when the subject is repeatedly and purposefully stressed. Even extreme forms of psychological "readjustment" such as the Stockholm Syndrome can be explained within the framework of resocialization theory. Resocialization thus becomes a concept within which we can link the various descriptors of medical education (from "difficult," "challenging," and "exacting" to "intimidating," "traumatizing," and "abusive" – all underscored by sleep deprivation and fatigue) to the process of socialization. It is a process – for better and/or for worse – to change hearts *and* minds.

CONCLUSIONS

The above discussion of social/self-control and professionalism return us to the concept of socialization. Without attempting to truncate what is, after all, an exhaustively broad topic about the nature of social and occupational preparation, it remains vitally important that we periodically pause and ask ourselves; "What exactly are we talking about when we use the term medical education"? Do we consider education to be the impartation of basic knowledge, skills, and requisite behaviors – and there are medical school mission statements specifying just that – or do we include concepts such as beliefs, normative behaviors, or perhaps even values, and proceed to talk about professionalism as identity? In many respects, the choice remains medicine's given its continued control over the selection and training of future physicians.

The Carnegie Foundation's comparative study of professional education in medicine, nursing, law, engineering, and clergy is quite specific in noting that the "common aim of all professional education [to be] specialized knowledge and professional identity."[36] Do we agree? An affirmative or negative answer has important implications for how we structure and deliver medical training.

Socialization, at root, is learning to be an insider and in this chapter we have focused on one set of social process involved in what it means to become and be an insider as professional. While I do not wish to disparage the training of knowledge and skills, it should be fairly clear from our brief review of the socialization literature that socialization is, at root, more about deep than surface learning and more about identity transformation than practices of situational adjustment. When we talk about socialization, the behaviors of record are normative not idiosyncratic and the attitudes of import have to do with core beliefs and values rather than the more ephemeral aspects of social life such as the all time favorite *American Idol* winners, or even something directly germane to the world of medicine such as how one feels (e.g., attitudes) about physician pay for performance. Finally, while the process of socialization need not be thought of as unequivocally top down and prescripted (except in special circumstances such as resocialization), it always involves core attributes of what it means to be an in-group member.

With all of this in mind, a particular challenge for medical educators today, given the presence of medicine's professionalism project, is to wrestle with and reconcile the ambiguous and discordant conceptions of the physician as professional that still exist within the broader medical culture of medicine and then to infuse these newer understandings into a series of learning environments that are intentionally designed to reinforce and promote the types of physicians as professionals we wish to produce. Until recently, becoming a professional was thought to be (if it was thought about at all) little more than a byproduct of an educational process. One *was* a professional by virtue of *becoming* a physician. Medical educators no longer can accept this rather benign, passive, and essentially insipid view of professionalism.

A related challenge for educators is the clash between the altruism centric view of professionalism, at least as represented within medicine's current professionalism project, and the questioning by medical students of core definitional attributes. While I do not mean to imply that meanings about professionalism are literally "up for grabs," I do believe there is a legitimate sociological question as to whether the professionalism proffered by the "old guard" ultimately is reconcilable with newer and emergent forms of professionalism.[3]

The generational battles about "old-school" versus "lifestyle" professionalism are not the only site of epistemological conflict around what it means to be a physician. The most visible debate today, both in the public media and in the medical literature, revolves around conflicts of interest.[70] There are deep schisms within medicine about what situations, behaviors, and values represent "genuine" conflicts of interest. While conflict of interest does not subsume the full range of professionalism issues, this broad category of issues does speak, front and center, to a core principle, at least within the nostalgic professionalism literature, claimed by organized medicine, namely "the primacy of the patient," the placing of patient welfare above all other considerations (a.k.a. altruism). Parallel discussions revolve around the integrity of medical research and scientific data.[71,72] Finally, it is important to acknowledge that there are an appreciable number of physicians who unequivocally insist that medicine no longer is a profession, that it has become a business, and therefore the whole professionalism initiative is nothing more than an exercise in nostalgia and the final grasping of a form of occupational colonialism.

Issues of medical education, socialization, and professionalism are, of course, a great deal more complicated and nuanced than the characterizations represented in this chapter. In some very real respects, I have been unfairly restrictive in both my questions and my answers. Nonetheless, I believe the issue as framed ("What does it mean to be a physician as professional?") is more foundational than asking how to best define or measure professionalism. At root, we want our definitions and measures to reflect core meanings rather than to dictate them ex post facto.

Finally, there is the issue of authenticity. When we label something "professional" are we referring to the product of deep or of surface learning? The issue is not one of semantics or aesthetics. Medicine trains for the usual and commonplace as well as the unusual and idiosyncratic. It is *relatively* easy to *be* professional, and even easier to *appear* so, within the usualness of everyday medical life. All medical settings, including those infused with crisis (e.g., the ER and ICU), have routines that fill the vast majority of "what goes on." At the same time, every work setting has its "black swans,"[1] the unanticipated and often unanticipatable events that truly stretch the boundaries of an occupation's knowledge, skills, and values. This is why training in professionalism functions – and should function – at the level of socialization and at the level of values and identity. Case studies are important pedagogical tools. They help students to grasp particulars. So too is the situated learning that takes place on the job as individuals "learn the ropes" and "the way things are done around here." However, medical practice is riddled with the unexpected. This is the nature of the beast. This is why, when the unusual surfaces, the hope is that practitioners will return to their knowledge base and tease out *new* answers, return to their skill sets and come up with *innovative* procedures, and return to what they *truly* value and *be* physicians as professionals.

Efforts to lay bare the variety and types of learning that go on during this transformation of lay outsiders to medical insiders is an iterative process. We may seek to move some aspects of the informal and hidden curriculum more under the spotlight of formal educational activities, but there will always be those aspects of any occupational learning, particularly workplace learning, that remain counter to and even antithetical to what is being formally proffered. Counterfactuals are part of the richness, and messiness, of social life. Nonetheless, the omnipresence and often countervailing nature of the informal and hidden curriculum does not mean we do not continually and reflectively ask ourselves; "What does it mean to be a physician as professional," and then to fold our answers back into the structure and process of medical training. After all, the iterative process of linking reflection with subsequent action speaks to a type of integrity that is the hallmark of what it means to be a profession.

REFERENCES

1. Taleb, NN. *The Black Swan: The Impact of the Highly Improbable.* New York: Random House; 2007.
2. Wear, D, Kuczewski, MG. The professionalism movement. Can we pause? *Am J Bioeth.* 2004;4:1–10.
3. Castellani, B, Hafferty, F. Professionalism and complexity science: a preliminary investigation. In Wear, D, Aultman, JM (eds.). *Medical Professionalism: A Critical Review.* New York: Springer; 2006:3–23.
4. Cohen, JJ. Professionalism in medical education, an American perspective: from evidence to accountability. *Med Educ.* 2006;40:607–617.
5. Horton, R. *What's Wrong with Doctors. The New York Review of Books.* www.nybooks.com/articles/20214. Accessed October 1, 2007.
6. Cruess, RL. Teaching professionalism: theory, principles, and practices. *Clin Orthop Relat Res.* 2006;449:177–185.
7. Cruess, RL, Cruess, SR. Teaching professionalism: general principles. *Med Teach.* 2006;28:205–208.
8. Goldie, J, Dowie, A, Cotton, P, Morrison, J. Teaching professionalism in the early years of a medical curriculum: a qualitative study. *Med Educ.* 2007;41:610–617.
9. O'Donnell, JF. Competencies are all the rage in education. *J Cancer Educ.* 2004; 19:74–75.
10. Goldstein, EA, Maclaren, CF, Smith, S, Mengert, TJ, Maestas, RR, Foy, HM, Wenrich, MD, Ramsey, PG. Promoting fundamental clinical skills: a competency-based college approach at the University of Washington. *Acad Med.* 2005;80:434–433.
11. Riesenberg, LA, Rosenbaum, PF, Stick, SL. Competencies, essential training, and resources viewed by designated institutional officials as important to the position in graduate medical education. *Acad Med.* 2006;81:426–431.

12. Litzelman, DK, Cottingham, AH. The new formal competency-based curriculum and informal curriculum at Indiana University School of Medicine: overview and five-year analysis. *Acad Med.* 2007;82:410–421.

13. Hafferty, FW. Professionalism and commercialism as antitheticals: a search for 'unprofessional commercialism' within the writings and work of American medicine. In Parsi, K, Sheehan, M (eds.). *Healing as Vocation: A Medical Professionalism Primer.* New York: Rowen and Littlefield; 2006:35–59.

14. ABIM Foundation, ACP-ASIM Foundation, and European Federation of Internal Medicine. Medical professionalism in the new millennium: a physician charter. *Ann Intern Med.* 2002;136:243–246.

15. Arnold, L. Assessing professional behavior: yesterday, today, and tomorrow. *Acad Med.* 2002;77:502–515.

16. Blank, L, Kimball, H, McDonald, W, Merino, J, for the ABIM Foundation ACPF, and European Federation of Internal Medicine (EFIM). Medical professionalism in the new millennium: a physician charter 15 months later. *Ann Intern Med.* 2003;138:839–841.

17. Coulehan, J. Viewpoint: today's professionalism: engaging the mind but not the heart. *Acad Med.* 2005;80:892–898.

18. Ginsburg, S, Regehr, G, Lingard, L. Basing the evaluation of professionalism on observable behaviors: a cautionary tale. *Acad Med.* 2004;79(10 suppl.): S1–S4.

19. Inui, TS. *A Flag in the Wind: Educating for Professionalism in Medicine.* Washington, DC: Association of American Medical Colleges; 2003.

20. Papadakis, MA, Teherani, A, Banach, MA, Knettler, TR, Rattner, SL, Stern, DT, Veloski, JJ, Hodgson, CS, Kohatsu, ND. Disciplinary action by medical boards and prior behavior in medical school. *New Engl J Med.* 2005;353:2673–2682.

21. Stern, DT, ed. *Measuring Medical Professionalism.* New York: Oxford University Press; 2005.

22. Reynolds, PP. Reaffirming professionalism through the educational community. *Ann Intern Med.* 1994;120:609–614.

23. Rothman, DJ. Medical professionalism–focusing on the real issues. *N Engl J Med.* 2000;342:1284–1286.

24. Swick, HM, Szenas, P, Danoff, D, Whitcomb, ME. Teaching professionalism in undergraduate medical education. *JAMA.* 1999;282:830–832.

25. Swick, HM. Toward a normative definition of medical professionalism. *Acad Med.* 2000;75:612–616.

26. Wear, D, Aultman, JM. *Professionalism in Medicine: Critical Perspectives.* New York: Springer Verlag; 2006.

27. Wynia, MK, Latham, SR, Kao, AC. Medical professionalism in society. *New Engl J Med.* 1999;341:1612–1616.

28. Cruess, RL, Cruess, SR. Professionalism must be taught. *BMJ.* 1997;315:1674–1677.

29. Rowley, BD, Baldwin, DC Jr., Bay, RC, Cannula, M. Can professional values be taught? A look at residency training. *Clin Orthop Relat Res.* 2000;378:110–114.

30. Martin, J, Lloyd, M, Singh, S. Professional attitudes: can they be taught? *Clin Med.* 2002;2:217–222.

31. Stern, DT. *Can Professionalism be Taught. American Medical Association Journal of Ethics.* http://virtualmentor.ama-assn.org/2003/12/toc-0312.html. Accessed October 1, 2007.

32. American Medical Student Association (AMSA). *AMSA'S 2007 PharmFree Score-card.* Washington, DC: American Medical Student Association; 2007.

33. Goldstein, E, Maestas, RR, Fryer-Edwards, K, Wenrich, MD, Oelschlager, A-MA, Baernstein, A, Kimball, HR. Professionalism in medical education: an institutional challenge. *Acad Med.* 2006;81:871–876.

34. Hafferty, FW. What medical students know about professionalism. *Mt Sinai J Med.* 2002;69:385–397.

35. Smith, LG. Medical professionalism and the generation gap. *Am J Med.* 2005;118:439–442.

36. Sullivan, WM, Colby, A, Wegner, JW, Bond, L, Schulman, LS. *Educating Lawyers: Preparation for the Profession of Law.* San Francisco, CA: John Wiley & Sons; 2007.

37. Atherton, JS. *Learning and Teaching: Deep and Surface Learning.* www.learningandteaching.info/learning/deepsurf.com. Accessed October 1, 2007.

38. Tierney, WG. Organizational socialization in higher education. *J Higher Educ.* 1997;68:1–16.

39. Wentworth, WM. *Context and Understanding: An Inquiry into Socialization Theory.* New York: Elsevier; 1980.

40. Fineberg, IC, Wenger, NS, Forrow, L. Interdisciplinary education: evaluation of a palliative care training intervention for pre-professionals. *Acad Med.* 2004;79:769–776.

41. Schein, EH. *Organizational Culture and Leadership.* 2nd ed. San Francisco, CA: Jossey-Bass; 1992.

42. Van Maanen, J, Barley, SR. Occupational communities: culture and control in organizations. In Staw, BM, Cummings, LL (eds.). *Research in Organizational Behavior.* Vol 6. Greenwich, CT: JAI Press; 1984:265–287.

43. Pellegrino, ED. The medical community as a moral community. *Bull N Y Acad Med.* 1990;66:221–232.

44. Hafferty, FW, Franks, R. The hidden curriculum, ethics teaching, and the structure of medical education. *Acad Med.* 1994;69:861–871.

45. Hays, K. *Practicing Virtues: Moral Traditions at Quaker and Military Boarding Schools.* Berkeley, CA: University of California Press; 1994.

46. Janowitz, M. *The Professional Soldier.* New York: Free Press of Glencoe; 1960.

47. Leahy, JF. *Honor, Courage, Commitment: Navy Boot Camp.* Annapolis, MD: Naval Institute Press; 2002.

48. Lipsky, D. *Absolutely American: Four Years at West Point.* Boston, MA: Houghton Mifflin Co.; 2003.

49. Kleinman, S. Women in seminary: dilemmas of professional socialization. *Sociol Educ.* 1984;57:210–219.

50. Foster, CR, Dahill, L, Golemon, L, Tolentino, BW. *Educating Clergy: Teaching Practices and Pastoral Imagination.* San Francisco, CA: Jossey-Bass; 2005.

51. Quine, L. Workplace bullying in junior doctors: questionnaire survey. *BMJ.* 2002;324:878–879.

52. Kassebaum, DG, Cutler, ER. On the culture of student abuse in medical school. *Acad Med.* 1998;73:1149–1158.

53. Freidson, E. *Professionalism: The Third Logic.* Chicago, IL: University of Chicago Press; 2001.

54. Starr, PE. *The Social Transformation of American Medicine: The Rise of a Sovereign Profession and the Making of a Vast Industry.* New York: Basic Books; 1982.

55. Starr, P. Social transformation twenty years on. *J Health Polit Policy Law.* 2004;29:1005–1019.

56. Epstein, RM. Mindful practice. *JAMA.* 1999;282:833–839.

57. Niemi, PM. Medical students' professional identity: self-reflection during the preclinical years. *Med Educ.* 1997;31:408–415.

58. Sobral, DT. An appraisal of medical students' reflection-in-learning. *Med Educ.* 2000;34:182–187.

59. Wong, A. Mindfulness–rediscovering satisfaction and meaning in medical education. *Univ Toronto Med J.* 2003;80:265–267.

60. Harvill, LM. Anticipatory socialisation of medical students. *J Med Educ.* 1981;56:431–433.

61. Hochschild, AR. *The Managed Heart: Commercialization of Human Feeling.* Berkeley, CA: University of California Press; 1983.

62. Feldman, DC. Socialization, resocialization, and training: reframing the research agenda. In Goldstein, IL & Associates (eds.). *Training and Development in Organizations.* San Francisco, CA: Jossey-Bass; 1989:376–415.

63. Goffman, E. *Asylums: Essays on the Social Situations of Mental Patients and Other Inmates.* Garden City, NY: Doubleday; 1961.

64. Morrison, L. Resocialization In Ritzer, G (ed.). *Blackwell Encyclopedia of Sociology.* Blackwell Publishing, 2007. Blackwell Reference Online. http:// www.blackwellreference.com/subscriber/tocnode?id=g9781405124331_chunk_ g978140512433123_ss1-59. Accessed October 1, 2007.

65. Collins, MJ. *Hot Lights, Cold Steel: Life, Death and Sleepless Nights in a Surgeon's First Years.* New York: St. Martin's Press; 2005.

66. Gawande, A. *Complications: A Surgeon's Notes on an Imperfect Science.* New York: Metropolitan Books; 2002.

67. Transue, ER. *On Call: A Doctor's Diary.* New York: St. Martin's Press; 2004.

68. Hafferty, FW. *Into the Valley: Death and the Socialization of Medical Students.* New Haven, CT: Yale University Press; 1991.

69. Sinclair, S. *Making Doctors: An Institutional Apprenticeship (Explorations in Anthropology).* New York: Berg; 1997.

70. Brennan, TA, Rothman, DJ, Blank, LL, Blumenthal, D, Chimonas, SC, Cohen, JJ, Goldman, J, Kassirer, JP, Kimball, HR, Naughton, J, Smelser, N. Health industry practices that create conflicts of interest: a policy proposal for academic medical centers. *JAMA.* 2006;292:1044–1050.

71. Lo, B, Wolf, LE, Berkeley, A. Conflict-of-interest policies for investigators in clinical trials. *New Engl J Med.* 2000;343:1616–1620.

72. Stossel, TP. Regulating academic-industrial research relationships–solving problems or stifling progress? *N Engl J Med.* 2005;353:1060–1065.

PART THREE

Principles

Principles for Designing a Program for the Teaching and Learning of Professionalism at the Undergraduate Level

Richard L. Cruess, M.D., and Sylvia R. Cruess, M.D.

Until recent years, the subject of professionalism was not addressed formally in the medical curriculum. Students became professionals without being aware of it, with the assumption being that they patterned their behavior on that of respected role models.[1–3] It was only when both society and the profession came to believe that medicine's professionalism had been eroded by forces arising both inside and outside of the medical profession[4,5] that it was deemed necessary to teach professionalism as a distinct subject,[1,6–10] something that is now required by accrediting and certifying bodies.[11–14] Without question professionalism can be taught and learned in many different educational settings, using a variety of pedagogic tools and methods. However, as faculties of medicine have gained experience in teaching professionalism, common threads have emerged. It has become possible to outline a series of principles that can guide the actions of those designing, implementing, and administering programs aimed at promoting the acquisition of knowledge about professionalism and the behaviors characteristic of a professional. It is the goal of this chapter to outline these principles.

Any set of principles must be compatible with the complex nature of the medical curriculum through which individuals become transformed from members of the lay public into skilled professionals. There has not always been unanimity of opinion on how best to organize the teaching of professionalism. In part, this relates to individual and institutional approaches to the issue, with two schools of thought being predominant. Those who emphasized the need for detailed knowledge of the subject have tended to stress formal instruction, making the nature of professionalism explicit.[6,15,16] They generally define professionalism, list its attributes, and emphasize the role of trust, stressing its importance to medicine's relationship to society. They outline the obligations that medicine must meet in order to maintain its professional status. Others believed that the teaching of professionalism should be approached primarily as a moral endeavor, emphasizing altruism and service and stressing the importance of role modeling, efforts to promote self-awareness, community service, and other methods of acquiring experiential knowledge.[17–22]

While it would be wrong to overemphasize the differences between these two approaches, they did exist. There is now an emerging consensus that both groups are correct.[7–9,23,24] Professionalism must be taught explicitly as incoming medical students, residents, and faculty do not fully understand its nature and have not acquired a comprehensive knowledge about it during their education and training.[25,26] More significantly, the well-documented failures demonstrated by physicians show that they do not fully understand either its nature or the obligations associated with contemporary professionalism.[27–29] Furthermore, if physicians as rational beings are to incorporate a set of values into their day-to-day life, they should be able to articulate them, along with the reasons for their existence.

However, when the teaching of professionalism is limited to formal didactic sessions outlining the "cognitive base," without question, the impact will be minimal. Learners will not have the opportunity to reflect on the issues, to incorporate the attitudes and behaviors of professionalism into their daily lives, and to move to higher levels of both knowledge and performance.[7,8,17,21,24] Professionalism is fundamental to the process of socialization (see Chapter 3) during which individuals acquire the values, attitudes, interests, skills, and knowledge – the culture of the groups of which they seek to become a member.[4,30,31] For this reason, the acquisition of both explicit and tacit knowledge of professionalism must take place in parallel with the growth of knowledge in other areas. A balance should be struck between teaching the cognitive base explicitly and providing opportunities where reflection and learning can occur in an authentic context.

PRINCIPLES

Teaching the cognitive base of professionalism is not difficult. Establishing an environment where the process of socialization in its most positive sense can take place is much more challenging. The following principles can serve to assist those attempting to ensure that learners both understand professionalism and that they are properly indoctrinated into the "unwritten rules of studenthood and medical practice."[31] These principles encompass two large areas of activity. First, faculties of medicine and their associated teaching institutions must take a series of decisions that will indicate support in a public way for the teaching of professionalism, provide the resources required by the program, and create an environment that will allow the program to flourish. Second, a curriculum must be created that ensures that students and residents can be taught and learn the essence of professionalism.

The principles that are discussed here are drawn from the personal experience of the authors and their colleagues as well as that of others as reported in the literature. Of necessity, there will be some overlap among the principles as actions taken in one specific area of the complex process of contemporary medical education will rarely have results confined to that area. Nevertheless, it is felt that identifying and addressing each of the issues independently can assist those who are establishing programs on teaching professionalism.

Institutional Support

It is difficult to mount a major change in any organization unless there is strong support from its leadership[4,6,32–38] and educational institutions are no exception. Those directing medical schools and hospitals must first recognize the importance of professionalism and publicly signal their support. Financial and human resources are required and time for teaching must be allocated within the curriculum. Experience has demonstrated that the additional time required for new activities can be modest. Those faculties who have reported on their experiences have shown that there are many learning experiences already taking place throughout the curriculum that are devoted to the teaching of professionalism without being specifically identified as such. They can, with some reorientation, be included in an overall program.[35–40]

The active support of the dean and associate deans as well as influential department chairs is the key to the success of any significant curricular reform and establishing a program on the teaching of professionalism does constitute a major change.[4,6,32,37]

Allocation of Responsibility

Closely linked to the issue of institutional support is the need to allocate responsibility for establishing and directing a program for the teaching and learning of professionalism.[31–33,36–41] The decision as to who will be responsible is of some importance for symbolic as well as practical administrative reasons. Teaching programs on professionalism cross departmental and disciplinary lines and should be present throughout the continuum of medical education. An individual and/or a committee should be responsible for guiding the design, implementation, direction, and evaluation of these programs. This is a task that requires a feeling for the internal dynamics of the faculty, a comprehensive knowledge of professionalism based on contemporary literature, and both tact and diplomacy. The individual should command respect, have easy access to senior administration, be provided with adequate resources, and have the skills and knowledge to both create and administer the program and serve as its champion.

In addition to appointing the leader/champion, most faculties choose to establish a committee or working group composed of knowledgeable individuals from the academic units where the majority of the teaching will take place as well as local experts on professionalism and its evaluation.[35–41] The committee's function is to advise the individual responsible, participate in planning, assist in the administration, and provide leadership in the locales were the actual teaching and learning takes place.

The Environment

The institutional culture either can support professional behavior or subvert it. Medical education is carried out in a milieu that is heavily influenced by the atmosphere created within medicine's institutions and by the health care system.[4,5,7,8,23,42–45] There is a "formal curriculum" outlined in the mission statement of the institution and its course objectives.[44,45] This states what the faculty believes that they are teaching. It includes structured teaching, clinical exposure, and organized activities designed to promote self-reflection. The teaching of professionalism must be a prominent part of all these activities.

There is also an extremely powerful "informal curriculum" consisting of unscripted, unplanned, and highly interpersonal forms of teaching and learning that take place among and between faculty and students. This occurs in corridors and elevators, cafeterias, and social settings – indeed in any situation in which teachers and learners are together. Students, residents, and peers are always learning.[7] Teachers and role models at several levels, from peers to senior physicians, participate and can have a profound effect for good or ill on the attitudes of students and residents.[46] According to most reports, the implications of this for medical education are significant because the influence of the informal curriculum is all too often negative.[7,8,20–22,41,45] Virtually, every observer, including the students themselves,[33] have commented on the fact that students and residents are exposed to behaviors that are antithetical to professionalism and that this is a contributing factor in the well-documented cynicism that develop in both groups.

Finally, there is a hidden curriculum, consisting of a set of influences that are rarely articulated and that function at the level of the organizational structure and culture and that are the end result of a host of administrative decisions and policies. In order to create a hidden curriculum that actually promotes professionalism, the leadership of a faculty or academic health center must take decisions that indicate that they give priority to patient care, strive for excellence, and provide the financial and infrastructure support for those who teach. All members of the health care team should understand their role in creating an environment that both supports and rewards professional behavior and has a strong base in moral values, which is apparent to students.[21] This is where the active and visible support of the dean and other faculty leaders can exert a very positive effect.[34] These issues are discussed in Chapter 6.

The incentives and disincentives built into any institutional culture may require change, along with other factors including economic and structural policies established at the organizational level.[24,33,34,37,38]

It is difficult to overemphasize the fact that, to be successful, any program on teaching professionalism must recognize the need to evaluate and, if necessary, alter the formal, the informal, and the hidden curriculum in order to create an environment that supports rather than subverts the acquisition of professional values by students, residents, and faculty. These issues are addressed in Chapter 6.

The Cognitive Base

Students and residents must understand the nature of professionalism, the profession's historical roots, its strong moral base, and the reason society supports the privileged position of the professions. The obligations necessary to sustain professional status and professionalism's relationship to medicine's social contract with society should be presented. As outlined in Chapter 1, this constitutes the cognitive base of professionalism.

The definition and description are an important first step and are of paramount importance as they set the expectations for students and faculty.[1,6,24,34,47] Therefore, each institution should agree on the substance of the cognitive base and this must remain consistent throughout the continuum of medical education. There is now a rich literature to assist in choosing a definition. Utilizing this literature is important as it documents the fact that medicine itself does not define professionalism. Society does, delegating authority to the medical profession through licensing laws and by legislation establishing the regulatory framework.[6,3,5,48]

The definition chosen does not just dictate what must be taught and learned, it determines what will be evaluated in students and residents, and also in faculty members.

There is not one definition for first-year students and another for those in the final year. The same is true for residents, faculty members, and practicing physicians. For this reason, a definition should be chosen that can serve at the undergraduate and postgraduate levels as well as during continuing

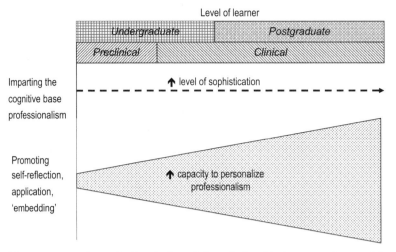

Figure 4.1. A schematic description of the relationship between the cognitive base and reflection. The cognitive base of professionalism should be presented to students on a regular basis throughout the curriculum. Students, residents, and practitioners have an increasing capacity for reflection on professionalism as they gain in experiential learning. Stage-appropriate opportunities for reflection should therefore be provided.

professional development. The cognitive base presented to students early in the curriculum should be reinforced throughout the course of medical education (Figure 4.1). It is possible to present different aspects of professionalism at different stages of training, stressing definitions and attributes early, and proceeding to emphasizing the social contract at a later stage. Opportunities for reflection always should be linked to instruction in the cognitive base.

Finally, all institutions affiliated with an academic center should be encouraged to use the same language, although they may choose different pedagogic approaches to teach and ensure that the cognitive base is learned.

The definition chosen should be one which encompasses all aspects of medical professionalism. Leaving out any part at any level – for example, self-regulation – will send a signal that this is not important. In addition, professionalism is integral not only to medicine's relationship to patients and their families but also to society in general. The expectations that both patients and society have of physicians as professionals must be a part of what is taught.

Finally, the definition of professionalism chosen must not represent the "nostalgic professionalism" of yesteryear.[49] Rather, it should reflect a professionalism that is suited to the present day practice of medicine.[49–52]

Experiential Learning and Self-Reflection

Professional identity arises "from a long term combination of experience and reflection on experience."[30(p63)] A major objective of medical education should be to provide stage-appropriate opportunities for gaining experience and reflecting upon it.[18,53,54] There must be structured opportunities allowing students, residents, and indeed practitioners to discuss professional issues in a safe environment, personalize them, and hopefully internalize appropriate values and behaviors over the course of education and training.[7,8,17,20,24,40,55–62] In this way, individuals develop their professional identity over a time, changing from novices into skilled professionals. Much of what is learned joins a larger body of knowledge described as tacit: that which one "knows but cannot tell."[63] While tacit knowledge is difficult to teach, it can be learned.[64] It is best learned not in the lecture hall, but by situated learning that encourages self-reflection and promotes "mindfulness"[17] or "reflective practice" (see Chapter 2).[65]

Experiential learning and reflection on the experience gained has always been inherent in medical education. The challenge in designing a program on teaching professionalism is to ensure that learners at all levels relate their experiences to professionalism and reflect upon these experiences in the context of medical professionalism. The objectives are twofold. The first is for professional behavior to "become manifest in lived experiences of physicians."[21(p893)] This is an important part of the process of socialization where the impetus for professional behavior comes from within the individual.[42] The second objective is to have the learners reflect upon the many threats to their professionalism that they will face as they function in today's complex health care systems. This should allow them to develop and articulate their own personal attitudes and solutions to situations involving conflicting values and obligations and to do so in a safe and supportive environment.

For this to occur, learners must first gain experience. This can occur in real-life situations taking place in clinical rotations or practice, in community service, or during activities specifically designed for the purpose. The key is to promote reflection upon these experiences. Reflection has been defined as "a purposeful form of thought provoked by unease in learners when they recognize that their understanding is incomplete."[66] It has been suggested that four things prompt reflection. First, there must be something upon which to reflect. The experiences listed above serve this purpose. Second, there must be time for reflection and this must be built into the curriculum on a regular basis. Third, there must be role models who are trained to promote reflection in learners. This again highlights the importance of faculty development for the role models. Finally, there must be motivation to reflect. In some, this motivation comes from within[67] but others require an external stimulus[61,62,66] Giving both importance and credit to reflective exercises is therefore necessary.

There is a large literature on reflection and mindfulness.[3,7,10,17–22,30,35,36,50,55,57,58,62,64,67–75] Virtually, all observers stress the extreme importance of highly personal activities, a safe environment, and interaction between individuals, either on a one-on-one basis or in small groups facilitated by a respected role model. Each faculty or teaching institution must decide which methods best suit its culture and its resources. The methods available include discussions of meaningful personal experiences in medicine, the use of vignettes, discussion of literature or films, the production and analysis of narratives, organized advisory groups, tutorials, mentors, portfolios in a variety of forms, an analysis of critical incidents, morning report, courses in the humanities, events drawn from community service, interprofessional teaching sessions, or any other strategy that can lead a learner to examine their own responses to dilemmas or difficult situations.[8,17–19,21,22,39,40,55–58,62,66,68–75]

These structured activities should be planned so that students and residents will, during the course of their reflection, address the major issues at the interface between medicine and society that are potential causes of tension. Thus, altruism, generational issues, the role of the individual in self-regulation, conflicts of interest, end-of-life issues, ethical concerns, as well as the traditional role of the healer must be included. The importance of medicine as a moral endeavor should be stressed and, while there are clearly situations for which there is no satisfactory answer, issues of right and wrong must be included.[21,22]

The capacity for self-reflection of a final-year student will be greater than that of one in the first year because they have acquired more experiential knowledge.[7,30,55] This is illustrated in Figure 4.1. Therefore, the activities devoted to self-reflection should be different depending upon the stage of training and should wherever possible be context specific, relating to activities that are taking place at that stage.

While all aspects of a program on teaching professionalism are important, those devoted to providing experiential learning and reflection upon what has been learned pose the greatest challenge and should be given the highest priority.

Role Modeling

Role modeling has been defined as that process whereby faculty members exhibit knowledge, attitudes, and skills; demonstrate and articulate expert thought processes; and manifest positive professional behaviors and characteristics.[76] This process involves both conscious and unconscious activities.[77] In fact, it is this mix of the conscious and the unconscious, the explicit and the implicit, that makes role modeling so complex. While the conscious portion is important to learning, the student's unconscious incorporation of observed behaviors is essential for role modeling to be effective.

Role models remain a very potent means of transmitting those intangibles that have been called the art of medicine and that are important components of professionalism.[22,78–82] They are also central to the development of the sense of collegiality that serves to obtain agreement on the common goals of the profession and encourage compliance with them.[83] The peer pressure of respected role models remains an enormously powerful tool.[82] Conversely, the destructive effects of role models who fail to meet acceptable professional standards can be equally strong.[20,22,33,79,84,85] Negative role modeling is pervasive and constitutes a significant issue for faculties of medicine.

Physicians model a broad range of the attributes of professionalism including clinical expertise, self-awareness and reflection, empathy and respect, attitudes toward patients and peers, personal qualities, and beliefs and values.[78,79] Each attribute may be demonstrated in an exemplary fashion; unfortunately, each attribute may also be modeled in a negative manner, causing a student to acquire attitudes or behaviors that are incompatible with good medical practice.

Role modeling takes place during instruction in the formal curriculum and the conduct of teachers at this level can have a profound effect. A teacher who demonstrates passion and enthusiasm for what he does can be extremely effective, while one who fails to do so misses a valuable opportunity.

Role models at several levels, from peers to senior physicians, function in the informal curriculum[7,45] and many of the corrosive effects of negative role modeling are experienced here.[80,86] The influence of the hidden curriculum on role modeling can also be profound. It is here where many of the barriers to effective role modeling are found. For example, an institutional culture that promotes overwork, leaving insufficient time for harried clinical teachers to promote the type of reflective practice needed to promote best practices among students, is detrimental to effective role modeling. Similarly, a culture that tolerates inadequate clinical care or poor interpersonal relationships inhibits positive modeling, as do administrative decisions that fail to demonstrate appreciation and support – both financial and nonfinancial – of those who are attempting to be exemplary.

Thus, an essential component of any teaching program on professionalism is the recognition of the importance of role modeling and a means of acknowledging those serving as good role models, including financial remuneration where appropriate. This requires valid and fair methods of evaluating the performance of faculty, the provision of opportunities for self-improvement through faculty development,[36,37] and other means to ensure that the institutional environment supports good role modeling and does not contain barriers to this essential method of transmitting the knowledge, skills, and the values of the profession. Finally, those who consistently demonstrate that they are detrimental to the professional development of students and residents must be relieved of their contact with them.

Faculty Development

Faculty development has been defined as that broad range of activities that institutions use to renew or assist faculty in their roles.[87] It is a planned program, or set of programs, designed to prepare institutions and faculty members for their various roles (see Chapter 9).[88] Comprehensive faculty development programs cannot focus solely on individual faculty members; they must also address the increasingly complex institutions in which teaching and learning occur.[89,90] They thus have the capacity to improve the knowledge and skills of faculty members and, acting through these individuals, to both improve role modeling and to alter the formal and the informal curricula.

To achieve consensus and ensure that faculty have the necessary knowledge and skills to both teach and role model professionalism, faculty development is a powerful tool.[36,37,45] For role models to be effective, they must understand the role that they are modeling. This starts with faculty agreement on definitions of professionalism and its characteristics, as well as on standards of behavior. The role must be made explicit to the role model as well as to the student.

Well-planned faculty development programs can be beneficial in several areas that impact on the teaching of professionalism. They are often instruments to effect change, leading to a revised curriculum. Programs can also produce a core group of knowledgeable individuals capable of not only teaching and modeling professional behavior but also, through peer pressure, assisting in changing the environment. Faculty development can be targeted at the entire faculty, bringing together individuals from various departments and disciplines to achieve a broad consensus. It can also be aimed at individual departments or academic units who are to have a major role in the teaching of professionalism. For those faculties establishing tutorial or mentorship programs as a part of their efforts to teach professionalism, ongoing faculty development of the tutors provides invaluable support.[37]

Faculty development programs can be constructed around several themes. The first and most obvious is "How to Teach Professionalism." This avoids any implication that faculty members are not themselves professional. In the process of developing teaching techniques appropriate to the individual or the school, professionalism as a subject must be addressed directly. The same is true of programs addressing "How to Evaluate Professionalism in

Students/Residents/Faculty Members" or "Role Modeling Professionalism." This allows the institutional definition and approach to teaching to be disseminated widely. Those who have completed the programs become more knowledgeable and, hopefully, more effective role models. The net result is a positive influence on the informal and hidden curriculum.

Continuity

It has become evident that professionalism must be taught in an integrated fashion throughout both the undergraduate and postgraduate curriculum.[7,8,24,30,37,38,41,55,56,70,71,73,74,91–93] The literature is quite consistent, indicating that virtually all faculties of medicine addressing this issue have chosen to give a longitudinal course with major components being present during each year of instruction.[35,37,38,40,41,55,69,71] As the objective is to teach the cognitive base and to internalize the values of the profession, both formal instruction and opportunities for self-reflection appropriate to the stage of training should be provided in all major teaching units. In this way, the growth of both explicit and tacit knowledge of professionalism will take place in parallel with growth of knowledge in other areas. Professionalism must be a part of all medicine and taught in an integrated fashion throughout the curriculum.

There are two reasons why it is not sufficient to provide opportunities for learning the cognitive base as an introductory learning experience. First, the professionalism that can be learned by students in the first year is less sophisticated and nuanced than that which can be presented during the final two years when the complexities of the relationships between physicians and patients and between medicine and society are grounded in personal experience. Second, students at all levels must be constantly reminded of the nature of professionalism and of its importance to medicine.

As an example of how one faculty has chosen to ensure that the nature of professionalism is examined on a regular basis in order to both reinforce learning and provide parallel opportunities for reflection on the issue, at McGill University[36,39] the first lecture on the first day of instruction has for many years presented the definition of professionalism and the characteristics of the professional. It is then followed by a small-group discussion led by trained facilitators using vignettes appropriate to the learner's level of knowledge (see Appendix C) in which the various attributes are identified so that students become familiar with the vocabulary. This definition is repeated in the second year at which time the characteristics of professional are linked to the obligations expected of physicians and the concept of professionalism as being the basis of medicine's social contract with society is introduced. Once again, there are small-group discussions using more sophisticated vignettes and analyses. In the third year, students meet in small groups with their mentors to discuss examples of exemplary or deplorable professional behavior, which they themselves have personally experienced. Finally, at the end of the fourth year, an eight-hour seminar series is given with an introductory didactic session which once again defines professionalism. However, now the emphasis is on the details of the social contract. Students in small groups read precirculated articles from the literature on medicine's social contract and present them to their colleagues under the guidance of a trained group leader. The objective is to encourage reflection and to have every student examine their own personal relationship to the profession and society, attempting to determine how they will meet the expectations of both patients and society and to think about what they expect of society. The entire class is brought together for these required sessions that are highlighted in the calendar as "Flagship Activities."

Evaluation

There are three levels of evaluation that should take place in any program on teaching professionalism. First, it is fundamental to evaluate the knowledge and performance of learners at all levels. Second, as the importance of the hidden curriculum has become recognized, it is apparent that the professionalism of the faculty must also be assessed. Finally, the program itself must be evaluated.

Evaluating the knowledge and performance of learners consists of two separate tasks.[93] Any systematic evaluation of professionalism should include an assessment of the knowledge of the learner as well as of their professional behaviors (see Chapter 7).

As there is a cognitive base to professionalism, it is relatively easy to measure knowledge of this subject using conventional assessment tools such as multiple choice or short answer questions. It is more challenging to ascertain whether learners have acquired the values and attitudes characteristic of the professional as these cannot be reliably assessed.[93-97] However, there are observable behaviors that reflect these values and attributes and they can be assessed. Because this assessment is potentially "high stakes," the tools used must be valid and reliable.

Formative evaluations with feedback on a regular basis are essential tools to assist students and residents in becoming professional. However, summative assessment must also be carried out. Professionalism is so fundamental to medicine's relationship to society that evidence that its cognitive base has been learned and its values internalized and reflected by behaviors must be recorded.[16,28,52] The public needs to be assured of the competence and character of graduates of both undergraduate and postgraduate programs.

Medicine as a profession is granted the privilege of self-regulation that requires that it sets and maintains standards.[4–6,98] Regular and rigorous evaluation is essential to meet this obligation, with summative evaluation providing evidence of the profession's accountability in this domain. This issue has been given added urgency by studies indicating that lapses in professional behavior observed in medical school are associated with subsequent unprofessional conduct in practice.[99,100]

Students have noted that a principal barrier to the learning of professionalism is unprofessional conduct by faculty members.[33] There is too often a major discrepancy between what faculty members teach and what they actually do. This is one of the major reasons why there are calls for the assessment of the "learning environment" as a part of accreditation.[14] While most faculties have policies in place to evaluate teaching and courses by students, specific evaluation of the professionalism of the teachers is rarely carried out and there are no reported validated tools to assist in this activity. In spite of this, an attempt should be made to evaluate the professionalism of faculty using whatever tools are available.[33,92]

As is indicated in Chapter 7, remediation should be linked to evaluation and there must be consequences to consistently poor performances.[93,95]

Finally, as is true of all educational activities, evaluation of the program itself must be carried out to ascertain if the goals of the faculty are actually being achieved. Obviously, an assessment of the performance of the learners is fundamental to this activity, Surveys of patients and other health professionals, peer review, and in the long term following students into practice and the assessment of their performance in practice by licensing bodies and professional associations are methods that can be used.[99,100]

An Incremental Approach

The experience of those who have instituted integrated programs on professionalism suggests that it is not possible to design and implement all aspects of the program simultaneously. Because many steps are required to have a successful program that operates throughout the continuum, an incremental approach appears to be preferable.[36–38,40,71,72,74,92] The naming of those responsible, educating the leaders as to the nature of professionalism, developing a definition and achieving buy-in from the faculty and students, promulgating this information through faculty development, and designing and introducing formal teaching and opportunities for experiential learning at all levels of instruction takes time.

Establishing a major program on teaching professionalism involves changing complex organizations that are inherently conservative. Many faculties have benefited from the experience gained in the world of business by utilizing either consultants or techniques developed in schools of business administration and there is a literature that can be of assistance.[32,37,70,101] Chapters 6 and 9 include the experiences of two faculties in doing this.

SUMMARY

This chapter has attempted to provide guidelines to assist those instituting programs on teaching professionalism. The theoretical background and experiences of those who have successfully instituted such programs are contained in other chapters of this book. The teaching of professionalism starts with the recognition that there is a cognitive base that must be taught explicitly. This must then be reinforced throughout the curriculum through experiential learning and reflection in order for the student to internalize it. A strong institutional commitment to supporting the teaching program throughout the educational process is required and a supportive environment must be created. The professionalism of all students, residents, and faculty must be evaluated, as must the program of instruction itself. Opportunities for remediation and improvement of both students and faculty are also necessary.

Coulehan[21] has exhorted us to engage the mind as well as the heart as we teach professionalism, an approach to medicine that has been with us for generations. Osler wrote that "the practice of medicine is an art, not a trade; a calling, not a business: a calling in which your heart will be exercised equally with your head."[102] Teaching the cognitive base of professionalism addresses the head and, if it is well done, the practicing physician should better understand the role they must play in medicine and in society. However, in order to be an authentic physician, this knowledge must reach the heart, becoming a part of one's being. Hopefully, the principles outlined in this chapter can assist those who wish to reach both the head and the hearts of students at all levels.

REFERENCES

1. Cruess, SR, Cruess, RL. Professionalism must be taught. *BMJ*. 1997; 315: 1674–1677.
2. Cote, L, Leclere, H. How clinical teachers perceive the doctor-patient relationship and themselves as role models. *Acad Med*. 2000; 75: 1117–1124.
3. Hensel, WA, Dickey, NW. Teaching professionalism: passing the torch. *Acad Med*. 1998; 73: 865–870.

4. Sullivan, W. *Work and Integrity: The Crisis and Promise of Professionalism in North America*. 2nd ed. San Francisco, CA. Jossey-Bass, 2005.

5. Freidson, E. *Professionalism: The Third Logic*. Chicago, IL: University of Chicago Press, 2001.

6. Cruess, RL, Cruess, SR. Teaching medicine as a profession in the service of healing. *Acad Med*. 1997; 72: 941–952.

7. Inui, TS. *A Flag in the Wind: Educating for Professionalism in Medicine. Association of American Medical Colleges*. Washington, DC: Association of American Medical Colleges, 2003.

8. Cohen, JJ. Professionalism in medical education, an American perspective: from evidence to accountability. *Med Educ*. 2006; 40: 607–617.

9. Ludmerer, KM. Instilling professionalism in medical education. *JAMA*. 1999; 282: 881–882.

10. Gordon, J. Fostering students' personal and professional development in medicine: a new framework for PPD. *Med Educ*. 2003; 37: 341–349.

11. Bataldan, P, Leach, D, Swing, S, Dreyfus, H, Dreyfus, S. General competencies and accreditation in graduate medical education. *Health Aff*. 2002; 21: 103–110.

12. Royal College of Physicians and Surgeons of Canada. The CanMeds roles framework. 2005. http://rcpsc.medil.org.canmeds/index.php. Accessed February 5, 2007.

13. General Medical Council. *Good Medical Practice*. London, 2006.

14. Liaison Committee on Medical Education. Functions and structure of a medical school: standards for accreditation of medical education programs leading to the M.D. degree. Washington. Liaison Committee on Medical Education: Publisher: Liaison Committee on Medical Education. June, 2007.

15. Swick, HM. Towards a normative definition of professionalism. *Acad Med*. 2000; 75: 612–616.

16. ABIM (American Board of Internal Medicine) Foundation. ACP (American College of Physicians) Foundation. European Federation of Internal Medicine. Medical professionalism in the new millennium: a physician charter. *Ann Intern Med*. 2002; 136: 243–246. *Lancet*. 359: 520–523.

17. Epstein, RM. Mindful practice. *JAMA*. 1999; 282: 833–839.

18. Novak, DH, Epstein, RM, Paulsen, RH. Toward creating physician-healers: fostering medical students' self-awareness, personal growth, and well-being. *Acad Med*. 1999; 74: 516–520.

19. Branch, WT, Kern, D, Haidet, P, Weissman, P, Gracey, CF, Mitchell, G, Inui, T. Teaching the human dimensions of care in clinical settings. *JAMA*. 2001; 286: 1067–1074.

20. Coulehan, J, Wiliams, P, Van McCrary, S, Belling, C. The best lack all conviction: biomedical ethics, professionalism, and social responsibility. *Camb Q Healthc Ethics*. 2003; 12: 21–38.

21. Coulehan, J. Today's professionalism: engaging the mind but not the heart. *Acad Med*. 2005; 80: 892–898.

22. Huddle, TS. Teaching professionalism: is medical morality a competency? *Acad Med*. 2005; 80: 885–891.

23. Fox, RC. Medical uncertainty revisited. In Bird, CE, Conrad, P, Fremont, AM, eds. *Handbook of Medical Sociology.* 5th ed. Upper Saddle River, NJ: Prentice Hall, 2003: 309–425.

24. Cruess, R, Cruess, S. Teaching professionalism: general principles. *Med Teach.* 2006; 28: 205–208.

25. Hafferty, FW. What medical students know about professionalism. *Mt Sinai J Med.* 2002; 69: 385–397.

26. Barry, D, Cyran, E, Anderson, RJ. Common issues in medical professionalism: room to grow. *Am J Med.* 2000; 108: 136–142.

27. Smith, R. All changed, changed utterly. British medicine will be transformed by the Bristol case. *BMJ.* 1998; 316: 1917–1918.

28. Irvine, D. *The Doctor's Tale: Professionalism and Public Trust.* Abington, UK. Radcliffe Medical Press, 2003.

29. Freidson, E. *Professionalism Reborn: Theory, Prophecy, and Policy.* Cambridge, UK: Polity Press, 1994.

30. Hilton, SR, Slotnick, HB. Proto-professionalism: how professionalization occurs across the continuum of medical education. *Med Educ.* 2005; 39: 58–65.

31. Hafferty, FW. Professionalism-the next wave. *NEJM.* 2006; 355: 2151–2152.

32. Kotter, JP. Leading change: why transformation efforts fail. *Harvard Bus Rev.* 1995; 73: 59–67.

33. Brainard, AH, Bilsen, HC. Learning professionalism: a view from the trenches. *Acad Med.* 2007; 82: 1010–1014.

34. Brater, DC. Infusing professionalism into a school of medicine: perspectives from the Dean. *Acad Med.* 2007; 82: 1094–1097.

35. Smith, KL, Saavedra, R, Raeke, JL, O'Donell, AA. The journey to creating a campus-wide culture of professionalism. *Acad Med.* 2007; 82: 1015–1021.

36. Steinert, Y, Cruess, SR, Cruess, RL, Snell, L. Faculty development for reaching and evaluating professionalism: from programme design to curricular change. *Med Educ.* 2005; 39: 127–136.

37. Steinert, Y, Cruess, RL, Cruess, SR, Boudreau, JD, Fuks, A. Faculty development as an instrument of change: a case study on teaching professionalism. *Acad Med.* 2007; 82: 1057–1064.

38. Wasserstein, AG, Brennan, PJ, Rubenstein, AH. Institutional leadership and faculty response: fostering professionalism at the University of Pennsylvania School of Medicine. *Acad Med.* 2007; 82: 1049–1056.

39. Cruess, R. Teaching professionalism. *Clin Orthop Relat Res.* 2006; 449: 177–185.

40. Goldstein, EA, Maestas, RR, Fryer-Edwards, K, Wenrich, M, Oelschlager, A-MA, Baerstein, A, Kimball, H. Professionalism in medical education: an institutional challenge. *Acad Med.* 2006; 81: 871–876.

41. Fryer-Edwards, K, Van Eaton, E, Goldstein, EA, Kimball, HR, Veith, RC, Pelligrini, CA, Ramsey, P. Overcoming institutional challenges through continuous professional improvement: the University of Washington Experience. *Acad Med.* 2007; 82: 1073–1078.

42. Hafferty, FW. Reconfiguring the sociology of medical education: emerging topics and pressing issues. In Bird, CE, Conrad, P, Fremont, AM, eds. *Handbook*

of Medical Sociology. 5th ed. Upper Saddle River, NJ: Prentice Hall, 2003: 238–257.

43. Sullivan, W. What is left of professionalism after managed care. *Hastings Cent Rep.* 1999; 29: 7–13.

44. Hafferty, FW, Franks, R, The hidden curriculum, ethics teaching, and the structure of medical education. *Acad Med.* 1994; 69: 861–871.

45. Hafferty, FW. Beyond curriculum reform: confronting medicine's hidden curriculum. *Acad Med.* 1998; 73: 403–407.

46. Stern, DT. In search of the informal curriculum. Where and when professional values are taught. *Acad Med.* 1998; 73: S 28–30.

47. Stern, DT, Papadakis, M. The developing physician: becoming a professional. *NEJM.* 2006; 355: 1794–1799.

48. Hafferty, FW, McKinley, JB. *The Changing Medical Profession: An International Perspective.* Oxford: Oxford University Press, 1993.

49. Castellani, B, Hafferty, FW. The complexities of medical professionalism: a preliminary investigation. In Wear, D, Aultman, JM, eds. *Professionalism in Medicine: Critical Perspectives.* New York: Springer, 2006: 3–25.

50. Frankford, DM, Konrad, TR. Responsive medical professionalism: integrating education, practice, and community in a market driven era. *Acad Med.* 1998; 73: 138–145.

51. Rosen, R, Dewar, S. *On Being a Good Doctor: Redefining Medical Professionalism for Better Patient Care.* London: King's Fund, 2004.

52. Royal College of Physicians of London. *Doctors in Society: Medical Professionalism in a Changing World.* London: Royal college of Physicians of London, 2005.

53. Dreyfus, HL, Dreyfus, SE. *A Five Stage Model of the Mental Activities Involved in Directed Skill Acquisition.* Unpublished manuscript supported by the Air Force Office of Scientific Research under contract F49620-79-C-0063 with the University of California, Berkeley.

54. Leach, DC. Professionalism: the formation of physicians. *Am J Bioethics.* 2004; 4: 11–12.

55. Maudsley, G, Strivens, J. Promoting professional knowledge, experiential learning, and critical thinking for medical students. *Med Educ.* 2000; 34: 535–544.

56. Wear, D, Castellani, B. The development of professionalism: curriculum matters. *Acad Med.* 2002; 75: 602–611.

57. Baernstein, A, Fryer-Edwards, K. Promoting reflection on professionalism: a comparison trial of educational interventions for medical students. *Acad Med.* 2003; 78: 742S–747S.

58. Larkin, GL. Mapping, modeling, and mentoring: charting a course for professionalism in graduate medical education. *Camb Q Healthc Ethics.* 2003; 12: 167–177.

59. Mamede, S, Schmidt, HG. The structure of reflective practice in medicine. *Med Educ.* 2004; 38: 1302–1308.

60. Benbassat, J, Baumal, R. Enhancing self-awareness in medical students: an overview of teaching approaches. *Acad Med.* 2005; 80: 156–161.

61. Sobral, DT. Medical students' mindset for reflective learning: a revalidation study of the reflection-in-learning scale. *Adv Health Sci* Ed. 2005; 10: 303–314.

62. Albanese, MA. Creating the reflective lifelong learner: why, what, and how. *Med Educ.* 2006; 40: 288–290.

63. Polanyi, M. *Personal Knowledge: Towards a Post-Critical Philosophy.* Chicago, IL: University of Chicago Press, 1958.

64. Schon, DA. *Educating the Reflective Practitioner: Toward a New Design for Teaching and Learning in the Professions.* San Francisco, CA: Jossey-Bass, 1987.

65. Schon, DA. *The Reflective Practitioner: How Professionals Think in Action.* New York: Basic Books, 1983.

66. Grant, A, Kinnersley, P, Metcalf, E, Pill, R, Houston, H. Students' views of reflective learning techniques: an efficacy study at a UK medical school. *Med Educ.* 2006: 40: 288–290.

67. Dewey, J. *How We Think.* Boston, MA: Heath. 1933.

68. Markakis, KM, Beckman, HB, Suchman, AL, Frankel, RM. The path to professionalism: cultivating humanistic values and attitudes in residency training. *Acad Med.* 2000; 75: 141–150.

69. Kuczewski, MG, Bading, E, Langbein, M, Henry, B. Fostering professionalism: the Loyola model. *Camb Q Healthc Ethics.* 2003; 12:1161–1166.

70. Suchman, AL, Williamson, PR, Litzelman, DK, Frankel, RM, Mossbarger, DL, Innui TS and the Relationship-Centered Care Initiative Discovery Team. Toward an informal curriculum that teaches professionalism. Transforming the social environment of a medical school. *J Gen Intern Med.* 2004; 19: 501–504.

71. Christianson, CE, McBride, RB, Vari, RC, Olson, L, Wilson, HD. From traditional to patient-centred learning: curriculum change as an intervention for changing institutional culture and promoting professionalism in undergraduate medical education. *Acad Med.* 2007; 82: 1079–1088.

72. Dobie, S. Reflections and on a well traveled-path: self-awareness, mindful practice, and relationship-centered care as foundations for medical education. *Acad Med.* 2007; 82: 422–427.

73. Goldie, J, Dowie, A, Cotton, P, Morrison, J. Teaching professionalism in the early years of a medical curriculum: a qualitative study. *Med Educ.* 2007; 41: 610–617.

74. Kalet, AL, Sanger, J, Chase, J, Keller, K, Schwartz, MD, Fishman, ML, Garfall, AL, Kitay, A. Promoting professionalism through an online professional development portfolio: successes, joys, and frustrations. *Acad Med.* 2007; 82: 1065–1072.

75. Swick, HM. Professionalism and humanism beyond the academic health center. *Acad Med.* 2007; 82: 1022–1028.

76. Irby, DM. Clinical teaching and the clinical teacher. *J Med Educ.* 1986: 61; 35–45.

77. Epstein, RM, Cole, DR, Gawinski, BA, Piotrowski-Lee, S, Ruddy, NB. How students learn from community-based preceptors. *Arch Fam Med.* 1998; 7: 149–154.

78. Wright, SM. Examining what residents look for in their role models. *Acad Med.* 1996; 71: 290–292.

79. Wright, SM, Wong, A, Newill, C. The impact of role models on medical students. *J Gen Int Med.* 1997; 12: 53–56.

80. Wright, SM, Kern, DE, Kolodner, K, Howard, DM, Brancati, FL. Attributes of excellent attending-physician role models. *NEJM*. 1998; 339: 1986–1993.

81. Wright, SM, Carrese, JA. What values do attending physicians try to pass on to house officers. *Med Educ*. 2001; 35: 941–945.

82. Kenny, NP, Mann, KV, MacLeod, HM. Role modeling in physicians' professional formation: reconsidering an essential but untapped educational strategy. *Acad Med*. 2003; 78: 1203–1210.

83. Ihara, CK. Collegiality as a professional virtue. In Flores, A, ed. *Professional Ideals*. Belmont, CA: Wadsworth, 1988: 56–65.

84. Feudtner, C, Christakis, DA, Christakis, NA. Do clinical clerks suffer ethical erosion? Student perceptions of their ethical environment and personal development. *Acad Med*. 1994; 69: 670–679.

85. Reddy, ST, Farnan, JM, Yoon, JD, Leo, T, Upadhyay, GA, Humphrey, HJ, Arora, VM. Third-year medical students' participation in and perceptions of unprofessional behaviors. *Acad Med*. 2007; 82 S10: S35–S39.

86. Baldwin, DC, Daugherty, SR, Rowley, BD. Unethical and unprofessional conduct observed by residents during their first year of training. *Acad Med*. 1998; 73: 1195–1200.

87. Centra, JA. Types of faculty development programs. *J Higher Ed*. 1978; 49: 151–162.

88. Bland, CJ, Schmitz, CC, Stritter, FT, Henry, RC, Aluise, JJ. *Successful Faculty in Academic Medicine: Essential Skills and How to Acquire Them*. New York: Springer-Verlag, 1990.

89. Steinert, Y. Faculty development in the new millennium: key challenges and future directions. *Med Teacher*. 2000; 22: 44–50.

90. Wilkerson, L, Irby, DM. Strategies for improving teaching practices: a comprehensive approach to faculty development. *Acad Med*. 1998; 73: 387–396.

91. Rudy, DW, Elam, CL, Griffith, CH. Developing a stage-appropriate professionalism curriculum. *Acad Med*. 2001; 76: 503.

92. Hickson, GB, Pichert, JW, Webb, LE, Gabbe, SG. A complimentary approach to promoting professionalism: identifying, measuring, and addressing unprofessional behaviors. *Acad Med*. 2007; 82: 1040–1048.

93. Stern, D T (ed.). *Measuring Medical Professionalism*. New York: Oxford University Press, 2005.

94. Arnold, L. Assessing professional behaviors: yesterday, today, and tomorrow. *Acad Med*. 2002; 77: 502–515.

95. Arnold, L. Responding to the professionalism of learners and faculty in orthopaedic surgery. *Clin Ortop Relat Res*. 2006; 449: 205–213.

96. Epstein,, RM, Hundert, E. Defining and assessing professional competence. *JAMA*. 2002; 287: 226–235.

97. Epstein, RM. Assessment in medical education. *NEJM*. 2007; 356: 387–396.

98. Stevens, R. Public roles for the medical profession in the United States: beyond theories of decline and fall. *Milbank Q*, 2001; 79: 327–353.

99. Papadakis, MA, Teharani, A, Banach, MA, Knettler, TR, Rattner, SL, Stern, DT, Veloski, JJ, Hodson, CS. Disciplinary action by medical boards and prior behavior in medical school. *NEJM*. 2005; 353: 2673–2682.

100. Kirk, LM, Blank, LL. Professional behavior—a learner's permit for licensure. *NEJM*. 2005; 353: 2709–2711.

101. Kirch, DJ, Grigsby, RK, Zolko, WW. Reinventing the academic health center. *Acad Med*. 2005; 80: 980–989.

102. Osler, W. *Aequanimitas, with Other Addresses to Medical Students, Nurses and Practitioners of Medicine*. 3rd. ed. Philadelphia, PA: P. Blakiston, 1932.

5   Resident Formation – A Journey to Authenticity: Designing a Residency Program That Educes Professionalism

David C. Leach, M.D.

> Hope is not the same as optimism. An optimist ignores the facts in order to come to a comforting conclusion. But a hopeful person faces the facts without blinking – and then looks behind them for potentials that have yet to emerge – knowing that the human experiment would never have advanced were it not for the possibilities, however slim, that lie hidden behind the facts.[1]

In May, 2002, Parker Palmer facilitated a retreat for residency program directors who had received the Accreditation Council for Graduate Medical Education's (ACGME's) Parker Palmer Courage to Teach Award. During the retreat, a case was presented, a case in which a liver transplant donor had died while in intensive care. He died despite the fact that the surgery had gone smoothly and despite the fact that his wife, who was with him throughout the entire postsurgical period, insisted repeatedly and to no avail that her husband was going downhill fast. Three months later, the state health commissioner issued an incident report saying, "The hospital allowed this patient to undergo a major high-risk procedure and then left his postoperative care in the hands of an overburdened, mostly junior staff, without appropriate supervision." On the day the donor died, a first-year surgical resident with twelve days of experience in the transplant unit had been left alone to care for thirty-four patients. She could not – and did not – monitor every patient with the care and precision required.

The doctors at the retreat discussed the case in small groups and almost universally came to the conclusion that system issues were to blame. The analysis was impersonal and abstract. Culpable parties were the hospital, the system of supervision, inexperience, and staffing. During the debriefing Parker asked a question that brought the group to deep silence: "Who is the moral agent in this story?" We were not used to thinking in terms of moral agency. The group agonized over both the question and the fact that we, by habit, had avoided asking the question. Parker then inquired, "What if

Table 5.1. ACGME description of professionalism[2]

Residents must demonstrate a commitment to carrying out professional responsibilities, adherence to ethical principles, and sensitivity to a diverse patient population.

Residents are expected to:

Demonstrate respect, compassion, and integrity; a responsiveness to the needs of patients and society that supersedes self-interest; accountability to patients, society, and the profession; and a commitment to excellence and ongoing professional development.

Demonstrate a commitment to ethical principles pertaining to provision or withholding of clinical care, confidentiality of patient information, informed consent, and business practices.

Demonstrate sensitivity and responsiveness to patients' culture, age, gender, and disabilities.

residents were expected to be the moral agents of the institutions in which they work and learn?"

ACGME's statement about professionalism (Table 5.1) includes, "Residents are expected to demonstrate respect, compassion, and integrity; a responsiveness to the needs of patients ... that supersedes self-interest; accountability to patients ... and the profession; a commitment to excellence and ongoing professional development."[2] Parker encouraged us to go further – both then and in 2006 in his lecture: "The New Professional: Education for Transformation." In the latter he said, "I applaud all of this, of course, in our technocratic culture it is courageous to build values like these into accreditation standards. But there is something implicit in that statement that I believe should be made explicit: you cannot be faithful to a one-on-one ethic of doctor-patient relationships until you take it one more step – to an ethic that challenges the institutional conditions that demean or damage or destroy those relationships, sometimes with deadly results."

This was a new twist. Is it possible to design a residency program in which the resident, like the canary in the coal mine, detects and warns others when institutional conditions (relationships) are toxic to professional values? Is it possible to use the resident's own formation, their own journey to authenticity, to enable an institutional journey to authenticity?

The true professional is one who does not obscure grace with illusions of technical prowess, but one who strips away all illusions to reveal a reliable truth in which the human heart can rest.[3]

Residency programs themselves are a bit of an illusion; they are an artificial construct of the mind. The only things real in a residency program or an academic health center for that matter are the people in them and the relationships they have with one another, relationships that can either inhibit or facilitate the development of professionalism, relationships that mark the program or institution as professional or unprofessional. Parker was really asking us to change the nature of our relationships in ways that would foster professionalism. He was asking us to empower and listen deeply to the consciences of our novices, those who have not yet adjusted their moral sensibilities to accommodate institutional mores.

The task in designing a residency program that fosters professionalism requires creating an ecology that will support life; one that will enable fundamental human values to be preserved and nourished, that will not diminish but acknowledge and support both the patients and the professionals engaged in the work at hand. The forms of medicine have changed dramatically. Technology, delivery systems, payment systems, the range of professionals delivering care, consumerism, alternative medicine, and so forth, all have modified the experience for both patient and provider. Many advances enhanced medicine's potential to be more effective; however, they have also threatened medicine's ability to be faithful, faithful to its traditional and oft-espoused values. To design for professionalism requires being clear about values and form. Dee Hock has said, "Substance is enduring; form is ephemeral. Preserve substance; modify form; know the difference."[4] If we want to preserve and nurture values and yet be malleable as to form we can look to the traditional values of medicine as expressed in documents such as the Physician Charter[5]; yet, we can also look to the human heart. When people work in an environment in which daily behaviors are in conflict with deeply held values they wither, the patients wither, and the residents in formation in such an environment wither with them. This chapter will explore how the relationships in an academic institution and within its residency programs might be designed in ways that allow the profession to be both more effective and more faithful, in ways that foster professional life and the benefits thereof.

Pfeffer and Sutton[6] are critical of the way we use facts, accept dangerous half-truths, and adopt total nonsense in our organizations. They offer five questions to consider before trying a new idea or practice.

1. What assumptions does the idea or practice make about people and organizations? What would have to be true about people and organizations for the idea or practice to be effective?
2. Which of these assumptions seem reasonable and correct to you and your colleagues? Which seem wrong or suspect?

3. Could this idea or practice still succeed if the assumptions turned out to be wrong?

4. How might you and your colleagues quickly and inexpensively gather some data to test the reasonableness of the underlying assumptions?

5. What other ideas or management practices can you think of that would address the same problem or issue and be more consistent with what you believe to be true about people and organizations?

Ten design interventions are offered in this chapter. I offer them based on the following nine assumptions:

1. People are basically good. Given the option, they would rather help than hurt patients and each other. The basic tenets of professionalism are attractors to the human spirit unless the institutional ecology disables, frustrates, and renders unachievable respectful behaviors and relationships.*

2. The formation of the professionalism in resident physicians depends on the development of the resident as a person. The resident's journey to authenticity as a physician and as a person depends on both them and others paying attention to the individual and collective journeys to authenticity. This is a journey related to, but not limited to, competence.

3. Three things are inextricably linked: patient care, health professional formation, and health system performance.[7] A prerequisite to good resident education is good patient care; a prerequisite for both is a system designed to enable, assure, and improve both.

4. Professionalism is about relationships: the doctor-patient relationship, the doctor-colleague relationships, and the profession-society relationships. Residents learn from encounters with patients but also from encounters with a wide variety of other professionals.

5. During residency, residents learn about social justice and the profession's attitude about equitable health care. They are taught to see or to

---

* Some would claim this assumption as false and provide substantial evidence for their case. Self-interest is frequently expressed as an organizing principle, small pleasures can derive from petty behaviors that diminish others, and defensive scapegoating is a modus operandi in many institutions. Yet, I contend that this assumption is a form of hope rather than optimism – as distinguished by Parker Palmer's quote at the very beginning of this chapter. I think that while such behaviors are manifest, there is abundant evidence that people yearn to be freed from the prison that petty behaviors impose and that they want very much to express professional behaviors as defined in the competencies.

not see inequities in care. They are taught that this is or is not part of the social contract.

6. The Dreyfus Model of skill acquisition[8] applies to the acquisition of professionalism. This model describes the progression of learners from novice and advanced beginners (rule-based behavior) to competent, proficient, expert, and master (increasingly dependent on both rules and context). Accordingly, it is important that residents learn the rules of professionalism and then apply those rules in various and ever more complex situations.

7. Residents are currently socialized to cope with broken systems; if they were taught to master systems, the aims of professional formation would be furthered. An unwritten curriculum exists in which residents get high marks for getting things done in a broken system and are given little or no guidance about how to fix the broken system. While not universal, large numbers of residents in the various specialties are abandoned and left like the children in Golding's novel *The Lord of the Flies*[9] to cope as best they can. As in the novel, the mores that develop under conditions of abandonment are the antithesis of professionalism.

8. Enabling professionalism requires more than the science of disease biology; it also requires relieving patients and their families of the burdens of illness. Human suffering demands more than sympathy ("I'm sorry you hurt."); it demands empathy and compassion. Patients need to have their subjective feelings recognized, validated, and honored; they need both the resident's objectivity and their companionship in subjectivity. Naming the disease is not always the same as naming the hurt.

9. Many of the features of residency programs that are now good will be part of the new world.

THE CONTEXT OF THE WORK

Residency is an intense experience. The learning curve is steeper than at any other time in a physician's life; the difference in skill and knowledge between a first-year resident and a chief resident is profound. It is also a time in which the habits of a lifetime are developed. The experiences of residency are seared into the brain with an intensity and vividness that is unusual. Many physicians can describe patients seen during residency thirty or more years after the encounter. It is a time when professionalism and all things move from the abstract to the concrete. It is a time captured in stories rather than goals and objectives.

The context in which health care and resident formation occur does not make the task of fostering professionalism easy. Relentless pressures of time and economics, fragmentation of care and the relationships supporting care, increasing external regulation, exciting but disruptive new knowledge and technologies, and above all the broken systems of health care dominate conversations and characterize the external environmental context.

The internal context is also daunting. Justifiable lack of trust pervades the system. Beth McGlynn estimates that only about 54 percent of the time do patients receive care that is known to be best, a number that falls to 2–3 percent when evidence-based guidelines are bundled. At some level, we know this to be true and yet hospital Web sites proudly announce that they provide the best care with the best doctors, the best technology, and so forth. Some Web sites are so detached from acknowledging human suffering that they make it seem like a hospital might be a fun place to visit. As a profession we have tolerated that messaging, forgetting Hannah Arendt's adage that every time we make a promise we should plan for the forgiveness we will need when that promise is broken.[10]

The hospital bill, at least in the United States, is frequently not interpretable by the hospital's own administrative staff let alone patients. Paul O'Neill said he knows of no other industry that regularly accepts a 38 percent reimbursement on amounts billed, a percentage that he states is the national average.[11] We all know how the number is derived. In the United States, hospitals actively negotiate with several insurers in ways designed to cover their costs. Inflated bills and discounted deals, while cumbersome, work fine as long as the aggregate reimbursements cover expenses and some margin. The system works fine, until a patient shows up with no insurance and with no one to negotiate for a discounted rate. The undiscounted fees are billed to those least able to pay. The hospital bill is about as far away from "respect, compassion, and integrity; a responsiveness to the needs of patients . . . that supersedes self-interest; accountability to patients . . ." as one can get.

It is hard to foster professionalism when such incongruities between espoused and evident behaviors are so apparent. I call this the "Abraham Verghesse problem." At a spectacular forum hosted by the American Board of Internal Medicine in the summer of 2005 the audience was, with some pride, celebrating the accomplishments of the Physician Charter on Medical Professionalism.[5] This well-written document, endorsed by many, clarifies principles and commitments in very important ways. Yet, in the midst of the celebratory speeches, Abraham Verghesse stood up and said that his medical students shrugged that the principles in the charter were self-evident, it was why they went into medicine, why were so many making such a fuss about it? Dr. Verghesse then said, "Perhaps we pay so much attention to the words because there is no other evidence that the phenomena exists." Everyone became silent.

Creating institutions and residency programs that foster behaviors more congruent with professional values requires that the humans in the institution or program have access to their own inner wisdom and bring that wisdom to the work at hand.

There is a pervasive form of modern violence to which the idealist . . . most easily succumbs: activism and overwork. The rush and pressure of modern life are a form, perhaps the most common form of its innate violence. To allow oneself to be carried away by a multitude of conflicting concerns, to surrender to too many demands, to commit oneself to too many projects, to want to help everyone in everything is to succumb to violence. The frenzy of the activist neutralizes his (or her) work . . . It destroys the fruitfulness of his (or her) work, because it kills the root of inner wisdom which makes the work fruitful.[12]

MOVING FROM FRENZY TO WISDOM: DESIGNING TO EDUCE LATENT WISDOM

Educe: vt (L educere to draw out); 1: to bring out as something latent; syn evoke, elicit, extract, extort, to draw out something hidden.[13]

The task of designing a residency program to educe professionalism requires that we move from frenzy to wisdom and create an environment in which they can move from frenzy to wisdom.

Design Feature 1: Work with rather than against Human Nature

Residents and all humans come equipped with three faculties that are naturally aligned with the goals of professionalism: the intellect, the will, and the imagination. The object of the intellect is truth, that of the will goodness, and that of the imagination beauty. The job of a good doctor boils down to discerning and telling the truth, putting what is good for the patient before what is good for the doctor, and making clinical judgments that are – in a way – beautiful – are harmonious with the particular needs of the patient as well as the generalizable scientific evidence at hand.

This construct invites a new frame for organizing experiences: how good a job did I do in discerning and telling the truth, in putting the patient's interest first, in accommodating the particular realities of the patient's situation in my clinical judgments?

Residents have two primal fears: they do not want to hurt anyone and they do not want to appear stupid. They are on a journey, a journey to authenticity, to become authentic physicians. It is a journey in which they discover both clinical wisdom and themselves. It is a journey that no one can take for them or spare them but we can help them. It is a journey that is surrounded by external drama but that actually proceeds from the inside out. Residency should build on the bedrock of the intellect, will, and imagination and offer experiences that strengthen and test these capacities.

So how might one design a program that would allow residents to proceed on such a journey?

It begins by the program director, faculty, and others committing their whole selves to the task. It begins when they discover and nurture their true self. That sounds silly – a true self – as opposed to a series of false selves; however, it is not uncommon to offer the world only part of ourselves. We put on a persona and wear it like a suit of clothes. It enables us to be facile in dealing with the outside world; it is a protective mask. There are problems with this approach. It turns out that patients do better if the whole doctor shows up – not just the intellect, not just the head and the hands, but also the heart. Likewise, residents learn by mimicking and if they see their whole mentor show up rather than just the intellect, they become more complete and their faculties are all more fully developed.

This journey to authenticity is not being taken by the resident and faculty alone. The profession of medicine is on the same journey. To the extent that our profession discerns and tells the truth about health care, to the extent that it puts what is good for the patient and the public before what is good for the doctor, and to the extent that it is creative and generative – it is an authentic profession. For us authenticity is a verb, not a noun. It is not a state of rest; it requires constant vigilance.

Design Feature 2: Enable Reflective Practice

Competence is the habitual demonstration of reflective practice[14]; competence in professionalism involves habitual reflection on relationships, encounters with patients, colleagues, and society. This type of reflection cannot be mandated but can be supported and enabled by systems that allow residents to keep track of their experiences with patients and others, a system that fosters and teaches self-reflection, that offers shared learning experiences with others and that supports the needed clarifying conversations about those experiences, and that enables some experiences to be formally evaluated. Experiences that may be especially fruitful sources of reflection about professionalism include the noncompliant patient, cross-cultural issues, critical incidents, informed consent, interprofessional conversations, promises made and kept/not kept, end-of-life care, and others.

ACGME is developing a learning portfolio that is designed to support reflection.[15] It is based on the premise that resident learning begins with experience rather than with goals and objectives. A drop-down menu of educational experiences is followed by prompts and textboxes for self-reflection as well as opportunities to share reflections with others selected by the resident. Being mindful of one's formation enables the true purposes of residency to emerge.

Design Feature 3: Community Reflection

Good reflection requires both solitude and community: solitude to organize thoughts about experiences, and community to clarify if those thoughts hold up under scrutiny. It is in reflection and in conversation that professionalism both develops and is made manifest. Our society highly values individualism and materialism; professionalism requires community and attachment to traditional values. Transparent community reflections about the values being espoused and expressed on a daily basis are crucial if the redesigned residency is to foster truth telling. Each institution should have a visible social contract with the community it serves – a contract not written by the public relations department but by the health professionals themselves. While morals may be an individual responsibility, mores express the aggregate community moral compass and should be transparent. A "Professionalism Morbidity and Mortality Conference" that cuts across departmental boundaries is an example of a community reflection. The recently released "Good Medical Practice – USA" document is another example of such a contract. Developed by several organizations this document includes both patient expectations of their doctors and doctors' expectations of each other.[16]

Design Feature 4: Validating and Mining the Resident's Feelings

Embedded in the higher education process is a systematic discounting of the subjective; it is thought to be a source of bias and unreliability. And yet, the journey to authenticity as a physician requires more than simply attention to the objective details in our world. Compassion, empathy, and deep respect are all dependent on the truths revealed by the human heart. Parker Palmer argues that residents are moral agents,[1] agents that can keep the health care system honest about its dealings with the ill. As such they should be taught, not to distrust their hearts, but to depend on them and to acquire the discipline of discernment that they offer. Instead of quietly discounting their own hearts, they should be taught to share the disease and clarify how this can be used to improve the community. The perverse goal of teaching young professionals of good conscience to distrust their conscience cannot be part of the new design.

Design Feature 5: Attention to Group as well as Individual Formation

Professionalism requires deep attention to small group dynamics. The assumption that the doctor-patient relationship is a one-to-one relationship is flawed. In fact it is more like a twenty-to-one relationship – with several types of doctors, nurses, and other health professionals each operating with the assumption that they are in a one-to-one relationship with the patient. This leaves the patient to sort out conflicting signals, priorities, and plans. Needed is clarity for all about the roles, authorities, and functions of the various members of the team. Yet, the journey to authenticity has been viewed as an individual journey. New educational models that will enable the emergence of authentic truths discovered by small groups are required. Simple techniques such as nominal group, rank ordering, the ladder of inference, appreciative inquiry, affinity diagrams, and so forth.[17] should be learned and practiced by residents. Groups that can and will tackle the large barriers imposed by institutional life are important. Attention to small group formation will enable and strengthen attempts at individual formation.

Design Feature 6: Getting Discretion and Discipline Right

It is commonly said that the most important thing offered by physicians is their individual judgment. Reserving the autonomy needed for individual judgments is considered a hallmark of professionalism. Yet, as medicine has moved from best guess to credible evidence-based protocols, and as the extent of medical error and its consequences became apparent to both the profession and the public, system approaches to enhance safety were developed and are needed. Almalberti[18] has demonstrated that safe systems can only be achieved if individual actors constrain the autonomy of inappropriate discretion and dependably offer the evidence-based disciplined behavior of better, safer care. He reports that only two types of health care offer safety that is in any way comparable to the safety levels of the commercial airline industry or the nuclear power industry: class I anesthesia and blood banking. In both these examples, individual doctors have yielded some of their autonomy to common protocols that make it very difficult to make a mistake. Designing residency programs for professionalism now means fostering a deep understanding about the proper use of discretion and the proper adherence to evidence-based discipline in the care of patients including the use of guidelines.

Design Feature 7: Simulation

The use of simulated encounters to foster health professional learning is about respect – for the patient, for one's colleagues, and for oneself. Basic clinical skills should be taught as far away from the patient as possible; gone are the days when a sweaty resident and a sweaty patient both endured first attempts at procedures. Technology now enables residents to learn and practice skills; to approach the patient armed with confidence and experience. It should be deployed wherever possible. In addition to procedural simulations, the resident's journey to competence in professionalism benefits from team rehearsals, in situ simulations, and cognitive simulation. Communication within teams is also about respect. Reducing uncertainty by clarifying roles and expectations under rehearsal conditions enhances patient safety and takes team competence to a higher level. In situ simulation brings a simulated encounter into the real workplace and exposes habitual communication patterns and team dynamics as well as overall system performance. Most in situ scenarios involve cross-departmental boundaries and make apparent the cumulative effects of several interprofessional conversations and behaviors. Cognitive simulation as developed by Usha Satish[19] has been used to study residents in different specialties. As residents progress from first year to chief residents, what they think increases tremendously; however, how they think changes not at all. Residents in different specialties think differently, but during their training their decision-making style does not change. In her previous experience with Fortune 500 CEOs, Usha reports that the best CEOs had a wide repertoire of decision-making styles at their disposal depending on the circumstances. Residents lack this flexibility and approach each problem stereotypically. Using simulation offers a remarkable opportunity to broaden their approach to decision making in ways that allow more respect for the patient's particular circumstances to be expressed.

Design Feature 8: Social Justice

Every resident encounters the poor. Many academic health centers include care of the poor in their mission statements; they are frequently the backbone of such care in their communities. Yet, widespread disparity exists in everything across the larger society. Clarity about the profession's responsibility to have an opinion about disparity is lacking. We have been ineffective at best and silent at worst about whether health care is a right or a privilege. We have confined our response to individual patients and only those who by whatever mechanism get in the door to see us.

If residents are to be the moral agents of the system this must change. They, more than most, are charged with mobilizing endless social service consults to somehow get resources to those lacking any. The larger social system of health care is a valid element of all curricula – in its explicit absence the implicit is all we can offer.

Design Feature 9: Linking Evaluations to System Improvement

The current system has compartmentalized education and patient care and this is a missed opportunity. It came about because it has been very important to clarify that residents are students and not employees. It assumes that the intense pressures of service would compromise and diminish the educational agenda. This is half-true and the existing accreditation system frequently cites programs for just that. Yet, there are some wonderful examples of a different model. A combined preventive medicine residency program at Dartmouth is limited to Dartmouth residents in any one of the nine categorical programs and combines with the categorical program to add two years to training during which the resident gains a masters degree and becomes board eligible in preventive medicine as well as the categorical program. Preventive medicine as a stand-alone specialty has not been growing; yet, this new approach has generated real excitement, has become the largest in the country, and is growing. Limited to Dartmouth residents, the program is approved for forty positions. There is early evidence that residents are applying to the categorical programs just to get into the combined program. The practicum year is an attractor. During that year, the resident must fix a system problem. Dartmouth regularly puts its clinical outcomes on a public Web site (www.dartmouth-hitchcock.org). The CEO and the program director ask the resident to identify an area in which Dartmouth can improve, for example, the treatment of community-acquired pneumonia, and the resident, reporting directly to the CEO, improves health. The CEO is very enthusiastic and has given financial support to the program because it enables him to achieve the common goal of improving Dartmouth's clinical outcomes and enhancing resident education. The resident's grade depends to some extent on improving, for example, the treatment of community-acquired pneumonia.

Medical students and residents are not naive; they know that they will be expected to repair and redesign the current system. Empowering them to do so by formal didactics and experiences in system improvement makes them better professionals and moves the agenda from whining to improving – a tangible expression of professionalism.

Design Feature 10: Residents as Future Stewards of Professionalism

The task is not finished in this generation. If we are to preserve the substance of medicine, we must prepare residents to adapt to an unknown future. Some will be familiar with the Star Trek series. In the earliest version, medicine was represented by Doctor McCoy, an irascible Georgia family practitioner who felt intensely protective of his patients and distrusted the fancy technology available on the Starship Enterprise. Star Trek: The Next Generation, the next iteration brought Beverly Crusher, a woman, a physician deeply skilled in interpersonal relationships and very fluent and comfortable with technology. Subsequently, Star Trek: Voyager found the doctor replaced by a hologram, absolutely current with medical knowledge and technology but somewhat lacking in bedside manners.

Science fiction aside, a commitment to professionalism requires that we prepare this generation of residents to adapt to a very different world than we are now experiencing. They must learn how to build a system of medical education that yields fidelity as well as effectiveness and to do so as unimaginable realities emerge. The human heart will be a constant even in the world of holograms and robots, but only if it is invited and nourished as a source of compassion and empathy. Designing a learning environment that fosters the human requires attention to experiences, reflection on experiences in solitude and in community, and learning and formal assessment of learning. It means learning how to design for authenticity. It means that the profession now as it goes about the work of redesign also keeps notes to share with those who follow.

CONCLUSIONS

In the end, professionalism is determined by individual responses to vocation; it is about character development. The work of medicine is such that it is impossible to do without being shaped by it. Institutions are also shaped by the work and the mores associated with it. Professional formation of both the individual and the institution are inevitably coupled with the quality of patient care. If we accept Parker Palmer's adage that professionals strip away illusions to reveal truth, then the place to begin is with transparency: telling the truth about patient outcomes. Telling the truth on Web sites, in conversations, in disclosure statements, in advertising, and everywhere can strip away the illusions that now exhaust us and make professionalism nothing more than an aspiration, a set of words incongruent with evident behaviors.

While I have argued that individual formation is informed by more than self-interest, arguing that institutions are not primarily motivated by self-interest is much more daunting. I am reminded of G. K. Chesterton's statement that "Certain theologians dispute the doctrine of original sin, which is the only part of Christian theology which can really be proved."[20] The evidence of the habitual and aggressive pursuit of institutional self-interest is incontrovertible. Yet, we mistake concept for reality if we consider that institutions are real. In fact they, like residency programs, are nothing more than the people in them and the relationships they have with one another. Institutions are impenetrable, unresponsive, and self-interested only if we are impenetrable, unresponsive, and self-interested. We project our darkness onto our institutions and declare it the other. As in the classic psychiatric transference reaction, we attribute to our institutions what lives in our own hearts. To quote Parker Palmer, "We need professionals who know the difference between the treasure embodied in their profession and the earthen vessels that hold it. We need professionals who are 'in but not of' the institutions in which they work. We need professionals whose allegiance to professional values liberates them to become constructive critics of the contexts in which their work is done."[1] The journey to authenticity for us, our learners, and our institutions begins by telling the truth. Transparency makes the illusions of the institution as other unsustainable; it also makes for really good conversations. It is an essential element of the new professionalism and residency offers the crucible in which the purification can begin.

REFERENCES

1. Palmer, PJ. Education for the new professional. Marvin Dunn Memorial Lecture. ACGME Educational Workshop; March 4, 2006; Orlando (FL).
2. Accreditation Council for Graduate Medical Education (ACGME). Outcome Project: Competencies[cited March 15, 2006]. Available from: www.acgme.org/outcome/comp/compFull.asp.
3. Palmer, PJ. *The Active Life*. San Francisco (CA): Jossey-Bass; 1999.
4. Hock, D. *The Birth of the Chaotic Age*. San Francisco (CA): Berrett-Koehler; 1999.
5. *Medical Professionalism in the New Millennium: A Physician Charter*. ABIM Foundation. www.abimfoundation.org/professionalsim/pdf_charter/ABIM_CharterIns.pdf Published in the *Ann Int Med*; 136:243–246, February 2002.
6. Pfeffer, J, Sutton, R. *Hard Facts, Dangerous Half-Truths, and Total Nonsense*. Boston (MA): Harvard Business School Press; 2006.
7. Batalden, PB, Davidoff, F. What is "quality improvement" and how can it transform healthcare? *Qual Saf Health Care*. 2007 Feb;16(1):2–3.

8. Dreyfus, H. *On the Internet*. London: Routledge; 2001.

9. Golding, W. *The Lord of the Flies*. New York: Penguin; 1999.

10. Arendt, H. Labor, work, action. In Baehr, P, editor. *The Portable Hannah Arendt*. New York: Penguin Books; 2003: 167–181.

11. O'Neill, Paul. *Personal communication*, March, 2004.

12. Merton, T. *Conjectures of a Guilty Bystander*. New York: Image; 1968.

13. *Webster's New Collegiate Dictionary*. Springfield (MA): G. & C. Merriam; 1981.

14. Leach, D. Presentation on the ACGME portfolio. *Organization of program director associations*; November 17, 2006; Rosemont (IL).

15. Accreditation Council for Graduate Medical Education (ACGME). The ACGME Learning Portfolio: Experience, Reflect, Learn, Assess [cited 2007 Nov 27]. Available from: http://www.acgme.org/acWebsite/portfolio/learn_cbpac.asp

16. National Alliance for Physician Competence. Good medical practice—*USA* [cited 2007 Nov 27]. Available from: http://www.gmpusa.org/

17. Scholtes, P, Joiner, B, Streibel, B. *The Team Handbook*. 3rd ed. Madison (WI): Oriel Inc.; 2003.

18. Almalberti, R, Auroy, Y, Berwick, D, Barache, P. Five system barriers to achieving ultrasafe health care. *Ann Intern Med*. 2005;142(9):756–764.

19. Satish, U, Streufert, S. Value of a cognitive simulation in medicine: towards optimizing decision making performance of healthcare personnel. *Qual Saf Health Care*. 2002;11(2):163–167.

20. Chesterton, GK. *Orthodoxy*. New York: Bantam Doubleday Dell; 1991.

6 Supporting Teaching and Learning of Professionalism – Changing the Educational Environment and Students' "Navigational Skills"

Thomas S. Inui, M.D., Ann H. Cottingham, M.A.R., Richard M. Frankel, Ph.D., Debra K. Litzelman, M.D., Anthony L. Suchman, M.D., and Penelope R. Williamson, Sc.D.

> Medical schools must insure that the learning environment for medical students promotes the development of explicit and appropriate professional attributes (attitudes, behaviors, and identity) in their medical students.
>
> Liaison Committee on Medical Education, Standard MS-31-A: effective July 1, 2008

Professionalism and professional standards in medicine are an active domain of discourse today.[1] The reasons are many. Public concern over the sheer cost of medical care and the growth of un-insurance are daily news fare as are questions about patient safety and quality of care. Concern about how advances in biomedical science will be put to use are also visible.

The definition and meaningfulness of "professionalism" are also open for discussion. Sociologists have described professions as learned (highly knowledgeable) and self-regulating domains of work.[2,3] Others have described professionalism as values-based domains of competency, or the moral core of medicine.[4,5] Many approaches to education and training in professionalism are also apparent. Organizational and programmatic experimentation has been fueled by residency program requirements for education in professionalism endorsed by the Accreditation Council for Graduate Medical Education (ACGME), and explicit attention to this area of education by the National Board of Medical Examiners (NBME) and the Association of American Medical Colleges (AAMC).[7] Some state associations of medical schools, for example, the Associated Medical Schools of New York,[6] have seized the initiative and formed "learning networks" to pursue curriculum and organizational development in this domain.

In the explosion of literature focused on educating for professionalism, much expository text has been devoted to exploring the various qualities of "the good physician." Statements from the AAMC (expressed as educational objectives for schools of medicine), the NBME (identifying the domains of

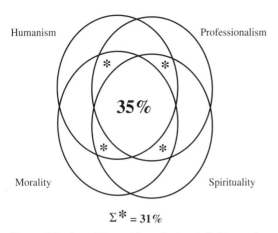

Figure 6.1. A problem with exclusive definitions: the semantic domains overlap.

professionalism), and the ACGME (unbundling the domains of profession-alism intended to be part of the curriculum in residency programs) all offer relevant perspectives.[4] All these organizational statements resonate remarkably with one another, emphasizing the importance of such attributes as respect-fulness, skill and knowledge, commitment to excellence, caring, compassion, superb communication, integrity, honesty, accountability, dutifulness, and al-truism. Inui[4] and Swick[8] speculate that this high degree of congruence arises because the authors and organizational sponsors of these consensus state-ments share a view of medicine as a virtuous activity, a moral enterprise in which individuals in the profession do their best to act from shared root values. These include acting on a secure foundation of truth/science, building thera-peutic alliances, curing whenever possible, providing care and comfort, accept-ing differences and being empathic, taking right action/avoiding error, and being self-sacrificing when necessary to preserve patients' interests (altruism).

Baldwin and colleagues[9,10] suggest that the qualities and root values of the good physician may not be unique to the domain of professionalism in med-icine. Instead, after several studies intended to explore the associations be-tween the behaviors of the good physician and several different domains (professionalism, humanism, morality, and spirituality in medicine), they conclude that many of these qualities – attributes such as altruism, compas-sion, dedication to excellence, dutifulness, respectfulness, accountability, in-tegrity, and responsibility – are empirically linked to two or more of these domains. Of 52 terms typically used to describe professionalism, more than one-third (35 percent) were also believed by students, residents, and practi-tioners to be attributes of humanism, morality, and spirituality in medicine, and an additional 31 percent were seen as associated with three of these four "ism" domains (Figure 6.1).

Baldwin's work leads us to a possible conclusion. "Educating for professionalism in medicine" is the same as educating for humanism, moral action, or spirituality in medicine – in effect, supporting the development of "character and conscience" in the future physician. If we hope, and expect, physicians to be exemplars of civil and moral behavior and to be sensitive to the spiritual dimensions of health in others, medical education must attempt to invoke and secure the same root values to support and guide their behaviors as we hope to invoke and secure for "professionalism in medicine".

> An obese patient had to have his groin examined. There was a very strong odor to which the doctor almost got sick. He told the patient how bad it smelled. I would have done my best to make it through the exam but not make the patient feel any worse about the smell because he knew about the smell but could do nothing to make it better.
>
> > [A third-year student on the internal medicine clerkship, IUSM, February 2004, checking off "Respect, Caring, Compassion, Communication"]

> I recently witnessed a situation in which a patient wanted to be discharged AMA. The patient was in severe failing health and was looking toward another operation due to infection. My team all gathered with him and tried to convince him to stay – educating him as to the possible results of his actions (death). The gentleman refused and refused to accept their advice. In the end, he is still going to leave AMA. Nobody on the team – frustrated as they were – even began to raise their voice or in any way show the man any disrespect. Interestingly, if the man stays it will cause much more work for our team and our team is post call and all are tired and want to go home. It would have been much easier to just accept the man's wishes and let him go – probably to soon die of sepsis. I feel that what I witnessed shows deep compassion for human life, even if only to lengthen it for a short time. My team showed that even though they were overworked and tired, they were willing to give up their time and efforts for someone that they did not know and would gain little or nothing personally by keeping him here. I notice a deep sense of sorrow after the incident. The rest of our rounds was much more quiet and reserved.
>
> > [A third-year student on the internal medicine clerkship, IUSM, February 2004, checking off "Altruism, Responsibility and Accountability, Respect, Honor and Integrity, Caring, Compassion, Communication, Leadership, Knowledge and Skills"]

And what form does such development of future physicians – teaching and learning for professionalism, character, and conscience in medicine – take today? One especially challenging aspect of education becomes apparent when we observe that students and graduate trainees learn most powerfully from the environment in which they are educated and less powerfully from readings or formal classroom-based content we provide.[11,12]

The good news – and the bad news – for educators is that students are learning all the time. The implications of this observation are several:

- As educators, we need to understand the acquisition of professional values as "learning from experience" rather than from didactics. In this context, we may need to examine and perhaps borrow approaches from other helping professions (e.g., preparation for careers as clergy) in which educators combine experience and reflection in order to foster moral growth and the deepening of values.
- As organizational leaders, we need to be mindful of the "lessons" imparted by the environments in which we educate and train physicians. These environments (physical and social) have been intentionally constructed – or come together willy nilly – for the sake of faculty convenience, medical care efficiency, and/or the support of subspecialty procedural practice, without explicit attention to the moral values they express.
- As educators and individuals who live and work in these organizational environments, we need to seriously contemplate how we learn and facilitate the learning of others. How are the essential values-relevant elements of our own experiences made clear and lifted up for individual and group reflection? How can we create and sustain a shared community mindfulness of professionalism and professional values in the larger academic community in which medical students learn?

Whatever approaches we take, none of this individual and community action can be simple or straightforward. Inui[4] has commented elsewhere that the actual lived experience of value-based action in the profession of medicine may be fairly described as "struggling to keep one's balance in precarious situations." These situations are ones in which our ideals might clearly be in play, but the nuances of context complicate choices, priorities, and actions. In our lived experiences, we find ourselves regularly compromising these ideals – often for good reason – such as when one ideal is counterpoised against another. Making such compromises, others (including our students) see us clearly as acting under conditions of irreducible uncertainty, swimming in a sea of conflicts, causing harm and incurring risk, appearing to be arrogant, making mistakes, hassled by the circumstances of daily work, and maximizing our income, rather than embodying our ideals.

Under these circumstances, students recognize a disturbing difference between the ideal-focused reading and lecturing they encountered early in their undergraduate medical education and the uninterpreted day-to-day stream of behaviors they see us exemplifying later. Our silence in the face of these situational challenges to values deepens the ambiguity of the situation and the learners' confusion. All this contributes to a discouraging "formative arc" of education. Available evidence indicates that our learners move:

- From being focused on the formal to being focused on the "informal curriculum" (from noting what we say to noting what we do);
- From being open minded and curious to being test driven and minimalistic, focused only on what they need to know to pass examinations;
- From being open hearted and idealistic to being well defended;
- From being altruistic to cynical, concluding that medicine is a field in which one must say one thing and do another;
- From being empathic to being task-driven, focused less on the patient's experience and more on getting their own work done;
- Backward, rather than forward in capacity for moral reasoning.

How could this retrogression be occurring, contrary to our best intentions? As Bryan[13] has suggested, our medical students may be climbing A.H. Maslow's "deficit needs" ladder, which emphasizes the needs to which all of us give highest priority, including physiological needs, personal safety needs, the need to feel as if we belong and are comfortably accommodated within our closest social circle, and preserving rudimentary self-esteem. This theoretic perspective comes alive if we think of our medical students' quick break for lunch, long hours leading to sleep deprivation ("physiological needs"), concerns about needle-stick incidents or scary walks at night to the parking lots surrounding our academic health centers ("personal safety needs"), love-hate relationships with their classmates in a highly competitive environment ("closest social circle needs"), and reiterating cycles of placement on the lowest rung of a competency ladder as they rotate from one radically different clinical experience to the next ("self-esteem needs"). As Bryan notes, is it then any wonder that our learners have no time for growth as civil characters with strong consciences in a process that Maslow (and before him Aristotle) described as "self-actualization?" And little wonder that they have difficulty getting beyond basic do's and don'ts of professional codes of behavior to "higher order" professionalism that might evoke their deeply held values, as they learn to navigate the increasingly complex circumstances they will face as physicians.

How can we – and our learners with us – break out of this discouraging developmental trajectory? To begin, we should recognize and affirm that we can pursue two parallel approaches to educating for professionalism in medicine during undergraduate medical education years.[4,12] The first approach emphasizes a clear understanding of the roles and responsibilities, indeed the social accountability, of medicine as a learned profession and the history of how this special group of privileged workers has shouldered these responsibilities. We can help students understand the principles and codes of acceptable behavior or commitments that have emerged from taking this responsibility and how these understandings inform choice making in the complex situations physicians face.[14] The second approach emphasizes the primacy of learning through reflection on experience (alone or with peers), learning to notice how values are served or abridged through choices and actions that were or were not taken. This second approach is one we have emphasized at Indiana University School of Medicine (IUSM)[15,16] where educating for professionalism occurs in the context of a fully implemented competency curriculum consisting of eight domains in addition to the domain of professionalism (communication skills, self awareness, moral and ethical reasoning, lifelong learning, community context, basic clinical skills, using science to guide decision making, and problem solving). These competencies are introduced during a week-long orientation in the first year and continue to be represented as dimensions of every course throughout the four years of medical school. The core elements of the curriculum, with particular attention to our explicit effort to integrate learning from the "informal" and "formal" curriculum has been recently well summarized by Litzelman and Cottingham.[15] One integrative activity in the professionalism competency curriculum uses medical student "journals" written during the internal medicine and surgery clerkships. Here, we capture student-level lived experience, create dialogic learning around these experiences, and build a stage-appropriate foundation of experiential learning for students who decide for themselves how general principles of behavior might assist them in making complex choices involving competing and sometimes conflicting values. The specifics of this approach are described in greater detail elsewhere.[16]

> I was presenting a patient and mentioned some arterial blood gas values. The team resident asked me to explain the test results. I was only able to give a cursory interpretation and then asked for help. Both the resident and the attending were very willing to help and genuinely felt that my request was valid. There have been times on other rotations when I have asked for help and have not gotten such a good reaction. I was not made to feel like I was stupid or witless – rather, I felt that I did a good thing in admitting my lack of specific knowledge and was taught in a way that was good for me. It was a great example of how to treat people with respect. This was an excellent case of modeled professional behavior.
>
>   [A third-year student on the internal medicine clerkship, IUSM, October 2004, checking off "Respect, Leadership, Knowledge and Skills"]

Our ward team and the ICU team were rounding together and we all entered a patient's room in the unit. There were at least 15 people in the room. The team discussed the patient, examined him, adjusted the ventilator settings and left – all totally oblivious to the family members who were also in the room. After we left, I noticed that the intern, who had just started on service that morning, stayed behind and knelt down beside the wife of the patient. She was explaining what the team had just done. No one else noticed what she had done, but I did, and I was very impressed by her behavior.

> [A third-year student on the internal medicine clerkship, IUSM, April 2004, checking off "Caring, Compassion, Communication, Leadership"]

In teaching from these narratives, our intent is to emphasize critical incidents[17] as a method for fostering mindfulness and growth in our students' capacity to recognize values embedded in actions. We also hope to demonstrate the capacity of physicians (even physicians in their formative years) to constructively engage with one another in community discussions of complex experiences in which such actions take place. In this dialogue, we are able to surface situations from a student's perspective, and in an age/stage-appropriate manner help them to identify behaviors that embody (exhibit) altruism, compassion, respect, duty, accountability, and so on. In effect, the students – in a process of experience followed by reflection in a community of peers – become able to locate the instincts and manifestations of character and conscience already within themselves that grow and mature into what others will recognize as professionalism later in their careers.

In these situations, students come to recognize the importance of certain questions that are transferable to other occasions – questions that may be useful to them as they sort out their own experiences later:

- What was it about this situation that attracted your attention?
- Why did this particular set of events unfold?
- Have any of the rest of you (student peers) seen something like this? What did it make you think at the time?
- How did you feel in the moment? Now?
- What were the choices in this situation?
- Would you make the same choices that you saw someone else make?
- If not, why not?
- In this situation what would you actually say if you wanted to change what was done?
- What are the risks of doing or saying something different? What are the risks of not doing something different?

In dialogues around questions like this, the students begin to understand that what they and others (including fellow students, attending physicians, other medical professionals and patients, and family members) hold most dear is the basis for moral action and right relationships. The process is similar to learning from sacred texts in which one asks questions such as, In this situation, where is the good (the valued, God)? Where am I in this story? and What, then, should I do?

Besides learning the value of community reflection on useful questions that may be applied to many situations, another, perhaps more explicit way to describe the set of capacities that students may acquire in this dialogic process is to say that we are attempting to inculcate "professional competence"[18] in our students. We hope that this competency allows them to interpret experience, make mindful choices, begin to become proactive in shaping their own thoughts and actions, and even begin to mindfully shape the thoughts and choices of others in their environments. This competency is founded on four constituent capacities:

1. Awareness and sensitivity – understanding ideals and values of the profession for self and others in situational context.
2. Judgment – having a capacity to distinguish reasons and values in a behavioral context.
3. Motivation – having the capacity to weigh and prioritize choices and actions on the basis of values in a situation.
4. Conduct – having the character, skills, and ability to habitually act on values, even in risky circumstances.

In effect, we attempt to teach our students how to navigate successfully through complex and risky situations. They, like us, are risk-aware. They worry about patient risk, but they also are concerned with risk of failure, humiliation, and poor academic assessment in hierarchical systems that dominate academic medical centers' cultures. In these choppy waters, they focus on their own day job, which is to learn and grow as future physicians who must angle for optimal evaluations as credentials for postgraduate training positions. The two forms of navigation we hope they will understand and master, speaking metaphorically, are historically identifiable as Euro-centric navigation and South-Pacific (Truk Islander) navigation.[19]

Voyages spanning over one-hundred miles of open ocean are still made in sailing canoes and longer ones were made in the past. The destination is often a tiny dot of land less than a mile across, and visible from any distance only because of the height of those coconut trees which may grow in its sandy soil. From a canoe, virtually at the level of the ocean's surface, even a forested island is visible only three or four miles away . . . to assure that the travelers will come close enough to their destination to sight it after covering miles of empty ocean, with shifting winds and currents, the crew usually rely on one of their number who has been trained in a variety of traditional techniques by an older master navigator, usually a relative of his. These techniques do not include even a compass, to say nothing of chronometer, sextant, or star tables . . .

Essentially, the navigator relies on dead reckoning. He sets his course by the rising and setting of stars, having memorized for this purpose the knowledge gleaned from generations of observation . . . Between stars, or when the stars are not visible due to daylight or storm, the course is held constant by noting the direction of the wind and the waves. A good navigator can tell by observing wave patterns when the wind is shifting its direction or speed and by how much. In a dark and starless night the navigator can even tell these things from the sound of the waves as they lap upon the side of the canoe's hull, and the feel of the boat as it travels through the water . . .

[Thomas Gladwin, 1964, Culture and Logical Process]

The European tradition of navigation is the alternative with which we are most familiar in the Western hemisphere, utilizing charts, chronometers, compasses, and sextants. The Portuguese or Spanish navigator successfully plotted and pursued his course across vast stretches of ocean, guided by celestial sightings and compass readings. Essentially, a rule and chart-based system of navigation with periodic checks on position by external criteria, the European navigation system is a metaphorical analog to proceeding through complicated situations in the life of medicine guided by codes of behavior and general principles. By contrast, the South Pacific islander navigation method uses strong impressions of situation and context, as well as intuition and judgment derived from experience and reflection. Situation and ephemera-centered (flotsam, jetsam, wave forms) as well as guided by a vision of the unseen goal, this method has also served sailors successfully in open-ocean navigation, even to the present day.

Our hope for our medical students is that they learn to use both forms of navigation to acquire skills and perspectives born of experience, a constructive pattern of sound behaviors (habits) that will become their manifest "character," and a set of personal values they are able to recognize and articulate as "constellations" to which they look for guidance. This process of learning to navigate complex, confusing, and risky situations is one that we know to be a core pedagogic method in the helping professions other than medicine. In seminarian preparation, for example, it is referred to as "formation," the process that permits an individual to mature and become the person who can successfully serve a calling.[4,20] The essential ingredients of formation are described as engaging in service, reiterating cycles of experience and reflection, growth in knowledge of self as well as the field of endeavor, and constant attention to one's inner life as well as the hustle and bustle in the life of action. In formation, one acquires the knowledge, skills, and technical expertise needed to render service but also persistently asks the question, "Whom am I becoming, as I move toward this life of service?"

In our view, success in educating for professionalism in medicine requires a fusion of two approaches. On the one hand, exposure in the formal curriculum emphasizes student engagement with evidence from research – scholarly work in various traditions that brings together systematic observations from history, social and behavior science, moral philosophy, the law, and spiritual traditions that provide depth to our accounts of duty, accountability, social expectation, general rules of conduct, and regulatory mechanisms. On the other hand, even with comprehensive knowledge from research, each student, trainee, and practitioner in his/her career also needs a rigorous and systematic process for learning from his/her experience of the informal curriculum (the organizational and social environment in which they are immersed). Testing general guidelines for behavior for "goodness of fit" in the complex situations that arise, sensing the force of potential regulatory mechanisms for social justice (litigious or otherwise) that may be invoked if the behaviors of the physician fail to meet expectations or breach expected conduct boundaries, and learning from what are observed to be conventional behaviors in the local and prevailing "community of medicine" are all necessary to understanding what will work in the local culture of medicine in which an individual is practicing. Fusing learning from both the formal and the informal curriculum produces practical knowledge and resourceful practical wisdom (*phronesis* in Greek, the synthesis of "theoretical mind" with "practical mind"). Metaphorically, this is precisely what we attempt to prepare our learners to do when using both star-guided navigation and wind and wave-guided navigation to explore their lived experience. The principal of altruism may be a sound general principle and "north star" for our actions, but under certain circumstances – pitted, for example, against other high values of our profession – it may assume a lesser priority than other considerations. Reading the waves, the wind, and observing the "flotsam and jetsam" in the specific situation as well as the identity of birds that fly by, we may decide that altruism should give way to maintenance of our integrity or to truth telling in a particular circumstance.

Using student journal entries to teach skills in how to mindfully "read and navigate" the life of medicine is an important objective for the professionalism curriculum at IUSM. However, in isolation, these skills are unlikely to flourish especially given the larger organizational context of most modern medical centers. At IUSM, we have also initiated and sustained a complementary program of organizational change intended to enhance the informal curriculum and stimulate more mindfulness about the learning environment we create in every moment so it will better embody the professional aspirations and values we hope our students will adopt. Described at greater length in previous publications,[15,21] these efforts have included an extensive process of "appreciative inquiry."

Appreciative inquiry is an organizational development method that involves interviewing and storytelling to draw out the best of an organization's experience.[22] It is a process designed to:

- Facilitate the discovery of factors that give life to an organization;
- Change the nature of conversations in an organization;
- Stimulate the evolution of a collective's "future vision"; and
- Set the stage for future strategic action.

The assumptions of appreciative inquiry are several. It assumes that (1) something is working well for every person or group in an organization and (2) that looking at what works well and doing more of it is more motivating and energizing than looking for what does not work and trying to do less. Triggered by an initial round of appreciative interviews at IUSM, capturing and reporting individual and social narrative has become an important mode of communication at our organization that powerfully expresses cultural meaning. The narratives from our internal medicine and surgical clerkships that punctuate this chapter are used for professionalism dialogues during clerkships, student intercessions, house staff orientations and retreats, departmental grand rounds, faculty development retreats and workshops, hospital staff physician meetings, and external professional meetings and workshops.

Appreciative narratives are both a point of departure and a way to consolidate learning. Many others in the environment have moved to use story gathering and social narrative as a tool for education, illustration, and tracking organizational performance. These include the Dean and Executive Associate Deans of the IUSM, Chair of the Department of Pediatrics, our hospital system executives, faculty and residents in the Emergency Department of our public hospital's Level One Trauma Center, the Gold Foundation Honor Society, the Community Service Learning Program, our hospital system's nursing executives, among others. Appreciative stories, solicited and lightly juried by students, are also collected into annual publications that become gifts to new matriculants and their families at our school's White Coat Ceremony. The stories also serve as core content for a column in our school e-newsletter that publishes narratives and brief commentaries as "Mindfulness in Medicine" columns.

What are these stories about? Elsewhere we have reported the content of the student narratives, certainly the most numerous stories and the ones that have been used most widely.[16] They report a slice of students' lived experience in hospitals and clinics. The larger corpus of narratives, written by the diverse community of people on our campus, brings into focus anything that might capture the imagination. They are "pixels" that taken together create a composite portrait of our academic medical center environment "through the fresh eyes" of our students, faculty, staff, nurses, administration, and (in some cases) patients. Students, of course, see almost everything and are honest witnesses to the ordinary life world of IUSM. Their plain-language narratives in booklets, newsletter columns, read at surgical grand rounds, and elsewhere are a mirror for us all. Positive stories inspire and motivate wonderfully. Negative stories – with explicit or implicit commentary – serve to remind and generate corrective energy for the next risk. Individually and collectively, these stories seem to have stimulated our community to mindful experimentation with daily actions that shift us toward civility, mutual respect; celebration of our best moments; explicit efforts to repair and avoid egregious behaviors; and educational innovation that opens "communities of learning." The stories have made visible what was previously not discussed. The ingrained habit of withholding comment about unprofessional behavior – of looking on in silence – is giving way to shared observations and reflection.

Many activities in the school have been transformed by the mindful use of narrative. Admissions interviews now take the form of real dialogue with applicants, who become acquainted (even at an admissions interview!) with the character of our community. Committee meetings are more personal and engaging and often facilitated with meeting process techniques that build member acquaintance and common understanding. Alumni look forward to news of the school in the form of student and faculty stories. In effect, the organization is becoming progressively entrained by its own emerging professional narrative.[23] The writing and retelling of narrative from our students, faculty, patients, and others seem to deepen the heuristic value of these narratives for individuals as well as building greater relationship-centered community through the use of organizational and personal narrative, deepening our professional culture.[24,25]

During my first week of my first medicine rotation at the VA I was lucky enough to have an intern that taught me some valuable lessons about medicine as well as integrity and accountability. Drug/Pharmaceutical representative lunches are carried out at the VA every Wednesday and during the week the representatives show up almost daily with all types of free stuff – from sodas and snacks to promises of dinners at St. Elmo's. These guys and gals spare no expense to gain even a lowly third year's attention and favor. In an unbiased way my intern challenged me to think about my stance on these representatives, their reason for being in our hospital and what ethical questions were raised by these practices by drug companies. In retrospect he gave me a choice to make my own conscious decision on an ethically-charged issue. It was a great lesson and I'll appreciate it for the rest of my career. I'm sorry his month with our team ended because we enjoyed boycotting the free food last Wednesday after we realized that as young physicians in training we couldn't passively participate in what these unethical solicitations represent.

> [A third-year student on the internal medicine clerkship, IUSM, June 2004, checking off "Responsibility and Integrity, Honor and Accountability, Leadership"]

At a macro organizational level, the emergence of a more aligned and relational community of action may have permitted some otherwise high-risk administrative transitions to take place at IUSM without bloodshed and loss of leadership momentum. These include the implementation of a mission-based budget allocation system, and a comprehensive reexamination of how the clinical research enterprise needs to be reformed in order to meet the challenge of NIH's Clinical Translational Sciences Award Program. We also feel that these efforts to deepen our shared professional culture have contributed to the recent substantial improvement in our graduating students' ratings of the quality of their educational experience (these ratings are now at unprecedented highs) and to the explosive growth in our out-of-state applicant pool (increased by more than 80 percent in the past four years). While we set out to transform our organizational environment for the sake of enhancing teaching and learning in professionalism, the resulting organizational transformation seems to have had many other useful consequences as well.

> My very first patient on the internal medicine rotation was an elderly gentleman who presented with altered mental status and ARF. During his stay with us, he was never coherent. In fact he went from mumbling a few nonsensible words at admission to becoming verbally unresponsive. Therefore, it was easy for staff and students alike to hurry in, do a brief physical exam on him and not think too much about it. Unfortunately, his condition continued to worsen while in the hospital, and he passed away on his second day with us.
> The next morning during rounds, my resident unexpectedly pulled out an old wrinkled piece of paper and solemnly began to read a poem. I cannot recall the name of the poem nor the author; however, I will never forget the message the poem was meant to convey to us that day. The poem spoke of a lost loved one. It spoke of anguish and loneliness. To us, this patient was just that . . . a patient. We spent so much time those two days frantically searching for a reason for his deteriorating health and following up hundreds of labs. But, to those loved ones who mourned by his bedside that last night, he was their everything.
> As a fresh medical student, this death had not gone unnoticed by me. I had been deeply touched seeing the family the night of the passing. I have not yet become desensitized to this fact of life. However, as the poem was being read, I could tell by the expressions of the interns present that perhaps they had not given as

much thought to this gentleman's passing. The poem served as a thought pro-
voking reminder that behind each patient we lose is a person who has lost their
East, their West … their everything.

[A third-year student on the internal medicine clerkship, IUSM, June 2004,
checking off "Respect, Honor and Integrity, Caring, Compassion, Communication"]

CLOSING COMMENTS

To improve the teaching of professionalism at IUSM, we have concluded that
our learners need formal didactics in combination with opportunities to
learn mindfully and, in community, from their experience. We have taken
as a central pedagogic thesis the need to prepare our learners in educational
methods that are best described as "formation," emphasizing reflection for
moral growth and development as integral to experience-based learning. We
acknowledge that this process of moral formation may be seen, alternatively,
as deepening the preparation of students for humanism, spirituality, and
professionalism in medicine but do not fret about this ambiguity since we
believe that all these domains are rooted in similar values. Opportunities to
journal and be in dialogue with one another as we build the narrative of our
organization seem to be instrumental in our progress. In addition to using the
usual quantitative metrics of academic organizational performance to track
our progress, we are using social narrative from all quarters to continuously
understand and learn from the lived experience of what is happening in our
environment. This social narrative serves both as a mirror for our community
and as a stimulus to organizational change. The gathering, retelling, and
sharing of narrative actually seems to move our organization in the direction
of a deeper values-based professional organizational culture, to the benefit of
our students, our staff, our patients, and ourselves. We have consciously tried
to inculcate deeper mindfulness of the choices we make and the values we
exemplify as we do our daily work in classrooms and clinics, hospital wards
and boardrooms, and in administrative offices, knowing that the "informal
curriculum" is not only how we teach most powerfully but also how we
conduct our daily lives and navigate our careers.

REFERENCES

1. Wear, D, Bickel, J. *Educating for Professionalism: Creating a Culture of Humanism in Medical Education*. Iowa City (IA): University of Iowa Press; 2000.
2. Freidson, E. Professionalism reborn: theory, prophecy and policy. In Dingwall, R,
Lewis, P, editors. *The Theory of Professions: State of the Art*. Chicago (IL): The
University of Chicago Press; 1994: 13–29.

3. Freidson, E. *Professionalism: The Third Logic on the Practice of Knowledge*. Chicago (IL): The University of Chicago Press; 2001.

4. Inui, TS. *A Flag in the Wind: Educating for Professionalism in Medicine*. Washington (DC): Association of American Medical Colleges; 2003.

5. Sullivan, WM. *Work and Integrity: The Crisis and Promise of Professionalism in America*. New York: HarperCollins Publishers; 1995.

6. Cohen, JJ. Ideas and ideals: the annual meeting addresses of AAMC president Jordan J. Cohen, M.D. In *Our Compact with Tomorrow's Doctors*. Washington (DC): Association of American Medical Colleges; 2006: 62–67.

7. Associated Medical Schools of New York Meeting. *Professionalism: I Know it When I Don't See It*. New York: Mount Sinai School of Medicine; 2005 December 16.

8. Swick, HM. Toward a normative definition of medical professionalism. *Acad Med*. 2000;75(6):612–616.

9. Baldwin, DC. Two faces of professionalism. In: Parsi, K, Sheehan, MN, editors. *Healing as Vocation: A Medical Professionalism Primer*. Lanham (NY): Rowman & Littlefield Publishers, Inc.; 2006: p. 103–119.

10. Baldwin, DC, Self, DJ. The assessment of moral reasoning and professionalism in medical education and practice. In Stern, DT, editor. *Measuring Medical Professionalism*. New York: Oxford University Press; 2006: 75–93.

11. Coulehan J. Viewpoint: today's professionalism: engaging the mind but not the heart. *Acad Med*. 2005;80(10):892–898.

12. Stern, DT, Papadakis, M. The developing physician – becoming a professional. *NEJM*. 2006;355(17):1794–1799.

13. Bryan, CS. Medical professionalism and Maslow's needs hierarchy. *Pharos Alpha Omega Alpha Honor Med Soc*. 2005;2(68):4–10.

14. Cruess, R, Cruess, S, Johnston, SE. Professionalism and medicine's social contract. *J Bone Joint Surg Am*. 2000;82-A(8):1189–1194.

15. Litzelman, DK, Cottingham, AH. The new formal competency-based curriculum and informal curriculum at Indiana University School of Medicine: overview and five-year analysis. *Acad Med*. 2007;4(82):410–421.

16. Inui, TS, Cottingham, AH, Frankel, RM, Litzelman, DK, Mossbarger, DL, Suchman, AL, Vu, TR, Williamson, PR. Educating for professionalism at Indiana University School of Medicine: feet on the ground and fresh eyes. In Wear, D, Aultman, JM, editors. *Professionalism in Medicine: Critical Perspectives*. New York: Springer; 2006: 165–184.

17. Branch, WT. Use of critical incident reports in medical education: a perspective. *J Gen Intern Med*. 2005;20(11):1063–1067.

18. Baldwin, DC, Bunch, WH. Moral reasoning, professionalism, and the teaching of ethics to orthopaedic surgeons. *Clin Orthop Relat Res*. 2000;(Number 378): 97–103.

19. Gladwin, T. Culture and logical process. In Goodenough, WH, editor. *Explorations in Cultural Anthropology: Essays in Honor of George Peter Murdock*. New York: McGraw Hill; 1964: 167–177.

20. Palmer, PJ. *The Courage to Teach: Exploring the Inner Landscape of a Teacher's Life*. 10th anniversary edition. San Francisco (CA): Jossey-Bass; 2007.

21. Suchman, AL, Williamson, PR, Litzelman, DK, Frankel, RM, Mossbarger, DL, Inui, TS; Relationship-Centered Care Initiative Discovery Team. Toward an informal curriculum that teaches professionalism: transforming the social environment of a medical school. *J Gen Intern Med*. 2004;19(5 Pt. 2):501–504.

22. Watkins, JM, Mohr, BJ. *Appreciative Inquiry: Change at the Speed of Imagination*. San Francisco (CA): Jossey-Bass/Pfeiffer; 2001.

23. Kelly, JR. Entrainment in individual and group behavior. In McGrath, JE, editor. *The Social Psychology of Time: New Perspectives*. Thousand Oaks (CA): Sage; 1988: 89–110.

24. Linde, C. The acquisition of a speaker by a story: how history becomes memory and identity. *Ethos*. 2000;28(4):608–632.

25. Dobie, S. Reflections on a well-traveled path: self-awareness, mindful practice, and relationship-centered care as foundations for medical education. *Acad Med*. 2007;82(4):422–427.

7 Assessment and Remediation in Programs of Teaching Professionalism

Christine Sullivan, M.D., and Louise Arnold, Ph.D.

A resident has been consistently late to required case conferences. This past week two patients complained that he was rude to them. Should his professionalism be assessed, and if so, how? Does he need remediation; and if he does, how can it be achieved? These questions beg answers because assessment of professionalism and remediation of professional lapses are fundamental to medical professionalism and because accrediting bodies expect teaching programs to address the professionalism of learners. Accordingly, this chapter will explore the role of assessing professionalism, methods for assessing professionalism of learners and faculty, and unresolved issues surrounding assessment of professionalism. The chapter will then address the process of remediation of unprofessional behavior, for identification of professional lapses of physicians and physicians in training demands a response. Since the environment of an institution or group can impact both the assessment of professionalism and the remediation of unprofessional behavior, the chapter will close with a description of methods for characterizing an environment's professionalism.

ASSESSING PROFESSIONALISM OF LEARNERS AND FACULTY

Assessment's Role

Assessment of medical professionalism can serve several purposes. In its summative form, it indicates whether learners and faculty have met professional standards and certifies that educational programs have complied with criteria for fostering professionalism. Because learning professionalism is

---

The authors thank Amrita Burdick, Clinical Medical Librarian at the University of Missouri-Kansas City School of Medicine, for assistance with the literature search for this chapter.

a process that can be prolonged and involves continual striving, its assessment must also be formative to guide an individual's professional development.[1] Further, assessment can convey to learners and evaluators the principles of professionalism and their importance. By educating learners and faculty about expectations for professional behavior, assessment can help prevent professional lapses.

Assessment Methods

Recent scholarship in assessing medical professionalism has generated the following benchmarks of effective assessment.[1-6] The purpose of the assessment must be clear with formative and summative assessment separated to enhance the perceived safety of the assessment and its acceptance among learners and faculty. The assessment should be comprehensive, yet practical, covering the requisite attitudes, knowledge, and behaviors appropriate to the stages of a medical career.[7] It should emphasize situations where the principles of professionalism conflict so that the recognition of the conflict, its resolution, and the reasoning behind the resolution can be examined. The assessment should be realistic and grounded in the context in which it occurs. It must involve professional judgment[8] and fair-minded subjectivity[9] because, ideally, learning professionalism entails the incorporation of values into one's identity as a professional.

Many tools, incorporating quantitative and/or qualitative approaches, are now available to assess professionalism[10]: its foundational components of communication and ethics and its central principles of excellence, humanism, accountability, and altruism.[7] These include standardized clinical encounters, high-fidelity simulations, portfolios, reflection, observations over short-defined periods, critical incidents and longitudinal observations, multisource assessments including peer assessments, written examinations, and measures of conscientious behavior. The selection of a tool should depend upon the purpose of the assessment and the measure's reliability, validity, and practicality. Table 7.1 summarizes major advantages and disadvantages of assessment methods available.

Standardized clinical encounters such as observed structured clinical examinations (OSCEs) assess learners' professionalism in test settings that approximate real situations. They allow examinees to demonstrate competence: what they know how to and what they can do in those settings. Administered in practice settings, unannounced, standardized encounters can also reveal examinees' performance: what they will do in their daily interactions with patients and professional colleagues.

Table 7.1. Advantages and disadvantages in using methods of assessing medical professionalism

Methods	Advantages	Disadvantages
Standardized clinical encounters	Can yield sound measures of competence, especially in communication, in settings that mirror the real world of medicine	Are resource intensive
High-fidelity simulations	Can measure teamwork and interprofessional communication	Require additional study to establish quality of the measurement
Portfolios	Are well suited to assessing complex phenomena such as professionalism; require examinees to decide how best to demonstrate their achievement	Are resource intensive
Reflection	Can provide insight into learners' attitudes, development of professional identity, and reasoning about professional dilemmas	Is not appropriate for summative assessment
Faculty observations of learners	Typically measure routine performances of learners in the real world of medicine; are easy to design and use	Can produce data with low reliability unless attention is paid to numbers of observations and observers, training of observers, and discussion of observations
Critical incident reports	Can predict future professional lapses	Provide information about only a few learners who are exemplars or who are deficient
Multisource assessments	Offer a more complete picture of learners' professionalism than that derived from a single source	Evaluators may be reluctant to address unprofessional behavior
Self-assessment	Can be a fruitful starting point for professional development	Accurate self-assessment is difficult to achieve
Peer assessment	Can provide unique information about learners' professionalism	Not suited to high-stakes assessment; peers may be reluctant to participate in assessment of each other
Knowledge tests	Have excellent face and content validity	Relationship between test scores and performance in the real world is unknown

In particular, standardized clinical encounters yield psychometrically acceptable assessments of communication skills of individual learners and faculty as well as groups of physicians working in teams.[11] The use of standardized encounters to measure candidates' communication skills as part of Step 2, Clinical Skills, of the United States Medical Licensing Examination is a testament to this technique's power. At the institutional level, too, OSCEs offer reliable and valid scores of residents' communication.[12]

OSCEs simulating reality-based dilemmas can test examinees' ethical reasoning and ethical behaviors.[13-15] These examinations can present the examinee with richer content than do other methods of assessing medical ethics. However, the large number of stations required to achieve high-stakes reliability of ethics OSCEs points to their best use as formative assessments.[16]

OSCEs have also assessed examinees' professionalism per se; one of its central principles, humanism, and dimensions of humanism including empathy, cultural sensitivity, respect/compassion, interpersonal skills such as patient rapport, and integrity.[17-24] These OSCEs can be psychometrically acceptable if attention is paid to case specificity. Further, OSCEs can pose value conflicts to examinees whose responses might reveal professional lapses[4] and the processes by which they resolve the conflicts.

In sum, OSCEs can reliably and validly measure the foundational skill of communication and the principle of humanism. They are ideal for testing competence[25] and even performance if unannounced standardized patients visit real practice sites.

High-fidelity simulations offer yet another approach to assessing professionalism in a setting that mirrors the complexity of medical practice in the real world. Instruments simulating crises have tested the teamwork and interprofessional communication of anesthesiologists, emergency medicine physicians, and surgeons.[11] For example, scenarios confronted emergency medicine residents with ethical dilemmas during crisis resource management courses; accompanying performance checklists identified areas in which residents' professionalism needed improvement.[26] The use of high-fidelity simulations in assessing professionalism and subsequent debriefing of examinees is ripe for further development.

Portfolios, "purposeful collections of evidence that learners gather to record and reflect on their progress and achievement in selected domains, . . . are well suited for . . . assessment of complex . . . competencies, including professionalism."[27] If properly designed, portfolios promote reflection that transforms the experience of clinical practice into learning.

Medical educators have implemented portfolios with medical students and residents.[27-31] Moreover, recertification processes in several specialties such as internal medicine include portfolios.

Working portfolios conveying process and progress are appropriate for formative assessment and are particularly applicable to assessing professionalism as a developmental process. In contrast, performance portfolios displaying final products are appropriate to summative assessment; they are unique among assessment tools because they require individuals to make decisions about how best to demonstrate their own achievement.[27] Some educators advise against the use of portfolios for summative assessment due to the paucity of reliability data. Several studies offer support for portfolios in summative assessment, if the number of portfolio entries is adequate, if there is agreement about standards for assessing portfolio contents, and if raters receive training and discuss differences in their scoring.[29,31]

Reflection as a tool for assessing medical professionalism is not confined to portfolios. Learning logs, assigned essays written during orientation or during clerkships, responses to ethical dilemmas, reports about critical incidents meaningful to the learner, narratives, and self-assessment exercises such as those included in the American Board of Internal Medicine (ABIM) recertification process can prompt learners to reflect upon professionalism.[16,32–36]

Reflection is a way to find meaning in events.[37] Thus, if subjected to rigorous content analysis, the products of reflection can afford understanding learners' attitudes toward the medical profession, the development of a professional identity, and learners' reasoning that underlies their behavior. Reflection is especially appropriate to assessing professionalism because it entails "[according to Coles] not so much getting the right answer but in deciding what is 'best' in the situation"[38] where principles of professionalism frequently conflict.

Faculty observation of learners can focus on a single performance as a basis for judgment or on impressions gathered about learners' routine performance over a particular time period. The Professionalism Mini-Evaluation Exercise is an example of faculty observation of a single performance.[39] Research suggests that it might be a psychometrically sound tool with the ability to promote self-reflection and awareness of the importance of professionalism among learners while taking context surrounding the behavior into account. Rating scales direct faculty observation of learners' routine performances related to professionalism.[40–44] These scales ask faculty to judge the occurrence of the behavior, the quality of the performance, and/or whether the performance was satisfactory or not.[45] Global performance rating scales are a predominant assessment method across the continuum of medical education. Although they are easy to design and use, global ratings, and faculty observations more generally, pose a number of problems, particularly if the assessment focuses on professionalism. Multiple observations, multiple observers, training of observers, and other strategies can increase the reliability and thus the value of the ratings.[1,45,46]

Critical incident reports and longitudinal observations are important variations of faculty observations of learners' professionalism. They are effective ways to assess professionalism.[47–53] At one school, a physicianship evaluation system, that monitors students' critical-incident reports longitudinally, predicted patterns of subsequent unprofessional behavior.[51] Domains of student behavior related to future disciplinary actions of state licensing boards included severe irresponsibility, resistance to self-improvement, and lapses in integrity.[52,53] Although these longitudinal critical incident reports identify learners with deficiencies, they do not provide information about the professionalism of the majority of learners.[1]

Multisource assessments or 360-degree evaluations are a way to expand the judgments of faculty about learners' professionalism to include perspectives of nurses, allied health care professionals, patients, patients' families, and the self. Typically, the multisource assessments rely on questionnaires to gather information in numerical and/or narrative form. Based on these tools, comparisons of ratings by nurses, patients, attending physicians, and/or program supervisors have produced profiles of the communication skills, professionalism, professional behaviors, humanism, responsibility, and psychosocial aspects of patient care of physicians and physicians in training.[5,54–58] Moderate correlations among ratings by an array of evaluators suggest that multisource evaluations might offer a more complete picture of learners' professionalism.[5] Reproducible results depend upon using a number of raters, for example, ten nurses and larger numbers for faculty and patients.[44] Learners have found the results of multisource evaluations useful but caution that the process itself can impact whether they will address others' unprofessional behavior.[59]

Self-assessments are frequently a part of 360-degree evaluations. Medical students and their evaluators found accurate self-assessments of personal and professional behaviors difficult to achieve.[60] Under certain conditions, self-assessments can match faculty expectations, especially if the standards are explicit.[61,62] Self-assessments can be a fruitful starting point for growth in professionalism. However, until there is clarity about the theoretical construct of self-assessment and how it is measured, its potential as an assessment technique cannot be fully realized in medical education,[63] particularly in assessing professionalism.

Peer assessment is another avenue for gaining a more complete picture of the professionalism of physicians and physicians in training because peers have better access to observing one another than do other evaluators. Studies show that peers can distinguish each others' technical knowledge/skills from their nontechnical knowledge/skills and that they can assess each others' communication, interpersonal skills, relations with patients, humanism, and work habits in reliable and moderately valid ways.[64,65] The choice of criterion variables to study their validity, however, remains problematic.[64]

Further, learners' refusal or reluctance to provide candid information about each other can compromise the psychometric characteristics of peer assessment.[64] In students' eyes, the conditions that would facilitate their honest participation in peer assessment include an assessment that is 100% anonymous, provides immediate feedback, focuses on unprofessional *and* professional behaviors, and uses peer assessment formatively while rewarding exemplary behavior and addressing serious repetitive professional lapses.[66] Students stressed that peer assessment must be embedded in a supportive environment.[66,67] Successful peer assessment programs in several institutions mirror some of these conditions.[68–70]

In sum, peer assessment should be part of comprehensive assessment of professionalism. It can yield psychometrically acceptable information as long as peers' concerns about the assessment are addressed. Peer assessment is best for formative decisions, at least in medical school and residency programs, since peers appear generally unwilling to participate in high-stakes assessments.[64]

Other Techniques Written examinations involving multiple-choice questions, case-based questions, and essays relevant to ethics, law, and professionalism have excellent face and content validity; but the connection between learners' performance on the examinations and performance in clinical settings is unknown.[16] High-quality instruments for measuring students' and residents' moral reasoning (which is related to clinical performance) are available.[6,71] Scales to measure empathy, teamwork, and lifelong learning can contribute to a multiscore profile of professionalism[72] as can scales tapping cultural competence.[6] Indicators of students' conscientious behavior such as completion of required course evaluations predicted professional behavior during the clinical years.[73]

Specific Approaches to Assessing Faculty's Professionalism

Assessment of faculty's professionalism is critical for countering learners' feelings that they are, unjustly, the only targets of assessment of professionalism. Besides routine instructor evaluations of professionalism that learners complete, special tools assessing instructors' professionalism have been developed. These primarily include rating forms,[74–76] but a novel objective structured teaching evaluation measures educators' responses to learners' lapses in professional behavior.[77] Instruments appropriate for assessing professionalism of practicing physicians by patients[6,78] can also be applied to faculty.

Assessment Issues and Recommendations

Despite the growth in the study of assessing professionalism, a number of issues remain unresolved. Critics claim that the discourse on medical professionalism has been too abstract[79] and that students' ideas about professionalism do not match the abstract conceptualizations of professionalism.[80,81] The movement toward concretizing professionalism as behaviors[82] rather than qualities can counteract the concern about abstraction, especially if evaluators have been involved in selecting the behaviors that will be assessed. Focus on assessing behaviors may also side step the issue of whether professionalism should be cast as a competency[8] or whether it is duty or virtue based.[83] Yet, an exclusive focus on behaviors runs the risk of declaring those individuals with professional behaviors but unprofessional attitudes as satisfactory and those individuals with unprofessional behaviors but professional attitudes as unsatisfactory.[84] This prospect calls for exploration of individuals' reasoning in working through professional dilemmas.

Another issue is the inclusion of altruism in the concept of professionalism. Altruism has become suspect.[85,86] Without it, the threat of commercialism to medical practice and the welfare of patients and society looms; and medicine as the profession we know becomes an occupation. Perhaps a reframing of altruism that views it as actions aimed at increasing the welfare of others, especially those in need,[87] instead of self-sacrifice, might address this concern.

The complexity of professionalism suggests that its assessment should yield a profile of an individual's performance in terms of professionalism's major principles such as altruism, accountability, humanism, excellence, and their dimensions. The practicality of compiling a profile is questionable even though instruments are available to measure each principle. Moreover, evaluators do not usually make distinctions among the principles of professionalism; rather, they categorize learners' performances into two factors: the technical and the nontechnical.[5,88] Thus, a profile may be foreign to the way evaluators think and behave. This issue is part of a larger question, recently raised, as to whether assessment of separate graduate medical education competencies is possible.[89] Perhaps a global assessment of professionalism of learners or faculty can serve as a screening mechanism with follow-up using instruments to target-specific principles of professionalism, as needed.

Finally, evaluators continue to be reluctant to fail individuals with unsatisfactory performance.[90] Their reasons are legion.[1,90] Several longitudinal systems for tracking students' unprofessional behavior, de-scribed above, seem to decrease faculty's reluctance to report professional lapses. Attention paid to best practices in designing and implementing an assessment system, described elsewhere, may also encourage evaluators to participate candidly in assessment.[1,3] Perhaps an institutional culture can encourage evaluators to participate fully in the assessment process if it is designed to build and sustain the professional character of learners and faculty so they may strive toward wisely applying the principles of professionalism.[1]

REMEDIATION

Defining the Professional Lapse

Assessment methods can identify professional lapses, but what can we and should we do with the information? With an emphasis on performance stand-ards, patient care, and the working environment, medical organizations and governing boards have defined the individual with unprofessional behav-ior.[91–104] These definitions should be considered when describing a profes-sional lapse. The incidence of unprofessional behavior and the effect or potential effect of such behavior on patient care and the work environment mandate our response.[91–93,105]

Identifying the Lapse

Assessment methods previously described in this chapter can assist in the recognition of substandard performance. Of special note, the most frequent methods used to identify professional lapses in residents are direct observa-tion and critical incident reports.[95] Research findings stress that early lapse identification is critical to modify behavior(s) before they become refractory to change.[53,94,100,106]

Investigating and characterizing the lapse is mandatory prior to reme-diation. Fact finding, consultation, and documentation are crucial to de-termine the reliability of the report as well as the seriousness of the lapse.[107] In reporting incidents and lodging complaints, and to encour-age such reporting, the complainant needs to feel secure that the incident is being handled in confidence and should receive follow-up that the complaint has been reviewed and addressed.[104] Determining the cause of the lapse can assist with the remediation process.[93] Reasons to con-sider include behavioral, interpersonal, and attitude issues; impairment including medical, psychological, psychiatric, or substance abuse; stress management; cognitive issues; and family issues.[95,108]

The following example illustrates the need to characterize the lapse. One physician is found to have abandoned a patient during an emergent condition, while another physician has been reprimanded for repeated lack of timely medical record completion. Both physicians demonstrate substandard responsibility, but the first clearly has a more egregious lapse. In this context, those deficiencies that compromise or could potentially compromise patient care and safety must be addressed immediately. It is paramount to characterize the severity of the issue; this will affect both the immediacy and the extent of intervention.[1,95,104,107,109,110] The mild-to-moderately severe lapse often presents more challenge to remediate as administrators struggle with choosing activities that are meaningful, appropriate, and not considered merely "punishment" for the individual with the lapse.[109] Once the lapse has been identified and characterized, it must then be addressed with the individual.

The Remediation Process

So, who addresses the lapse? For medical students, it is the clerkship director; for residents the program director; for practicing physicians it is the department chair, a hospital's credentialing/review committees, as well as state licensing boards. How do these administrators approach the individual with a lapse, and how can they develop a plan for remediation? We discuss these issues below.

The meeting with the individual serves as notification and sets the remediation in motion. For less serious lapses, the meeting may be an educational opportunity in which methods to correct the behavior are agreed upon.[1] Simply, it may serve as a "wake-up call" for the individual, and that may be the only step required.[104] More serious lapses, frequent and/or recurrent lapses, or failure to improve after a less formal intervention should be addressed more formally.[1,104] The meeting should be scheduled with the objectives clearly in mind; a witness and/or scribe for the meeting is recommended.[104] The individual may divulge issues not previously known that might affect the interpretation of and response to the lapse, and the administrator should be prepared to redirect the individual who displaces blame or makes excuses.[94,103,104,111] The meeting should serve to confront the behavior(s) but should do so in an atmosphere of genuine concern.[103] In sum, notification serves as a mechanism to describe the unacceptable behavior(s), counsel and educate regarding acceptable behaviors, and allow the individual to respond to the findings as well as to contribute to the remediation plan. After the conclusion of the meeting, the remediation plan should be formalized taking into consideration any information obtained and suggested by the individual.

The remediation plan should have goals and expectations transparent for the individual, the administrator, and the institution.[108,112,113] The goal of the remediation should be behavioral change.[106–108,112] The timeframe for remediation, the monitoring of the process, what defines success, and the consequences of failure should be specified and understood by all parties.[104,112–114] The timeframe should not be indefinite. Is a slow, steady improvement acceptable? In a case of patient harm or potential harm, should immediate improvement be required? What should be done if there is a relapse? Under extreme circumstances, and if the lapse is recurrent and/or severe, or the remediation plan is ignored or not successfully completed, then more severe action including practice restriction, suspension, leave of absence, or termination may be initiated following the guidelines of due process.[115,116]

The remediation plan should fit the problem.[1] Consider a student who has failed a clinical rotation secondary to professional issues; simply repeating the rotation does not sufficiently address the cause of the lapse. Thus, the activities that the individual must undertake and complete should reflect the nature and severity of the lapse and the individual involved. Performance feedback is an important aspect to consider as it can provide the individual with continuous quality improvement during the remediation process. Discussions with an assigned advisor, education, ongoing performance feedback, self-reflection, and referral for evaluation and counseling are some recommended remediation activities.[1,25,50,92,93,109] Sensitivity training, conflict resolution, team building, or interpersonal relationship training may be mandated, depending on the circumstance of the lapse.[109,110,112] Referral to physician health programs may be necessary in certain cases.[1,99,100]

Techniques for Remediation

Various therapeutic models exist that can be utilized in the process to remediate the professional lapse. Feedback intervention is a technique in which the knowledge of performance can affect actions.[117] Positive feedback intervention through reinforcement and negative feedback intervention through punishment may facilitate learning and improve performance when standard goals are defined.[117] Motivational interviewing requires the individual to identify and mobilize values and intrinsic goals to change behavior.[118] It enables the individual to resolve his/her ambivalence regarding behaviors/perceptions and thereby promotes willingness for change.[119] Cognitive behavioral therapy is utilized to treat a number of conditions ranging from depression, anxiety, panic disorder, social phobia, and posttraumatic stress disorder. [120] The primary objective of the technique is to recognize the effect that thinking has on mood and then to change the way a person feels by adapting how one thinks and behaves.[120–122] In both motivational interviewing and cognitive behavioral therapy, motivation to change is elicited from the individual, not imposed from without.

Another approach to consider is the process used in addressing medical errors and systems within health care. The fundamental technique is root cause analysis that seeks to identify and understand the incident/error, define the primary and contributing factors, and prevent future events.[123–127] The goal is to convert substandard performance to acceptable work habits through educating the health care team, clearly defining expectations, and requiring accountability.[128] With a systems approach to both the problem and the solution, the groundwork for changing the environment is established.[129,130] This approach brings to light that the environment can contribute to the professional lapse, that the environment and the individual should be investigated when determining the cause of the lapse, and that the environment as well as the individual should be considered when implementing a process to remediate the lapse.

Likelihood of Success

Success can be improved if the student, resident, or physician has insight and awareness into the problem and a willingness to change the negative behavior.[1,93,100,131,132] Acceptance of the principles of professionalism, understanding the actions that define professionalism, self-reflection, and performance feedback can facilitate change.[1,39,108,133] In remediating professional lapses in residents, assigning a mentor/advisor and frequent performance feedback sessions have been found to be the most helpful methods.[95] Involving the learner in the process, thereby facilitating accountability and responsibility in the remediation, can increase the likelihood of success.[108] Consistency in adhering to the plan is requisite for remediation.[108,109,112]

Conversely, negative predictors for success include the denial that a problem exists and a weak follow-up plan.[94,103] The severity of the "punishment" and the feeling that there is a lack of consistency with the process may result in failure to complete the remediation.[134] In cases of "burnout," prevention is crucial.[97]

Due Process

Adherence to the principles of due process is mandatory when implementing remediation. Elements of academic due process include 1) the early notification of concern(s)/lapse(s), 2) the opportunity for the individual to respond to the issue(s), and 3) a transparent definition of competency based on professional standards.[95] The remediation process should include a written document for the individual that specifies the lapse, the methods, and timetable to correct/remediate the deficiency; the consequences of noncompliance or unsuccessful completion; and the right to appeal the decision based on the policies of the institution.[114]

> *Legal considerations* may serve as a deterrent for implementing and monitoring remediation. Since professionalism is considered part of clinical competency, in most cases, disciplinary actions and dismissal can be considered academic.[50] Courts defer to the professional judgment of an institution's faculty and administrators in student/resident academic dismissals.[50] *Horowitz v Board of Curators of the University of Missouri (1976)* is a landmark case that upheld the dismissal of a medical student based on behaviors that violated academic standards.[116] The National Practitioner Data Bank, the Joint Commission of Accreditation of Healthcare Organizations, state licensing boards, and health maintenance organizations (HMOs) define procedures and mechanisms to report and respond to physician misconduct.[99] Hospitals are required to respond to the disruptive physician, and individual physicians must report their own misconduct to HMOs according to policies and mandates.[99] With a duty and sometimes a requirement to report, administrators should be reassured that as long as due process and professional standards are adhered to, the courts and organizations will uphold their decisions.

An Example of a Remediation Plan

An internal medicine resident received clinical evaluations from internal medicine and other specialty faculty who cited poor interpersonal skills and a lack of respect, sensitivity, and responsibility for patients. In an informal remediation process, the program director and resident discussed the issues and met on a monthly basis to discuss performance. The resident attended a required human resources communication skills seminar. The expectation for the resident was that there was to be no further mention of attitude or professional issues on clinical evaluations. Results indicated no change in behavior during the informal remediation; in fact, the resident received a formal patient complaint and failed an outside clinical rotation during the process.

A formal remediation plan was implemented. It involved performance feedback after each of the resident's clinics from faculty using an assessment tool developed to address behaviors previously identified as unacceptable, monthly meetings with the hospital's director of guest services to discuss the patient perspective and review typical patient complaints, monthly faculty advisor meetings, monthly resident self-reflection using a performance questionnaire, and a required session with the director of counseling, health, and testing at the university. The resident was required to successfully repeat the failed clinical rotation. Resident responsibilities in the process were to initiate the feedback process with faculty, schedule all meetings, provide the program director with weekly updates, and conduct monthly self-assessment. Continued unacceptable behavior would result in suspension or separation from the training program.

The formal process, lasting several months, was successful. All clinical evaluations showed acceptable professional behavior. The resident successfully repeated the failed rotation and even received a patient satisfaction letter. Multiple faculty provided assessments; and all assessed the resident's clinic performance as competent, with the assessments showing less fluctuation in performance over time. The resident complied with all the assigned responsibilities.

Six months postremediation, however, a faculty cited the resident for unacceptable interactions with a patient and the health care team. The program director discussed this report with the resident, reestablished a more frequent performance feedback process, and told the resident that any future similar incidents would result in separation from the program. The resident had no subsequent lapses identified.

Why did the informal remediation plan fail? The resident later confided that they did not "buy in" to the belief that a problem existed and did not take the mandated communication seminar seriously. Upon review, the program director concluded that the remediation failed because the feedback occurred only monthly, the consequences for unsuccessful remediation were not clear, and the resident was not accountable for carrying out the remediation.

In contrast, why did the formal plan work? The process included multiple learning opportunities. The resident said that the frequent feedback and feedback from multiple sources helped define acceptable behaviors, provided examples of how to demonstrate those behaviors, and reinforced acceptable performance of these behaviors during clinical work. The resident also confided the realization that their previous performance had been substandard and expressed a genuine desire to change. Self-reflection and responsibilities during the process provided a catalyst for change.

Why the relapse? Successful remediation should not be considered a "cure." Simply put, past behavior can predict the likelihood for future behavior. Individuals with professional lapses might be prone to relapse if they feel that they are no longer accountable for their behavior. The potential for relapse should be considered when addressing the professional lapse.

Issues and Recommendations

A number of obstacles to the remediation of the professional lapse remain. Among these is the failure to report. There exists an underlying belief that these lapses may not be "fixable." Even with successful remediation, a relapse may occur. Further, administrators may simply not know how to approach the lapse. We recommend a consistent, individualized, transparent approach in which the individual with the lapse has primary responsibility for carrying out the plan and receives frequent explicit feedback from multiple sources. In addition, we postulate that frequent ongoing performance feedback might serve as a mechanism for preventing a professional relapse by providing behavioral markers of improvement and thus continuing ongoing self-awareness. Table 7.2 offers a template for designing a remediation plan.

EVALUATION OF THE ENVIRONMENT

Because context plays a critical role in shaping behavior[135] and because the environments of institutions and groups can affect the type and quality of assessment of professionalism,[1,5,66,67] the professionalism of learners and faculty,[85,136,137] and the remediation of unprofessional behavior,[96,97,132] it is important to evaluate the environment systematically for its stance on professionalism. Some of the instruments available to characterize an environment's professionalism provide pictures of an institution's culture – its norms, values, and basic assumptions about organizational life; others describe the institution's climate, that is, the perceptions of the culture that institutional members hold.[138]

Surveys are the most ubiquitous type of environmental assessment instrument. Some surveys elicit perceptions of learners and faculty about professionalism. Others ask individuals about themselves and provide an aggregated picture of the professionalism of a group or institution. Still

Table 7.2. Designing a remediation plan

Remediation plan process	Definition
Define and characterize the professional lapse	Identify the lapse in terms of behavior(s) taking into account the severity, circumstance(s), and cause(s) of the lapse
Goal(s)	Define what constitutes successful remediation of the lapse, in other words, what specific behavior(s) should be modified and how
Consequences	Define at the outset what will happen if the remediation plan is ignored, not completed successfully, or if a relapse occurs
Requirements	Choose plan elements that can educate, modify, and monitor behavioral change. Requirements should include *activities* and *techniques* specific to the individual and the character of the lapse, *timeframe* for completion, and mechanism for *monitoring* and providing *feedback* to the individual during the process. *Due process* should be followed.

Adapted from Sullivan C, Arnold L, Yoder E, Raible M. Professionalism: assessment and remediation. Association of American Medical Colleges Annual Meeting, Group on Educational Affairs/Group on Student Affairs Mini-workshop Session, October 2006. Handout page 9.

others request institutional authorities for data either about their institutions or about their individual members.[139] The most relevant data about professionalism in the medical environment come from a survey that asked students and residents about the behaviors of residents at five institutions by operationalizing the ABIM elements of professionalism, but the internal consistency of only some of the survey items was acceptable.[140] Additional empirically driven surveys in medical education produce group data about a variety of environmental aspects such as patient centeredness[141] and mistreatment.[142] Other surveys, derived from social science theories on school climate, ethical climates, and organizations are also applicable to evaluating medical education environments for professionalism.[134,143–148] These tools describe the environment in terms of teamwork, warmth, humanism, respect, and social responsibility, for example.

Besides surveys, focus groups; content analyses of institutional stories, learners' essays and cases, institutional policies, and institutional responses to critical incidents; as well as naturalistic methods of observing daily activities of institutional members have produced insights into the formal, hidden, and unintended curricula relevant to professionalism.[136,149–153] For an environmental evaluation to be meaningful, however, powerful champions must take the lead in garnering support of faculty, staff, and learners; marshal resources for implementing the assessment; and have the skill to practice the principles of organizational change. A continuous quality improvement model might weaken resistance to undertaking an environmental assessment and using its results.

SUMMARY AND CONCLUSIONS

Assessment of medical professionalism and remediation of professional lapses are integral to teaching programs on professionalism. Although what is examined tends to be learned, what is not examined is a more potent message to learners and faculty when it comes to professionalism. Thus, a system for assessing medical professionalism, with the benchmarks mentioned at the outset of this chapter, needs to be a part of teaching programs. We reviewed specific assessment methods matched to the formative and summative purposes of assessment. With assessment in place and results generated, we suggested actions that need to be taken: recognition for exemplars of professionalism, ongoing development of learners' and faculty's professionalism, and remediation for individuals found to be deficient. We approached remediation as an educational process but recognized the need to specify consequences if remediation was unsuccessful. There remains the continuing challenge for learners and faculty alike to lay aside their reluctance to participate in assessing professionalism and to remediate professional lapses, understand and adopt the assessment and remediation methods that are available and effective, and continue to work toward improving the assessment and remediation processes. A more elusive goal remains: to alter the environments of teaching programs to promote professionalism without the risk of engendering cynicism and to prevent professional lapses in the first place through authentic supportive relationships among learners and faculty. Other chapters in this volume address these vital tasks.

REFERENCES

1. Arnold, L. Responding to the professionalism of learners and faculty in orthopaedic surgery. *Clin Orthop Relat Res.* 2006;449:205–213.
2. Veloski, JJ, Fields, SK, Boex, JR, Blank, LL. Measuring professionalism: a review of studies with instruments reported in the literature between 1982 and 2002. *Acad Med.* 2005;80:366–370.
3. Stern, DT. A framework for measuring professionalism. In Stern, DT, ed. *Measuring Medical Professionalism.* Oxford, UK: Oxford University Press; 2006: 3–13.
4. Ginsburg, S, Regehr, G, Hatala, R, McNaughton, N, Frohna, A, Hodges, B, Lingard, L, Stern, D. Context, conflict, and resolution: a new conceptual

framework for evaluating professionalism. *Acad Med*. 2000;75(10 suppl.): S6–S11.

5. Arnold, L. Assessing professional behavior: yesterday, today, and tomorrow. *Acad Med*. 2002;77:502–515.

6. Lynch, DC, Surdyk, PM, Eiser, AR. Assessing professionalism: a review of the literature. *Med Teach*. 2004;26:366–373.

7. Arnold, L, Stern, DT. What is medical professionalism? In Stern, DT, ed. *Measuring Medical Professionalism*. Oxford, UK: Oxford University Press; 2006:15–37.

8. Parker, M. Assessing professionalism: theory and practice. *Med Teach*. 2006; 28:399–403.

9. Huddle, TS. Teaching professionalism: is medical morality a competency? *Acad Med*. 2005;80:885–891.

10. Stern, DT, ed. *Measuring Medical Professionalism*. Oxford, UK: Oxford University Press; 2006.

11. Klamen, D, Williams, R. Using standardized clinical encounters to assess physician communication. In Stern, DT, ed. *Measuring Medical Professionalism*. Oxford, UK: Oxford University Press; 2006:53–74.

12. Yudkowsky, R, Downing, SM, Sandlow, LJ. Developing an institution-based assessment of resident communication and interpersonal skills. *Acad Med*. 2006;81:1115–1122.

13. Singer, PA, Robb, A, Cohen, R, Norman, G, Turnbull, J. Performance-based assessment of clinical ethics using an objective structured clinical examination. *Acad Med*. 1996;71:495–498.

14. Gallagher, TH, Pantilat, SZ, Lo, B, Papadakis, MA. Teaching medical students to discuss advance directives: a standardized patient curriculum. *Teach Learn Med*. 1999;11:142–147.

15. McClean, KL, Card, SE. Informed consent skills in internal medicine residency: how are residents taught, and what do they learn? *Acad Med*. 2004;79: 128–133.

16. Kao, A. Ethics, law, and professionalism: what physicians need to know. In Stern, DT, ed. *Measuring Medical Professionalism*. Oxford, UK: Oxford University Press; 2006:39–52.

17. Prislin, MD, Lie, D, Shapiro, J, Boker, J, Radecki, S. Using standardized patients to assess medical students' professionalism. *Acad Med*. 2001;76(10 suppl.):S90–S92.

18. Rogers, JC, Couts, L. Do students' attitudes during preclinical years predict their humanism as clerkship students? *Acad Med*. 2000;75(10 suppl.): S74–S77.

19. Hauck, FR, Zyzanski, SJ, Alemago, SA, Medalie, JH. Patient perceptions of humanism in physicians: effects on positive health behaviors. *Fam Med*. 1990;22: 447–452.

20. Schnabl, GK, Hassard, TH, Kopelow, ML. The assessment of interpersonal skills using standardized patients. *Acad Med*. 1991;66(9 suppl.):S34–S36.

21. Altshuler, L, Kachur, E. A culture OSCE: teaching residents to bridge different worlds. *Acad Med*. 2001;76:514.

22. Robins, LS, White, CB, Alexander, GL, Gruppen, LD, Grum, CM. Assessing medical students' awareness of and sensitivity to diverse health beliefs using a standardized patient station. *Acad Med.* 2001;76:76–80.

23. Klamen, DL, Williams, RG. The effect of medical education on students' patient-satisfaction ratings. *Acad Med.* 1997;72:57–61.

24. Van Zanten, M, Boulet, JR, Norcini, JJ, McKinley, D. Using a standardised patient assessment to measure professional attributes. *Med Educ.* 2005;39: 20–29.

25. Larkin, GL, Binder, L, Houry, D, Adams, J. Defining and evaluating professionalism: a core competency for graduate emergency medicine education. *Acad Emerg Med.* 2002;9:1249–1256.

26. Gisondi, MA, Smith-Coggins, R, Harter, PM, Soltysik, RC, Yarnold, PR. Assessment of resident professionalism using high-fidelity simulation of ethical dilemmas. *Acad Emerg Med.* 2004;11:931–937.

27. Fryer-Edwards, K, Pinsky, LE, Robins, L. The use of portfolios to assess professionalism. In Stern, DT, ed. *Measuring Medical Professionalism.* Oxford, UK: Oxford University Press; 2006:213–233.

28. Ben David, MF, Davis, MH, Harden, RM, Howie, PW, Ker, J, Pippard, MJ. AMEE medical education guide no. 24. Portfolios as a method of student assessment. *Med Teach.* 2001;23:535–551.

29. Rees, CE, Sheard, CE. The reliability of assessment criteria for undergraduate medical students' communication skills portfolios: the Nottingham experience. *Med Educ.* 2004;38:138–144.

30. Gordon, J. Assessing students' personal and professional development using portfolios and interviews. *Med Educ.* 2003;37:335–340.

31. O'Sullivan, PS, Cogbill, KK, McClain, T, Reckase, MD, Clardy, JA. Portfolios as a novel approach for residency evaluation. *Acad Psychiatry.* 2002;26: 173–179.

32. Niemi, PM. Medical students' professional identity: self-reflection during the preclinical years. *Med Educ.* 1997;31:408–415.

33. Niemi, PM, Vainiomaki, PT, Murto-Kangas, M. "My future as a physician"—professional representations and their background among first-day medical students. *Teach Learn Med.* 2003;15:31–39.

34. Lingard, L, Garwood, K, Szauter, K, Stern, D. The rhetoric of rationalization: how students grapple with professional dilemmas. *Acad Med.* 2001;76(10 suppl.): S45–S47.

35. Baernstein, A, Fryer-Edwards, K. Promoting reflection on professionalism: a comparison trial of educational interventions for medical students. *Acad Med.* 2003;78:742–747.

36. Charon, R. To render the lives of patients. *Lit Med.* 1986;5:58–74.

37. Branch, WT, Paranjape, A. Feedback and reflection: teaching methods for clinical settings. *Acad Med.* 2002;77:1185–1188.

38. Ginsburg, S, Lingard, L. Using reflection and rhetoric to understand professional behaviors. In Stern, DT, ed. *Measuring Medical Professionalism.* Oxford, UK: Oxford University Press; 2006:195–212.

39. Cruess, R, McIlroy, JH, Cruess, S, Ginsburg, S, Steinert, Y. The professionalism mini-evaluation exercise: a preliminary investigation. *Acad Med.* 2006; 81(10 suppl.):S74–S78.

40. American Board of Internal Medicine(ABIM). *Project Professionalism.* Philadelphia, PA: American Board of Internal Medicine; 1994.

41. Kreiter, CD, Ferguson, K, Lee, WC, Brennan, RL, Densen, P. A generalizability study of a new standardized rating form used to evaluate students' clinical clerkship performances. *Acad Med.* 1998;73:1294–1298.

42. Fontaine, S, Wilkinson, TJ. Monitoring medical students' professional attributes: development of an instrument and process. *Adv Health Sci Educ Theory Pract.* 2003;8:127–137.

43. Gauger, PG, Gruppen, LD, Minter, RM, Colletti, LM, Stern, DT. Initial use of a novel instrument to measure professionalism in surgical residents. *Am J Surg.* 2005;189:479–487.

44. Accreditation Council for Graduate Medical Education (ACGME) and American Board of Medical Specialties (ABMS). *Toolbox of Assessment Methods.* Version 1.1, September 2000. Chicago, IL: Accreditation Council for Graduate Medical Education and American Board of Medical Specialties. Available at www.acgme.org/Outcome/assess/Toolbox.pdf. Accessed June 22, 2007.

45. Norcini, J. Faculty observation of student professional behavior. In Stern, DT, ed. *Measuring Medical Professionalism.* Oxford, UK: Oxford University Press; 2006:147–157.

46. Boon, K, Turner, J. Ethical and professional conduct of medical students: review of current assessment measures and controversies. *J Med Ethics.* 2004;30: 221–226.

47. Rhoton, MF. Professionalism and clinical excellence among anesthesiology residents. *Acad Med.* 1994;69:313–315.

48. Phelan, S, Obenshain, SS, Galey, WR. Evaluation of the noncognitive professional traits of medical students. *Acad Med.* 1993;68:799–803.

49. Papadakis, MA, Osborn, EHS, Cook, M, Healy, K. A strategy for the detection and evaluation of unprofessional behavior in medical students. *Acad Med.* 1999;74:980–990.

50. Papadakis, MA, Loeser, H, Healy, K. Early detection and evaluation of professionalism deficiencies in medical students: one school's approach. *Acad Med.* 2001;76:1100–1106.

51. Papadakis, MA, Hodgson, CS, Teherani, A, Kohatsu, ND. Unprofessional behavior in medical school is associated with subsequent disciplinary action by a state medical board. *Acad Med.* 2004;79:244–249.

52. Teherani, A, Hodgson, CS, Banach, M, Papadakis, MA. Domains of unprofessional behavior during medical school associated with future disciplinary action by a state medical board. *Acad Med.* 2005;80(10 suppl.): S17–S20.

53. Ainsworth, MA, Szauter, KM. Medical student professionalism: are we measuring the right behaviors? A comparison of professional lapses by students and physicians. *Acad Med.* 2006;81(10 suppl.):S83–S86.

54. Brinkman, WB, Geraghty, SR, Lanphear, BP, Khoury, JC, Gonzalez del Rey, JA, DeWitt, TG, Britto, MT. Evaluation of resident communication skills and professionalism: a matter of perspective? *Pediatrics*. 2006;118:1371–1379.

55. Violato, C, Lockyer, J, Fidler, H. Multisource feedback: a method of assessing surgical practice. *BMJ*. 2003;326:546–548.

56. Ramsey, PG, Wenrich, MD, Carline, JD, Inui, TS, Larson, EB, LoGerfo, JP. Use of peer ratings to evaluate physician performance. *JAMA*. 1993;269:1655–1660.

57. McLeod, PJ, Tamblyn, R, Benaroya, S, Snell, L. Faculty ratings of resident humanism predict patient satisfaction ratings in ambulatory medical clinics. *J Gen Intern Med*. 1994;9:321–326.

58. Woolliscroft, JO, Howell, JD, Patel, BP, Swanson, DB. Resident-patient interactions: the humanistic qualities of internal medicine residents assessed by patients, attending physicians, program supervisors, and nurses. *Acad Med*. 1994;69:216–224.

59. Rees, C, Shepherd, M. The acceptability of 360-degree judgements as a method of assessing undergraduate medical students' personal and professional behaviors. *Med Educ*. 2005;39:49–57.

60. Rees, C, Shepherd, M. Students' and assessors' attitudes towards students' self-assessment of their personal and professional behaviours. *Med Educ*. 2005;39:30–39.

61. Gordon, MJ. A review of the validity and accuracy of self-assessment in health professions training. *Acad Med*. 1991;66:762–769.

62. Woolliscroft, JO, Ten Haken, J, Smith, J, Calhoun, JG. Medical students' clinical self-assessment: comparisons with external measures of performance and the students' self-assessments of overall performance and effort. *Acad Med*. 1993;68:285–294.

63. Eva, KW, Regehr, G. Self-assessment in the health professions: a reformulation and research agenda. *Acad Med*. 2005;80(10 suppl.):S46–S54.

64. Arnold, L, Stern, DT. Content and context of peer assessment. In Stern, DT, ed. *Measuring Medical Professionalism*. Oxford, UK: Oxford University Press; 2006:175–194.

65. Lurie, SJ, Lambert, DR, Nofziger, AC, Epstein, RM, Grady-Weliky, TA. Relationship between peer assessment during medical school, dean's letter rankings, and ratings by internship directors. *J Gen Intern Med*. 2007;22:13–16.

66. Arnold, L, Shue, CK, Kalishman, S, Prislin, M, Pohl, C, Pohl, H, Stern, DT. Can there be a single system for peer assessment of professionalism among medical students? A multi-institutional study. *Acad Med*. 2007;82:578–586.

67. Shue, CK, Arnold, L, Stern, DT. Maximizing participation in peer assessment of professionalism: the students speak. *Acad Med*. 2005;80(10 suppl.):S1–S5.

68. Dannefer, EF, Henson, LC, Bierer, SB, Grady-Weliky, TA, Meldrum, S, Nofziger, AC, Barclay, C, Epstein, RM. Peer assessment of professional competence. *Med Educ*. 2005;39:713–722.

69. Bryan, RE, Krych, AJ, Carmichael, SW, Viggiano, TR, Pawlina, W. Assessing professionalism in early medical education: experience with peer evaluation and self-evaluation in the gross anatomy course. *Ann Acad Med Singapore*. 2005;34:486–491.

70. Small, PA Jr., Stevens, CB, Duerson, MC. Issues in medical education: basic problems and potential solutions. *Acad Med.* 1993;68(10 suppl.):S89–S98.

71. Baldwin, DC Jr., Self, DJ. The assessment of moral reasoning and professionalism in medical education and practice. In Stern, DT, ed. *Measuring Medical Professionalism.* Oxford, UK: Oxford University Press; 2006:75–93.

72. Veloski, J, Hojat, M. Measuring specific elements of professionalism: empathy, teamwork, and lifelong learning. In Stern, DT, ed. *Measuring Medical Professionalism.* Oxford, UK: Oxford University Press; 2006:117–145.

73. Stern, DT, Frohna, AZ, Gruppen, LD. The prediction of professional behavior. *Med Educ.* 2005;39:75–82.

74. Szauter, K, Turner, HE. Using students' perceptions of internal medicine teachers' professionalism. *Acad Med.* 2001;76:575–576.

75. Ephgrave, K, Stansfield, RB, Woodhead, J, Sharp, WJ, George, T, Lawrence, J. The resident view of professionalism behavior frequency in outstanding and "not outstanding" faculty. *Am J Surg.* 2006;191:701–705.

76. Smith, CA, Varkey, AB, Evans, AT, Reilly, BM. Evaluating the performance of inpatient attending physicians. *J Gen Intern Med.* 2004;19:766–771.

77. Srinivasan, M, Litzelman, D, Seshadri, R, Lane, K, Zhou, W, Bogdewic, S, Gaffney, M, Galvin, M, Mitchell, G, Treadwell, P, Willis, L. Developing an OSTE to address lapses in learners' professional behavior and an instrument to code educators' responses. *Acad Med.* 2004;79:888–896.

78. Lipner, RS, Blank, LL, Leas, BF, Fortna, GS. The value of patient and peer ratings in recertification. *Acad Med.* 2002;77(10 suppl.):S64–S66.

79. Wear, D, Kuczewski, MG. The professionalism movement: can we pause? *Am J Bioeth.* 2004;4:1–10.

80. Ginsburg, S, Regehr, G, Stern, D, Lingard, L. The anatomy of the professional lapse: bridging the gap between traditional frameworks and students' perceptions. *Acad Med.* 2002;77:516–522.

81. Ginsburg, S, Stern, D. The professionalism movement: behaviors are the key to progress. *Am J Bioeth.* 2004;4:14–15.

82. National Board of Medical Examiners. Professional behaviors. Available at: http://professionalbehaviors.nbme.org/current-work.html. Accessed June 22, 2007.

83. Swick, HM, Bryan, CS, Longo, LD. Beyond the physician charter: reflections on medical professionalism. *Perspect Biol Med.* 2006;49:263–275.

84. Rees, CE, Knight, LV. The trouble with assessing students' professionalism: theoretical insights from sociocognitive psychology. *Acad Med.* 2007;82: 46–50.

85. Hafferty, F. Measuring professionalism: a commentary. In Stern, DT, ed. *Measuring Medical Professionalism.* Oxford, UK: Oxford University Press; 2006:281–306.

86. Johnston, S. See one, do one, teach one. *Clin Orthop Relat Res.* 2006;449:186–192.

87. Piliavin, JA, Charng, HW. Altruism: a review of recent theory and research. *Annu Rev Sociol.* 1990;16:27–65.

88. Silber, CG, Nasca, TJ, Paskin, DL, Eiger, G, Robeson, M, Veloski, JJ. Do global rating forms enable program directors to assess the ACGME competencies? *Acad Med.* 2004;79:549–556.

89. Margolis, MJ, Clauser, BE, Cuddy, MM, Ciccone, A, Mee, J, Harik, P, Hawkins, RE. Use of the mini-clinical evaluation exercise to rate examinee performance on a multiple-station clinical skills examination: a validity study. *Acad Med.* 2006;81(10 suppl.):S56–S60.

90. Dudek, NL, Marks, MB, Regehr, G. Failure to fail: the perspectives of clinical supervisors. *Acad Med.* 2005;80(10 suppl.):S84–S87.

91. Roberts, LW, Warner, TD, Rogers, M, Horwitz, R, Redgrave, G: Collaborative Research Group on Medical Student Health Care. Medical student illness and impairment: a vignette-based survey study involving 955 students at 9 medical schools. *Compr Psychiatry.* 2005;46:229–237.

92. Reamy, BV, Harman, JH. Residents in trouble: an in-depth assessment of the 25-year experience of a single family medicine residency. *Residency Educ.* 2006;38:252–257.

93. Williams, BW. The prevalence and special educational requirements of dyscompetent physicians. *J Contin Educ Health Prof.* 2006;26:173–191.

94. Wood, IK, Lazarus, C, Parmelee, DX. The challenging student or resident: strategies to recognize and effectively address disruptive behavior. *Acad Physician Sci.* April, 2007;7–9.

95. Yao, DC, Wright, SM. The challenge of problem residents. *J Gen Intern Med.* 2001;16:486–492.

96. Dyrbye, LN, Thomas, MR, Huntington, JL. Personal life events and medical student burnout: a multicenter study. *Acad Med.* 2006;81:374–384.

97. Thomas, NK. Resident burnout. *JAMA.* 2004;292:2880–2889.

98. American Medical Association. Physicians and Disruptive Behavior. Excerpts from AMA Policy Finder. 2004:1–9. Available at: www/ama-assn.org/ama/noindex/category/11760.html. Accessed June 27, 2007.

99. Meyer, DJ, Price, M. Forensic psychiatric assessments of behaviorally disruptive physicians. *J Am Acad Psychiatry Law.* 2006; 34:72–81.

100. Bohigian, GM, Croughan, JL, Bondurant, R. Substance abuse and dependence in physicians: the Missouri physicians' health program—an update (1995–2001). *Mo Med.* 2002;99:161–165.

101. House of Delegates of the Federation of State Medical Boards of the United States. The Special Committee on Evaluation of Quality of Care and Maintenance of Competence. 2006. Available at: www.fsmb.org/pdf/GPROL_essential_eleventh_edition.pdf. Accessed June 27, 2007.

102. Veldenz, HC, Scott, KK, Dennis, JW, Tepas, JJ, Schinco, MS. Impaired residents: identification and intervention. *Curr Surg.* 2003;60:214–217.

103. Winter, RO, Birnberg, B. Working with impaired residents: trials, tribulations, and successes. *Fam Med.* 2002;34:190–196.

104. Kissoon, N, Lapenta, S, Armstrong, G. Diagnosis and therapy for the disruptive physician. *Physician Exec.* 2002;28:54–58.

105. Healy, GB. Unprofessional behavior: enough is enough. *Laryngoscope.* 2006; 116: 357–358.

106. Marco, CA. Ethics seminars: teaching professionalism to "problem residents." *Acad Emerg Med.* 2002;9:1001–1006.

107. Grote, CL, Lewin, JL, Sweet, JJ, van Gorp, WG. Responses to perceived unethical practices in clinical neuropsychology: ethical and legal considerations. *Clin Neuropsychol.* 2000;14:119–134.

108. Hicks, PJ, Cox, SM, Espey, EL, Goepfert, AR, Bienstock, JL, Erickson, SS, Hammoud, MM, Katz, NT, Krueger, PM, Neutens, JJ, Peskin, E, Pushcheck, EE. To the point: medical education reviews—dealing with student difficulties in the clinical setting. *Am J Obstet Gynecol.* 2005;193:1915–1922.

109. Bennett, AJ, Roman, B, Arnold, LM, Kay, J, Goldenhar, LM. Professionalism deficits among medical students: models of identification and intervention. *Acad Psychiatry.* 2005;29:426–432.

110. Peltier, B. Response to unethical behavior in oral health care. *J Am Coll Dent.* 1998;65:19–23.

111. Engel, KG, Rosenthal, M, Sutcliffe, KM. Residents' responses to medical error: coping, learning, and change. *Acad Med.* 2006;81:86–93.

112. Larkin, GL, McKay, MP, Angelos, P. Six core competencies and seven deadly sins: a virtues-based approach to the new guidelines for graduate medical education. *Surgery.* 2005;138:490–497.

113. Pfifferling, J. The disruptive physician, a quality of professional life factor. *Physician Exec.* 1999;25:56–61.

114. Tulgan, H, Cohen, SN, Kinne, KM. How a teaching hospital implemented its termination policies for disruptive residents. *Acad Med.* 2001;76:1107–1112.

115. Youssi, MD. JCAHO standards help address disruptive physician behavior. *Physician Exec.* 2002;28:12–13.

116. Cobb, NH. Court-recommended guidelines for managing unethical students and working with university lawyers. *J Educ Soc Work.* 1994;30:18–31.

117. Kluger, AN, DeNisi, A. The effects of feedback interventions on performance: a historical review, a meta-analysis, and a preliminary feedback intervention theory. *Psychol Bull.* 1996;119:254–284.

118. Ruback, S, Sanboek, A, Lauritzen, T. An education and training course in motivational interviewing influence: GPs' professional behaviour—ADDITION Denmark. *Br J Gen Pract.* 2006;56:429–436.

119. Britt, E, Blampied, NM, Hudson, SM. Motivational interviewing: a review. *Aust Psychol.* 2003;38:193–201.

120. Butler, AC, Chapman, JE, Forman, EM, Beck, AT. The empirical status of cognitive-behavioral therapy: a review of meta-analyses. *Clin Psychol Rev.* 2006;26:17–31.

121. Blenkiron, P. Stories and analogies in cognitive behaviour therapy: a clinical review. *Behav Cognit Psychotherapy.* 2005;33:45–59.

122. Malik, ML, Beutler, LE, Alimohamed, S. Are all cognitive therapies alike? A comparison of cognitive and noncognitive therapy process and implications for the application of empirically supported treatments. *J Consult Clin Psychol.* 2003;71:150–158.

123. Friedman, AL, Greoghegan, SR, Sowers, NM, Kulkarni, S, Formica, RN Jr. Medication errors in the outpatient setting. *Arch Surg.* 2007;142:278–283.

124. Brown, M, Frost, R, Ko, Y, Woosley, R. Diagramming patients' views of root causes of adverse drug events in ambulatory care: an online tool for planning education and research. *Patient Educ Couns*. 2006;62:302–315.

125. Longo, DR, Hewett, JE, Ge, B, Schubert, S. The long road to patient safety: a status report on patient safety systems. *JAMA*. 2005;294:2858–2865.

126. Goel, A, MacLean, CD, Walrath, D, Rubin, A, Huston, D, Jones, MC, Niquette, T, Kennedy, AG, Beardall, RW, Littenberg, B. Adapting root cause analysis to chronic medical conditions. *Jt Comm J Qual Saf*. 2004;30:175–186.

127. Bagian, JP, Gosbee, J, Lee, CZ, Williams, L, McKnight, SD, Mannos, DM. The veterans affairs root cause analysis system in action. *Jt Comm J Qual Improv*. 2002;28:531–545.

128. Yates, GR, Bernd, DL, Sayles, SM, Stockmeier, CA, Burke, G, Merti, GE. Building and sustaining a systemwide culture of safety. *Jt Comm J Qual Patient Saf*. 2005;31:684–689.

129. Iedema, RAM, Jorm, C, Braithwaite, J, Travaglia, J, Lum, M. A root cause analysis of clinical error: confronting the disjunction between formal rules and situated clinical activity. *Soc Sci Med*. 2006;63:1202–1212.

130. Rex, JH, Turnbull, JE, Allen, SJ, Vande Voorde, K, Luther, K. Systematic root cause analysis of adverse drug events in a tertiary referral hospital. *Jt Comm J Qual Improv*. 2000;26:563–575.

131. Benbassat, J, Baumal, R. Enhancing self-awareness in medical students: an overview of teaching approaches. *Acad Med*. 2005;80:156–161.

132. Dyrbye, LN, Thomas, MR, Shanafelt, TD. Medical student distress: causes, consequences, and proposed solutions. *Mayo Clin Proc*. 2005;80:1613–1622.

133. Faustinella, F, Orlando, PR, Colletti, LA. Letters to the editor. Remediation strategies and students' clinical performance. *Med Teach*. 2004;26:664–665.

134. Bennett, RJ. Taking the sting out of the whip: reactions to consistent punishment for unethical behavior. *J Exp Psychol*. 1998;4:248–262.

135. Regehr, G. The persistent myth of stability on the chronic underestimation of the role of context in behavior. *J Gen Intern Med*. 2006;21:544–545.

136. Stern, DT. Values on call: a method for assessing the teaching of professionalism. *Acad Med*. 1996;71(10 suppl.):S37–S39.

137. Feudtner, C, Christakis, DA, Christakis, NA. Do clinical clerks suffer ethical erosion? Students' perceptions of their ethical environment and personal development. *Acad Med*. 1994;69:670–679.

138. Gershon, RRM, Stone, PW, Bakken, S, Larson, E. Measurement of organizational culture and climate in healthcare. *JONA*. 2004;34:33–40.

139. Baldwin, DC Jr., Daugherty, SR. Using surveys to assess professionalism in individuals and institutions. In Stern, DT, ed. *Measuring Medical Professionalism*. Oxford, UK: Oxford University Press; 2006:95–116.

140. Arnold, EL, Blank, LL, Race, KEH, Cipparrone, N. Can professionalism be measured? The development of a scale for use in the medical environment. *Acad Med*. 1998;73:1119–1121.

141. Haidet, P, Kelly, PA, Chou, C: Communication, Curriculum, and Culture Study Group. Characterizing the patient-centeredness of hidden curricula in medical

schools: development and validation of a new measure. *Acad Med*. 2005;80: 44–50.

142. Elnicki, DM, Linger, B, Asch, E, Curry, R, Fagan, M, Jacobson, E, Loftus, R, Ogden, P, Pangaro, L, Papadakis, M, Szauter, K, Wallach, P. Patterns of medical student abuse during the internal medicine clerkship: perspectives of students at 11 medical schools. *Acad Med*. 1999;74(10 suppl.):S99–S101.

143. Cavanaugh, S, Simmons, P. Evaluation of a school climate instrument for assessing affective objectives in health professional education. *Eval Health Professions*. 1997;20:455–478.

144. Agarwal, J, Malloy, DC. Ethical work climate dimensions in a not-for-profit organization: an empirical study. *J Bus Ethics*. 1999;20:1–14.

145. Ells, C, Downie, J, Kenny, N. An assessment of ethical climate in three health-care organizations. *J Clin Ethics*. 2002;13:18–28.

146. Vaicys, C, Barnett, T, Brown, G. An analysis of the factor structure of the ethical climate questionnaire. *Psychol Reports*. 1996;79:115–120.

147. Minvielle, E, Dervaux, B, Retbi, A, Aegerter, P, Boumendil, A, Jars-Guincestre, MC, Tenaillon, A, Guidet, B. Culture, organization, and management in intensive care: construction and validation of a multidimensional questionnaire. *J Crit Care*. 2005;20:126–138.

148. Scott, T, Mannion, R, Davies, H, Marshall, M. The quantitative measurement of organizational culture in health care: a review of the available instruments. *Health Services Res*. 2003;38:923–945.

149. Nestel, D, Robbe, IJ, Jones, KV. Personal and professional development in undergraduate health sciences education. *J Vet Med Educ*. 2005;32:228–236.

150. Coulehan, J. Today's professionalism: engaging the mind but not the heart. *Acad Med*. 2005;80:892–898.

151. Eggly, S, Brennan, S, Wiese-Rometsch, W. "Once when I was on call...," theory versus reality in training for professionalism. *Acad Med*. 2005;80:371–375.

152. Caldicott, CV, Faber-Langendoen, K. Deception, discrimination, and fear of reprisal lessons in ethics from third-year medical students. *Acad Med*. 2005;80:866–873.

153. Stern, DT. Practicing what we preach? An analysis of the curriculum of values in medical education. *Am J Med*. 1998;104:569–575.

8 Developing Professionalism across the Generations

Sharon Johnston, L.L.M., M.D., and Mark A. Peacock, B.A.

Maintaining, strengthening, and renewing professionalism is a responsibility for each generation of physicians. Medical professionalism has been called a dynamic social contract[1] derived from the interaction of many influences such as the tradition of healing, and scientific advances, society's needs and resources, cultural norms and major events, as well as the interests of members of the profession.[2,3] There are increasing calls for medicine to renew its professionalism and creatively adapt to social changes.[4,5] Over the past decade, the medical literature has evinced a growing interest in professionalism. This has concentrated largely on educating students and residents.[6–9] This focus on the newest members of the profession has brought to the forefront the existence of a generation gap in professional values between senior physicians and trainees.[10–12] Medical administrators and recruiters are also calling for greater efforts to bridge generational differences in the workplace to maximize productivity of this new cohort of physicians.[13–15]

Professionalism, reflective of the social contract between physicians and society, should be constantly reflected upon, renewed, and reaffirmed for existing members of the profession and developed for its newest members. One of the great challenges for the twenty-first-century medical profession is to adapt to internal and external changes and to influence the values of its members. Fostering shared yet continually developing values in an increasingly diverse profession and rapidly changing social and health care environment is a daunting task. This requires an intergenerational dialogue to bridge differences within the profession and, as a modernized definition of professionalism evolves, to avoid a mismatch between physician expectations of their professional role and society's expectations of its physicians.[4,16]

This chapter addresses one aspect of this challenge – the need to cultivate and maintain shared professional values across an expanding spread of generations of physicians in an era of increasingly rapid social change. It describes the strong commonalities between generations of physicians and highlights the recurring generational differences in values. It then presents two fundamental causes of these differences that must be understood in order to build shared values for the profession as a whole. Finally, it presents teaching strategies to enable students to begin developing their professional identity early and to encourage all physicians to engage in critical reflection on professionalism.

A DYNAMIC PROFESSION

The medical profession today is more diverse than ever.[17] The profession's evolution reflects the society from which its members come. In addition to growing ethnic, cultural, and gender diversity, the profession includes physicians who trained over more than a fifty-year span. The different generations within medicine represent subgroups, each of which shape the collective values.

A generation for the purposes of this discussion refers to a cohort of individuals born within a specific time frame. The different generations in North America have received many labels. We use the most common ones. The post-war generation born between 1927 and 1945 constitutes approximately 18 percent of practicing physicians in the United States and 12 percent in Canada. The baby boomers, born between 1946 and 1964 comprise 40 percent of US physicians and just over half of Canadian physicians. Born between 1965 and 1980, generation X makes up 40 percent of American physicians and one third of Canadian physicians. Most trainees and students are part of generation Y, born after 1980.

The global shared traits of a generational cohort result from being exposed to similar major social events and trends at a formative stage.[18] The generations and their predominant traits have been described elsewhere.[14,19–21] In the workforce, they are often distinguished by their relationship with authority, career expectations, learning styles, and approach to work-life balance. See Table 8.1 for a comparison of general cohort traits.

COMMON GROUND

Generational cohorts in medicine are not silos but rather share traits and overlapping features at the margins of each group. Thus, it is important to avoid stereotyping individuals from a particular generation. Furthermore, there are strong commonalties across all cohorts within medicine, due in part to the self-selection for medicine as premedical candidates across the generations have expressed similar reasons for choosing a medical career.[22] Admission committees have sought to select new members predicted to be

Table 8.1. Comparison of generation cohorts in medicine*

Generation cohort	Career expectations	Learning style	Professional influences
Post-war (1927–1945)	Dedication, institutional loyalty, hard work	Respect for authority and hierarchy, patience	Advances in diagnosis and treatments, Medicare & Medicaid
Baby boomers (1946–1964)	Driven, reward with hard work, career identity	Teamwork, respect skills/relationships, coaching	Growth of health care industry, from high trust to loss of autonomy
Generation X (1965–1980)	Skills and challenge, controllable lifestyle, no job security	Respect skills/knowledge, multitasking, independence, technology savvy, mentoring not supervision	Diversity, loss of autonomy, multiple stakeholders, medical technology
Generation Y (1980–1999)	Challenge, socially engaged, expect respect	Technology savvy, teamwork, fast pace, mentoring not supervision	Information technology, team work, diversity

* These categories are generalizations and there is overlap between groups.

most successful within the profession, thus reinforcing common values. However, most students applying for admission to medicine have a limited understanding of professionalism.[19] Nonetheless, certain elements are obvious to all well before admission. These include the need for hard work, service of patients, and desire to make a difference.[22]

Over the years, there has been very little debate on generational differences in most professional values. This might reflect in part to less attention being paid to professionalism and cohesive values, or an implicit sense that values were shared. For example, the principles of honesty and confidentiality are recited by all cohorts of physicians who take the Hippocratic Oath or a modern adaptation. Subsequent generations of medical students learn the importance of honesty and integrity in their explicit medical school curriculum.[23,24] Lapses in this commitment may span the generations equally.[25] The thirst for knowledge and a desire to understand and treat their patients is a trait shared by many generations of medical students.[26] Medical students continue to display a strong commitment to community service and show no less concern for equity.[27] In the absence of debate, and with evidence of common ground, we can assume significant similarities across the generations of physicians.

GENERATIONAL DIFFERENCES

Some generational differences in professional values do exist. The values conveyed in medical school fifty years ago have evolved. The core value of respect for patients, for example, has moved away from paternalistic benevolence and now reflects a greater emphasis on physician cultural competency and patient autonomy. Similarly, the concept of social responsibility has also progressed over the past century. Pressures on physicians to participate in allocating scarce health resources have challenged traditional notions of professionalism. Thus, today's medical students are developing their professional identities in a very different practice context and social setting than their mentors.

This pattern is not new. Career choices for students studied at one medical school from 1949 to 1976 mirrored evolving social values. The initial trend toward subspecialization shifted toward a greater interest in research careers than toward socially active fields of medicine, echoing wider social debates.[28] The younger generation believed that the older generation had lost touch with society and the social mission of medicine. This pattern revealed intergenerational differences in understanding professional values.[28]

Differences in professionalism have been noted with each new generation, often arising over perceived conflicts between lifestyle expectations and values such as altruism and commitment to patient care.[12,19,26,28,29] More than half a century ago, residents began demanding "reasonable work hours" and a salary. Their expectations raised concerns within the profession regarding their commitment to patient care and the professional values of the younger generation. Prior to World War II, interns and residents lived in the hospital and few were married. Some hospitals prohibited marriage. Yet, by the 1950s, most lived outside the hospital, receiving stipends instead of room and board, and an increasing number were married.[30] The older generation perceived a widening gulf between it and the younger generation over the latter's desire for a personal life distinct from a professional life and their rejection of "outdated" behavior guidelines.[30]

Different expectations for personal-professional life balance are seen most acutely between trainees and senior physicians, as the trainees' desire for more family or leisure time clashes with the long hours demanded for training and patient care. The current debate over an eighty-hour work week for trainees and the trend toward lifestyle specialties shows a repeating pattern of generational differences, largely over the issue of work-life balance.[31-33]

With time, of course, each new generation of medical trainees migrates to the ranks of senior physicians. Work patterns are changing as the younger generations progress in their careers, reflected in part in fewer hours worked or reduced patient visit volume.[34] However, the impact of such change or its significance for professional values is not fully understood. Nonetheless, some senior physicians are continually surprised at different lifestyle expectations from their juniors.

While the recurrent debate over a generation gap in professional values has focused mainly on the concept of altruism and work-life balance, the discussion on evolving professional values should expand beyond these issues. Moreover, senior physicians may observe significant changes in professionalism over their careers and should be prepared to reevaluate their own professional values and meaning of their work. Thus, efforts to redefine professionalism should include all physicians, not just trainees. Different generations should join the dialogue to learn from each other as well as to shape the collective values over time to reflect internal and external changes.[16] To facilitate intergenerational engagement, one must understand two key determinants of change in values within the profession: the impact of external social change on members and the natural internal socialization through career stages.

SOCIAL CHANGE

As the values of the wider society evolve, so to do the values of the medical profession. Many of the core principles of professionalism can be found in the Hippocratic Oath. Nonetheless, newer principles such as commitments to justice and to serve the public good have become an increasingly important part of the definition of professionalism[35] as both physicians and society have come to expect these values. The current discussion over physicians' social responsibility exemplifies this process of change.[36–38] This debate does not just happen within the medical literature or on single issues, but occurs over time, across generations, and beyond medical circles.

While all physicians contribute to the understanding of professionalism, the newest members have a unique role in shaping professional values early in their careers because they may understand dominant social norms more acutely than professional ones. A loosely age-matched group of individuals within the profession are a "younger generation" in part because their values have been shaped by the social events of the time more than their career.[39] Their common experience is mostly outside of medicine. Thus, each new generation of physicians contributes to negotiating the values, responsibilities, and privileges of professionalism with an ever-changing society.

The magnitude of difference between the newer and older generations in the profession depends on how pronounced are the societal changes from one generation to the next. Generational lifestyle expectations evolve as slowly or quickly as the surrounding social and cultural milieu change.[40] In stable or static societies, change may take lifetimes to occur. In more dynamic societies, generational differences may be observed within every decade.[40]

The generation gap in medicine began to receive a great deal of attention in the 1960s as society itself underwent significant transformation. The gap arises now as generation X students become physicians and members of generation Y become students.[12] These new physicians were raised during a period of unprecedented rapid social change, which is reflected in the increasingly shorter duration of generational cohorts and noticeable differences between them.[41]

The proportion of female physicians continues to rise and some gender differences in career interests and work patterns are evident. However, both men and women are showing similar declining interest in careers with "uncontrollable lifestyles," attaching a growing importance to family in making career choices.[21,42,43] This suggests a generational rather than simply a gender trend emanating from wider social changes in family structure and two working-parent families.

The influence of changing social values on new physicians as well as on the profession as a whole requires that physicians engage in a constant process of reflection and negotiation to assert their professional values, ensure their relevance to the collective and to society. Understanding students' and residents' prior socialization will facilitate the process of enabling and guiding them in developing their professional values as part of their career socialization.[44] It would be folly to try and preserve the professionalism of yesteryear – the "nostalgic professionalism" of Castellani and Hafferty.[16]

CAREER STAGE

While some generational differences in professional values result from social change, a significant portion of this difference may be related to career stage. Medical students *become* professionals as they learn their skills, responsibilities, and privileges. They are not professionals upon admission.[19,26,45,46] Thus, part of the generation gap over values such as altruism and lifestyle issues reflects the hierarchical training structure of medicine and the significant socialization process that occurs as students progress to residency and then to attending physicians.

Generational studies show that the loyalties and influences common to an age cohort are strongest early in life. With time, other affiliations such as career, community, or family assume greater importance at the expense of generational ties.[39] The values of the profession become more incorporated into an individual's identity the longer he or she is a member of the profession.[44,47] Conversely, professional identity will be weaker among the newest members.

As a medical student progresses to clerk, then intern, then senior medical resident, responsibilities and thus priorities shift from memorization and test taking, to self-focused skill mastery, to team "scutt work" and increasingly to patient welfare, team performance, education, and greater responsibility for patient outcomes. Residents may associate professionalism with a set of traits limited to their experience with patient care such as empathy, competence, and respect as opposed to values like altruism or justice.[48] Increasing levels of responsibility facilitate the development of professional values that require a broad, less self-centered outlook.[49,50] A senior practitioner may view professionalism in light of his most important concerns: the reputation of the profession, general career satisfaction, or the health problems of the community to which he or she belongs.[36] Thus, in comparing senior physicians to residents and students part of the generation gap may simply be incomplete professionalism.[46]

TEACHING STRATEGIES

As professionalism is dynamic, it must be developed across careers. Keeping values current and connected to societal needs is the responsibility not just of educators at academic medical centers but of all physicians and professional organizations. Currently, most efforts to develop professionalism focus on trainees – the newest members. This is understandable as the newest members have the most to learn in striving to become complete professionals. A student's basic character has been formed by the time he/she enters medicine, but his/her professional character begins to be shaped by the experience of medical school.[49] New generations of physicians must learn an initial "content" of professionalism. However, learning professionalism is an active process of developing a professional identity and requires skills to derive that identity from the content of professionalism and the experience of being a professional.

This active process happens over the long term and the profession must create strategies to enable the continuous development of professionalism for all physicians across their careers, not just for the first ten years. Thus, the next section focuses on strategies to cultivate professionalism across the generations for individuals and the profession as a whole. These strategies must be based on an understanding of how professionalism is learned and a professional identity developed.

The learning process for the newest members of the profession must start with an introduction to the "content" of professionalism, such as its definition and historical origin. Presenting the "content" of professionalism raises awareness to prepare students for the experience of the roles and expectations of being a professional. However, formal theory acquired through professional training is often not easily applied to concrete and "messy" situations of actual practice.[51] An individual's perception of their ability to deal with a situation shapes their actions.[51] A teaching methodology therefore must go beyond presenting content and must transmit skills that help build a sense of self-confidence in handling challenges to professional identity.

The development of a professional identity is a continuous and cyclical process that spans across career stages.[46,52] It is shaped by one's experience, specifically encountering the expectations of others and the act of resolving conflicts between what an individual understands as his or her role and the roles he or she observes or is expected to fill.[44] An experience such as responsibility for a new task, or recognition for a job well done, can reaffirm or undermine one's understanding of his or her professional identity. What is learned with each experience is applied to the next. Between each encounter, a learner must reflect, form an abstract conceptualization, and perform active experimentation to reaffirm professional identity or to adapt it to fit with a new concept.[53] Thus, physicians require skills to develop professionalism effectively through this cycle.

While all physicians need the same skills to develop their professionalism, the strategies to develop those skills will differ depending on career stage and generation. Teaching strategies should factor in differences in baseline understanding of professionalism, varying levels of experience, as well as generational learning styles shaped by distinct environments.

TEACHING STRATEGIES FOR MEDICAL STUDENTS

The content of professionalism should be introduced early to students using multiple pedagogical tools, as they begin acquiring the skills to develop their professionalism based both on formal content and on experiences. Increasingly, as these skills develop, the students' own experiences and complementary ones of their peers and senior physicians should guide learning. Student physicians increasingly should be empowered to develop their professionalism by evaluating and reflecting on the content of professionalism observed and experienced. The teaching of professionalism should recognize the preexisting identity of students and differences in social values to facilitate the integration of that personal identity into their professional one.

Table 8.2. Matching development strategies to generation groups

Teaching strategy	Younger students	Older physicians
Lectures	♦	
Case studies	♦	
Role modeling	♦	♦
Mentoring	♦	♦
Small-group discussions	♦	
Reflective practice	♦	♦
Technological tools	♦	
Journals		♦
Conferences		♦

Many methods are used to present the content of professionalism, as outlined in Table 8.2. All these methods must be rooted in a clear understanding of professionalism.[54] While professionalism is presented as both a current understanding and an evolving identity, it should not be defined differently from department to department or even institution to institution.

Lectures, case studies, and small-group discussions can introduce the content of professionalism and give it a context familiar to students at an early stage before they accumulate their own experiences. These methods inform students as to what constitutes professional behavior and attitudes, and provide basic knowledge as the foundation for the task of developing one's own professional identity. However, medical students are proto-professionals, becoming professionals,[46] and expectations of professionalism should reflect this immature level of identity. In order to engage students prior to experience giving meaning to their professional identity, career-stage relevant cases should situate professionalism in experiences students do or could imagine encountering.[41]

Role modeling and mentoring are additional ways of presenting the content of professionalism, and incorporating elements of experiential learning. Role modeling differs from mentoring in that it is less intentional and less formal.[49] It is also a ubiquitous learning tool as physicians from all generations can serve as role models. Role modeling can be a double-edged sword, however, as students can learn as much or more from negative role models as from positive ones.

Mentoring involves a more conscious effort to present the content of professionalism and guide identity development, making both more explicit.[55] Mentoring can adapt the presentation of the content of professionalism to facilitate learning from experiences or to complement experiences. This prepares students for the next career stage or even for experiences they might encounter long after completion of their formal training.

Facilitated discussions, whether as part of mentoring or small-group learning, can offer opportunities to present professionalism content, while also drawing out lessons from different experiences. In relating discussions to actual experiences, mentors can encourage and guide reflection on content. This is particularly valuable in addressing the hidden curriculum in medical education, the difference between what students are taught and what they learn.[56] Finally, such teaching exchanges allow for shared experience of students and teachers.[57] This is essential to foster a common understanding of professionalism in the current social context.

Providing feedback on demonstrated professionalism either formally or through mentoring and facilitated discussions further expands the understanding of professionalism and its application to different situations. Feedback can encourage the development of skills to form and reevaluate professional identity either strengthening the current understanding and resulting behavior or leading to a new interpretation and actions.

Reflective practice further serves to formalize the learning that takes place through experience. It is the critical review of experience.[58] It requires the ability to observe both one's surroundings and oneself,[59] and offers learners the opportunity to become participant/observers in their own learning. Reflective practice has used many tools such as storytelling and writing to encourage the cycle of learning and reshaping understanding and identity. Formalizing this process and investing time into it gives the process of identity development legitimacy ensuring it is valued as the important part of becoming and being a physician that it should be.

Since the process of identity formation for students takes place in many different settings, interactions through mentoring and facilitated discussions should include as diverse a representation of the roles of physicians as possible to match real-life experiences. Community physicians, and physicians in other professional leadership roles, should be involved in sharing experiences and guiding the development of professional identity for the newest members who will eventually take on such roles.[60]

The presentation of the content of professionalism and strategies to build the skills necessary to develop effectively a professional identity over the course of a career must take into account the different learning styles of a new generation and use the most effective methods for the target audience. Increasingly, this involves the use of information technology, and allowing students independently to find the content of professionalism.

The teaching of content such as values typically has relied heavily on interpersonal interaction. Information technology may seem out of place for this topic. However, the younger generation is increasingly adept at receiving content and learning with this medium. In fact, their comfort with technology leads to a perception that technology is underused in medical teaching.[61]

The use of information technology to teach values must be expanded by incorporating innovative approaches to allow for individual learning modules as well as group activities that are increasingly common in the everyday life of the younger generation. Traditional case-based teaching may take advantage of technology to create simulated experiences that can be shared, incorporating elements of interaction, and competition to motivate students to learn. Such methods may also further expose students to experiences beyond those immediately available at a single training institution. However, as identity formation is based on experiences and the cycle of learning from these, role modeling, mentoring, and old-fashioned personal interaction will remain critical in crafting identity formation.

STRATEGIES FOR OLDER PHYSICIANS

As the development of professionalism is an ongoing task over the course of a career, strategies to facilitate this process for senior physicians are also important. The same skills useful to students and residents in developing their professionalism may also be needed at later career stages. Thus, many strategies to facilitate the ongoing reflection on professionalism necessary for individuals, and the profession as a whole, are similar to those for the newest members of the profession. Just as teaching strategies for the younger generation must take into account their limited experience and different learning styles, so too strategies for more senior physicians must be attuned to accumulated experience and preexisting comfort with learning methods. In presenting professionalism to senior physicians, it is important to recognize that they have stronger predeveloped ideas of their professional identity when confronted with change or conflict between what they know as their role and what they observe or experience.

Thus, in reaching out to senior physicians, the presentation of content may encounter resistance if it conflicts with existing understandings. Strategies must thus reinforce the evolving nature of professionalism and need for adaptability and "keeping current." The continuing professional development of values and identity is similar to that for clinical knowledge and skills. Like the state of medical knowledge, social values change and doctors who are in constant contact with the public need to be aware of changing social norms.

Learning programs that stress physician knowledge alone have been shown insufficient to change practice behaviour.[62] Traditional continuing medical education lectures are therefore less likely to lead to meaningful reinterpretation of identity and values. Significant research is being done to understand how best to facilitate ongoing learning for physicians. Efforts to understand the best modalities for continuing professional development should receive attention similar to that given to updating clinical knowledge and skills. Innovative strategies relevant to senior physicians to enable reflective practice and create opportunities to guide the reframing of understanding when faced with conflicts between understanding and experience need to be crafted. These might use traditional media such as journals and conferences creating fora for discussion. Journal editors and professional societies leaders should be proactive in advancing the content of professionalism in these fora.

Encouraging intergenerational exchanges through discussions and inclusive participation on relevant panels or boards may create further opportunities for shared reinvention of professionalism allowing the accumulated experience within the profession to mix with the greater influence of social norms brought by younger members. Any teacher can be a student and any student can be a teacher. Within traditional academic institutions and in the wider practicing community such reciprocal learning should be encouraged.[63] Leadership is needed to create learning and development opportunities for individuals that will translate into advancing the whole profession's understanding of professionalism and relationship with the changing society it serves.

CONCLUSIONS

Medicine must continue its interest and investment in teaching evolving professionalism. Strengthening and renewing professionalism starts with effective learning in the first year of medical school but must extend over an entire career. Efforts to understand generational differences and build toward a shared and socially relevant understanding of professionalism are important as diversity within the profession and the pace of social change both rise. This challenge engages all physicians – no matter their generation. All physicians must participate in this dialogue.

REFERENCES

1. Cruess, RL, Cruess, SR, Johnston, SE. Professionalism and medicine's social contract. *J Bone Joint Surg Am.* 2000;82-A(8):1189–94.
2. Bucher, R, Strauss, A. Professions in process. *Am J Sociol.* 1961;66(4):325–34.
3. Royal College of Physicians. *Doctors in Society: Medical Professionalism in a Changing World.* London: Royal College of Physicians; 2005.
4. Mechanic, D. Managed care and the imperative for a new professional ethic. *Health Aff (Millwood).* 2000;19(5):100–11.

5. Sullivan, WM. Medicine under threat: professionalism and professional identity. *CMAJ*. 2000;162(5):673–5.

6. Cruess, RL, Cruess, SR. 1997. Teaching medicine as a profession in the service of healing. *Acad Med*. 1997;72(11):941–52.

7. Kuczewski, MG, Bading, E, Langbein, M, Henry, B. Fostering professionalism: the Loyola model. *Camb Q Healthc Ethics*. 2003 *Spring*;12(2):161–6.

8. Swick, HM, Szenas, P, Danoff, D, Whitcomb, ME. Teaching professionalism in undergraduate medical education. *JAMA*. 1999;282(9):830–2.

9. Wear, D, Castellani, B. The development of professionalism: curriculum matters. *Acad Med*. 2000;75(6):602–11.

10. Larson, DL. Bridging the generation X gap in plastic surgery training: part 1. Identifying the problem. *Plast Reconstr Surg*. 2003;112(6):1656–61.

11. Organ, CH Jr. The generation gap in modern surgery. *Arch Surg*. 2002 March;137(3):250–2. Erratum in: *Arch Surg* 2002 June;137(6):747.

12. Smith, LG. Medical professionalism and the generation gap. *Am J Med*. 2005 April;118(4):439–42.

13. Bickel, J, Brown, AJ. Generation X: implications for faculty recruitment and development in academic health centers. *Acad Med*. 2005;80(3):205–10.

14. Moody, J. Recruiting generation X physicians. Recruiting physicians today. *NEJM*. 2002 [cited November 27, 2007]. Available from: http://www.nejmjobs.org/rpt/recruiting-gen-x-physicians.aspx

15. Washburn, ER. Are you ready for generation X? *Physician Exec*. 2000;26(1): 51–7.

16. Castellani, B, Hafferty, FW. The complexities of medical professionalism: a preliminary investigation. In Wear, D, Aultman, JM, editors. *Professionalism in Medicine: Critical Perspectives*. New York: Springer; 2006: 3–25.

17. Association of American Medical Colleges. Diversity in the physician workforce: facts & figures, 2006 [monograph on the Internet]. Washington (DC): Association of American Medical Colleges; 2006 [cited November 27, 2007]. Available from: http://www.aamc.org/diversity/start.htm.

18. Kertzer, DI. Generation as a sociological problem. *Annu Rev Sociol*. 1983;9: 125–49.

19. Hafferty, FW. What medical students know about professionalism. *Mt Sinai J Med*. 2002;69(6):385–97.

20. Lancaster, LC, Stillman, D. *When Generations Collide*. New York: Harper Collins; 2002.

21. Zemke, R, Raines, C, Filipczak, B. *Generations at Work: Managing the Clash of Veterans, Boomers, Xers, and Nexters in Your Workplace*. New York: AMACOM; 2000.

22. Peck, J, Cooke, AI. *Characteristics of the 1998 MCAT Examinees*. Washington (DC): Association of American Medical Colleges; 2000.

23. Stern, DT. Practicing what we preach? An analysis of the curriculum of values in medical education. *Am J Med*. 1998;104(6):569–75.

24. Stimmel, B, Yens, D. Cheating by medical students on examinations. *Am J Med*. 1982;73(2):160–4.

25. Ginsburg, S, Regehr, G, Lingard, L. Basing the evaluation of professionalism on observable behaviors: a cautionary tale. *Acad Med.* 2004;79(10):S1–4.

26. Becker, HS, Hughes, EC, Geer, B, Strauss, AL. *Boys in White;[sic] Student Culture in Medical School.* Chicago: University of Chicago Press; 1961.

27. Eckenfels, EJ. Contemporary medical students' quest for self-fulfillment through community service. *Acad Med.* 1997;72(12):1043–50.

28. Funkenstein, DH. *Medical Students, Medical Schools and Society during Five Eras: Factors Affecting the Career Choices of Physicians 1958-1976.* Cambridge (MA): Ballinger Publishing Company; 1978.

29. Geokas, MC, Branson, BJ. Recruiting students for medicine. *Ann Intern Med.* 1989;111(5):433–6.

30. Ludmerer, K. *Time to Heal.* New York: Oxford University Press; 1999.

31. Newton, DA, Grayson, MS. Trends in career choice by US medical school graduates. *JAMA.* 2003;290(9):1179–82.

32. Ritchie, WP. Report of the American Board of Surgery retreat on graduate surgical education: current trends, future directions. Philadelphia (PA); American Board of Surgery; 2002.

33. Schwartz, RW, Haley, JV, Williams, C, Jarecky, RK, Strodel, WE, Young, B, Griffen, WO. The controllable lifestyle factor and students' attitudes about specialty selection. *Acad Med.* 1990;65(3):207–10.

34. Watson, DE, Slade, S, Buske, L, Tepper, J. Intergenerational differences in workloads among primary care physicians: a ten-year, population-based study. *Health Aff (Millwood).* 2006;25(6):1620–8.

35. Cruess, SR, Johnston, S, Cruess, RL. "Profession": a working definition for medical educators. *Teach Learn Med.* 2004;16(1):74–6.

36. Gruen, RL, Pearson, SD, Brennan, TA. Physician-citizens – public roles and professional obligations. *JAMA.* 2004;291(1):94–8.

37. Wear, D, Kuczewski, MG. The professionalism movement: can we pause? *Am J Bioeth.* 2004;4(2):1–10.

38. Whitehouse, PJ, Fishman, JR. Justice and the house of medicine: the mortgaging of ecology and economics. *Am J Bioeth.* 2004;4(2):43–45.

39. Esler, A. *Generations in History: An Introduction to the Concept.* Williamsburg (VA): Esler; 1982.

40. Goertzel, T. Generational conflict and social change. *Youth Soc.* 1972;3:327–52.

41. Johnston, S. See one, do one, teach one: developing professionalism across the generations. *Clin Orthop Relat Res.* 2006;449:186–92.

42. Lambert, EM, Holmboe, ES. The relationship between specialty choice and gender of U.S. medical students, 1990-2003. *Acad Med.* 2005;80(9):797–802.

43. Sanfey, HA, Saalwachter-Schulman, AR, Nyhof-Young, JM, Eidelson, B, Mann, BD. Influences on medical student career choice: gender or generation? *Arch Surg.* 2006;141(11):1086.

44. Pratt, MG, Rockmann, KW, Kaufmann, JB. Constructing professional identity: the role of work and identity learning cycles in the customization of identity among medical residents. *Acad Manage J.* 2006;49(2):235–62.

45. Fehser, J. Teaching professionalism: a student's perspective. *Mt Sinai J Med.* 2002;69(6):412–4.

46. Hilton, SR, Slotnick, HB. Proto-professionalism: how professionalisation occurs across the continuum of medical education. *Med Educ.* 2005;39(1):58–65.

47. Hafferty, FW. Reconfiguring the sociology of medical education: emerging topics and pressing issues. In Bird, C, Conrad, P, Fremont, A, editors. *Handbook of Medical Sociology.* 5th ed. New York: Prentice Hall; 2000: 238–56.

48. Brownell, AK, Cote, LM. Senior residents' views on the meaning of professionalism and how they learn about it. *Acad Med.* 2001;76(7):734–7.

49. Kenny, NP, Mann, KV, MacLeod, HM. Role modeling in physicians' professional formation: reconsidering an essential but untapped educational strategy. *Acad Med.* 2003;78(12):1203–10.

50. Slaby, AE, Schwartz, AH. Changing attitudes and patterns of behavior among emerging physicians. *Psychiatr Med.* 1971;(2):270–7.

51. Kaufman, DM. Applying educational theory in practice. *BMJ.* 2003;326(7382): 213–6.

52. Slotnick, HB. How doctors learn: education and learning across the medical-school-to-practice trajectory. *Acad Med.* 2001;76(10):1013–26.

53. Kolb, D, Fry, R. Toward an applied theory of experiential learning. In Cooper, C, editor. *Theories of Group Process.* London: John Wiley; 1975: 33–57.

54. Cruess, SR, Cruess, RL. 1997. Professionalism must be taught. *BMJ.* 1997; 315(7123):1674–7.

55. Rose, GL, Rukstalis, MR, Schuckit, MA. Informal mentoring between faculty and medical students. *Acad Med.* 2005;80(4):344–8.

56. Hafferty, FW. Beyond curriculum reform: confronting medicine's hidden curriculum. *Acad Med.* 1998;73(4):403–7.

57. Steinert, Y. Twelve tips for effective small-group teaching in the health professions. *Med Teach.* 1996;18(3):203–7.

58. Hilton, S, Southgate, L. Professionalism in medical education. *Teach Teach Educ.* 2007;23(3):265–79.

59. Epstein, RM. Mindful practice. *JAMA.* 1999;282(9):833–9.

60. Rosenfeld, JC, Sefcik, S. Utilizing community leaders to teach professionalism. *Curr Surg.* 2003;60(2):222–4.

61. Oblinger, D. Boomers, gen-Xers, and millennials: understanding the "new students." *EDUCAUSE Review Magazine* 2003;38(4):36–40,42,44–45.

62. Oxman, AD, Thomson, MA, Davis, DA, Haynes, RB. No magic bullets: a systematic review of 102 trials of interventions to improve professional practice. *CMAJ.* 1995;153(10):1423–31.

63. Lohman, H, Griffiths, Y. Coppard, BM, Cota, L. The power of book discussion groups in intergenerational learning. *Educ Gerontol.* 2003;29(2):103.

9 Faculty Development for Teaching and Learning Professionalism

Yvonne Steinert, Ph.D.

> The greatest difficulty in life is to make knowledge effective, to convert it into practical wisdom.
>
> Sir William Osler

The challenge of teaching and learning professionalism has been highlighted by many authors.[1–6] The increasing complexity of the practice of medicine, coupled with the entry of the state and corporate sector into the health care field, has drastically altered the relationship between the medical profession and the society it serves.[1] At the same time, role modeling, the traditional method for transmitting professional values from one generation to the next, is no longer sufficient.[2] Professionalism must be taught explicitly.

Despite consensus on the importance of teaching and learning professionalism,[7] many clinical teachers are not able to articulate the attributes and behaviors characteristic of the physician as a professional. Many faculty members are also not sure of how to best teach and evaluate this content area and may not be serving as effective role models. As a result, faculty development is needed to ensure the successful teaching and learning of professionalism.

To date, the literature on faculty development designed to support the teaching and evaluation of professionalism is limited.[8,9] The goal of this chapter is to outline the principles and strategies underlying faculty development programming in this area and to provide a case example from our own institution.

Faculty development refers to that broad range of activities institutions use to *renew* or *assist* faculty in their multiple roles.[10] That is, faculty development is a planned program designed to *prepare* institutions and faculty members for their various roles[11] and to *improve* an individual's knowledge and skills in the areas of teaching, research, and administration.[12] The goal of faculty development is to teach faculty members the skills relevant to their institutional and faculty position, and to sustain their vitality, both now and in the future.

In recent years, faculty development has become an increasingly important component of health sciences education.[13] Faculty development activities have been designed to improve teacher effectiveness at all levels of the educational continuum (e.g., undergraduate, postgraduate, and continuing medical education)[14] and diverse programs have been offered to health care professionals in a variety of settings. In this context, faculty development will refer to those activities designed to help educators in all settings (e.g., hospital, community, university) teach professionalism in a more effective and satisfactory manner and promote organizational change and development.

Wilkerson and Irby[15] have said that comprehensive faculty development programs should include both individual and organizational development. In the context of teaching and evaluating professionalism, both aspects are critical.

At the *individual* level, faculty development should:

- Address *attitudes* and beliefs that can impede the teaching and learning of professionalism.
- Transmit *knowledge* about the core content of professionalism as well as effective teaching and assessment practices.
- Develop *skills* in teaching and evaluating the behaviors that exemplify professionalism.

At the *organizational* level, faculty development should help to:

- Define a shared vision of professionalism and how it will be taught and evaluated.
- Create opportunities for teaching and learning professionalism.
- Address systems issues that can impede the teaching and learning of professionalism in the formal, informal, and hidden curriculum.[16]

WHY FACULTY DEVELOPMENT IS NEEDED

Teaching professionalism remains a challenge for many clinical and basic science teachers. Firstly, most physicians believe that they are "professional" and that teaching professionalism is intuitive. In fact, they often question why they need to learn about this content area. Secondly, as stated earlier, role modeling is no longer as effective a strategy as it once was. When both society and the profession itself were reasonably homogeneous, values were shared and could be transmitted effectively through role modeling.[1,2] The increasing complexity of the practice of medicine, the ethical dilemmas faced by contemporary physicians, and the diversity of the medical profession and society make this no longer true. Faculty must now be able to teach professionalism *explicitly* by articulating its core concepts and by demonstrating appropriate behaviors. In fact, it is the demonstration of these behaviors that is often lacking – and therefore challenging. Thirdly, teachers must be able to teach and evaluate this core competency. That is, they need to be aware of the most effective teaching and assessment strategies and realize that teaching and learning professionalism is not an "add on"; teaching must be integrated into the clinical and classroom setting. Finally, professionalism has to be valued by the organization, and teachers must identify opportunities to recognize the importance of teaching and learning professionalism in their institutional culture.

What are the implications of these challenges for faculty development? At an *individual level*, teachers need knowledge and skills in professionalism, knowledge and skills in teaching methods and evaluation strategies, and enthusiasm for teaching and learning. Faculty development programs therefore need to build motivation for learning, overcome resistance, and help teachers to make the implicit explicit. At a *programmatic level*, faculty developers and educators must build programs that focus on content and teaching methods, use appropriate faculty development methods and formats, focus on teaching and evaluating these competencies, and make learning pertinent and fun. Moreover, faculty developers need to assess teachers' needs, provide diverse programs, incorporate educationally useful theoretical frameworks (such as situated learning,[17] which is discussed in Chapter 2), remain relevant and practical, and evaluate effectiveness. Faculty developers also need to follow principles of adult learning and integrate faculty development for teaching and learning professionalism into ongoing programs. At a *systems level*, educators must address the organizational climate and culture, promote buy-in, identify opportunities for teaching and learning, determine the need for specialty-specific training, train the trainers, and facilitate dissemination.[8,14] At times, it will be more appropriate to work within the culture, responding to specific needs; at other times, organizational change will be needed to promote the teaching and learning of professionalism.[9]

GENERAL GUIDELINES FOR DESIGNING A FACULTY DEVELOPMENT PROGRAM

Guidelines for designing and delivering effective faculty development programs have been outlined in other venues.[13,14,18] A brief summary of these recommendations is warranted here, as awareness of these principles and strategies is fundamental to the design of any program.

Understand the Institutional/Organizational Culture

Faculty development programs take place within the context of a specific institution or organization. It is imperative to understand the culture of that institution and to be responsive to its needs. Professional development programs should also capitalize on the organization's strengths and work with the leadership to ensure success. In many ways, the cultural context can be used to promote or enhance faculty development efforts. For example, it has been noted that faculty development during times of educational or curricular reform takes on added importance.[19] It is also important to assess institutional support for faculty development activities, identify available resources, and lobby effectively. Faculty development cannot occur in a vacuum.

Determine Appropriate Goals and Priorities

In designing a faculty development program, it is imperative to clearly define program goals and priorities. What is the program trying to achieve – and why is it important to do so? It is equally important to specify program objectives, as they will influence the target audience (e.g., clinical teachers, program directors) as well as overall content and methodology. Determining priorities is not always easy, and it often involves consultations with diverse stakeholders. However, it is always essential to balance *individual* and *organizational* needs.

Conduct Needs Assessments to Ensure Relevant Programming

As outlined in Chapter 15, all continuing professional development activities should be based on the needs of the individual as well as the institution. Student needs, patient needs, and societal needs can also help to guide relevant activities. Assessing needs is required to refine goals, determine content, identify preferred learning formats, and assure relevance. It is also a way of promoting early "buy-in." Common methods for assessing needs include written questionnaires or surveys, interviews or focus groups with key informants (e.g., participants, students, educational leaders), observations of teachers "in action," literature reviews, and environmental scans of available programs and resources.[20,21] Whenever possible, educators should try to gain information from multiple sources and distinguish between "needs" and "wants." An individual teacher's perceived needs may clearly differ from those expressed by their students or peers.

Target Diverse Stakeholders

Rubeck and Witzke[19] have defined faculty development as the enhancement of faculty members' knowledge and skills so that they can make educational contributions that advance both the pedagogical program and the process of teaching and learning. This definition is particularly important in this context. In order for educational and curricular reform to occur, faculty development initiatives should target curriculum planners responsible for the design and delivery of educational programs focused on the teaching and learning of professionalism, administrators responsible for medical education and clinical practice as well as the institutions in which professionalism is displayed, and all health care professionals involved in teaching and learning. The latter group might include faculty members working in a university setting, clinical teachers of diverse backgrounds in the hospital and the community, and other members of the health care team.

Develop Different Programs to Accommodate Diverse Needs

One size does not fit all. Faculty development activities must be designed to accommodate diverse goals and objectives, content areas, and needs. In this context, it is also helpful to remember that faculty *development* can include faculty orientation, recognition, and support, and different programs will be needed to accommodate diverse objectives. For example, think tanks may be appropriate to promote buy-in, to develop consensus, and to design an educational blueprint.[8] Workshops may be more appropriate for knowledge and/ or skill acquisition. Program content and methods will also need to change over time to adapt to evolving needs.

Common faculty development methods and formats include faculty retreats and/or "think tanks", workshops and seminars, short courses, one-on-one consultations; role modeling and/or coaching, self-directed initiatives, and integrated longitudinal programs and fellowships.[22,23] The following section will briefly describe those formats that have particular appeal in this context.

Workshop, Seminars, and Short Courses

The literature describes workshops, seminars, and other short interventions as the most common formats of faculty development.[24] Workshops are most popular because of their inherent flexibility and promotion of active learning; moreover, faculty members value a variety of teaching methods within this format, including interactive lectures, small-group discussions and exercises, role-plays and simulations, and experiential learning.[23] Without a doubt, workshops play an important role in faculty development for the teaching and learning of professionalism.[8,9] At the same time, seminars and short courses have the added advantage of increased time and continuity.[23]

Integrated Longitudinal Programs

Some schools and universities have created integrated programs using a variety of faculty development methods in which faculty commit 10–20 percent of their time over one to two years in an attempt to increase their skills in particular faculty roles. The Teaching Scholars Program at McGill is one example of such a program.[25,26] By immersing themselves in educational content and methods for a year, faculty members can work on issues and topics of interest to them (e.g., the teaching and learning of professionalism). Integrated longitudinal programs have particular appeal in this context because teachers and faculty members can continue to practice and teach while improving their educational knowledge and skills. As well, these programs allow for the development of educational leadership and scholarly activity as well as teaching improvement.

Peer Coaching

Peer coaching as a method of faculty development has been described extensively in the educational literature, and more recently, in the health sciences.[27,28] Key elements of peer coaching include the identification of specific goals (e.g., improving specific teaching skills), focused observation of teaching by colleagues, and the provision of feedback, analysis, and support.[27] Peer coaching has particular appeal for the teaching and learning of professionalism because it occurs in the practice setting, enables individualized learning, and fosters immediate application.[14] It also models many aspects of professional practice.

Self-Directed Learning

It is surprising that self-directed learning initiatives are infrequently described in the faculty development literature. However, there is clearly a place for self-directed initiatives that promote "reflection in action" and "reflection on action,"[29] skills that are critical to the teaching and learning of professionalism. Self-directed learning activities have been used extensively in continuing medical education, and faculty development programs should build on these experiences. Westberg and Whitman[30] have also pointed out the need for more "state-of-the-art" resources to help faculty enhance their skills. Educational resources, such as those included in the appendices, can help to support teachers in this area.

Web-Based Learning

Web-based learning is intricately tied to self-directed learning initiatives, though all educational resources for independent learning do not need to be available online. As time for professional development is limited, and the technology to create interactive instructional programs is now in place, the use of computer-based faculty development should be explored.[31] It would also seem that online resources and learning programs could be considered as a supplement to centrally organized faculty development programs; they could also be used in a "staged approach," later in the development of teachers and faculty members. In many ways, web-based learning can allow for individualized programs targeted to specific needs and the sharing of resources, as long as educators do not lose sight of the value and importance of working in context, with colleagues.[14]

Incorporate Principles of Adult Learning and Instructional Design

Adults come to learning situations with a variety of motivations and expectations about teaching methods and goals. Key principles of adult learning[32] (outlined in Chapter 2) include the following:

- Adults are independent.
- Adults come to learning situations with a variety of motivations and definite expectations about particular learning goals and teaching methods.
- Adults demonstrate different learning styles.
- Much of adult learning is "relearning" rather than new learning.
- Adult learning often involves changes in attitudes as well as skills.
- Most adults prefer to learn through experience.
- Incentives for adult learning usually come from within the individual.
- Feedback is usually more important than tests and evaluations.

Incorporation of these principles into the design of a faculty development program can enhance receptivity, relevance, and engagement. In fact, these principles should guide the development of all programs, irrespective of their focus or format, as physicians demonstrate a high degree of self-direction and possess numerous experiences that can serve as the basis for learning.

Principles of instructional design (also outlined in Chapter 2) must be followed in the design and delivery of any faculty development program. For example, it is important to develop clear learning goals and objectives for a specific activity, identify key content areas, design appropriate teaching and learning strategies, and create appropriate methods of evaluation – of both the students and the curriculum. It is equally important to integrate educational theory with practice (e.g., situated learning) and to ensure that the learning is perceived as relevant to the work setting and to the profession.[33] Faculty development participants value interactive, participatory, and experientially based learning that relies on previous background and experience.[9,23]

A positive learning environment, which communicates respect and understanding of similarities and differences, and "equal" participation of all participants, is also essential, as is teacher "readiness," buy-in, and commitment.

Offer a Diversity of Educational Methods – In a Variety of Settings

In line with principles of adult learning, faculty development programs should try to offer a variety of educational methods that promote experiential learning, reflection, feedback, and immediacy of application.[23] As stated previously, common learning methods include interactive lectures, case presentations, small-group exercises and discussions, role-plays and simulations, videotape reviews, and live demonstrations. Practice with feedback is also essential, as is the opportunity to reflect on personal values and attitudes. Web-based modules and self-directed readings are additional methods to consider. Most importantly, whatever the method, the needs and learning preferences of the participants must be respected, and the methods should match the intended objectives. It is also helpful to remember that health care professionals learn best "by doing," and experiential learning should be promoted whenever possible.

Faculty development activities frequently take place in a centralized university or departmental setting. To be successful in this context, faculty development should occur where the teaching and learning of professionalism happens. Thus, some faculty development initiatives should move out of the university setting into the hospital and the community. Decentralized, site-specific activities have the added advantage of reaching individuals who may not otherwise attend faculty development activities, promoting experiential learning and developing a departmental or program-based culture of self-improvement.[34,35]

Promote Buy-In and Market Effectively

The decision to participate in a professional development program or activity is not as simple as it might at first appear. It involves the individual's reaction to a particular offering, motivation to develop or enhance a specific skill, being available at the time of the session, and overcoming the psychological barrier of admitting need.[19] Faculty developers face the challenge of overcoming reluctance and marketing their "product" in such a way that resistance becomes a resource to learning. In some settings, targeted mailings, professionally designed brochures, and product "branding" have been extremely valuable. In other contexts, continuing medical education credits, as well as free and flexible programming, help to enhance motivation and facilitate attendance. Buy-in involves agreement on importance, widespread support, and dedication of time and resources at both the individual and the systems level, and must be deliberately sought in all programming initiatives.

Evaluate – and Demonstrate – Effectiveness

Evaluation is the final step in instructional design and of critical importance in faculty development programming. At a minimum, a practical and feasible evaluation should include an assessment of the utility and relevance of the content, teaching and learning methods, and participants' intent to change. Moreover, as evaluation is an integral part of program planning, it should be conceptualized at the beginning of any program. It should also include qualitative and quantitative assessments of learning and behavior change, using a variety of methods and data sources.

In preparing to evaluate a faculty development program or activity, educators should consider the goal of the evaluation (e.g., program planning vs. decision making, policy formation vs. academic inquiry), available data sources (e.g., participants, peers, students, or residents), common methods of evaluation (e.g., questionnaires, focus groups, objective tests, observations), resources to support assessment (e.g., institutional support, research grants), and models of program evaluation (e.g., goal attainment, decision facilitation).[36–38] Each component requires careful planning and execution to ensure success. Kirkpatrick's hierarchy of evaluation[39] is also helpful in conceptualizing and framing the evaluation of effectiveness. This hierarchy includes the following levels:

- Reaction – participants' views on the learning experience.
- Learning – change in participants' attitudes, knowledge, or skills.
- Behavior – change in participants' behavior.
- Results – changes in the organizational system, the patient, or the learner.

Although program evaluation is fundamental to the design, delivery, and improvement of faculty development activities, it also helps to ensure scholarship in the teaching and learning of professionalism.

PRINCIPLES FOR DESIGNING FACULTY DEVELOPMENT PROGRAMS TO PROMOTE THE TEACHING AND LEARNING OF PROFESSIONALISM

Although the guidelines outlined above are all relevant to faculty development designed to promote the teaching and learning of professionalism, many of them are generic in nature. Based on our experience in the design and delivery of faculty development programs in this area over the past ten years,[8,9] we believe that certain principles and strategies emerge as critical to the success of programming in this area. They can also be conceptualized on two levels: 1) faculty development to promote teaching excellence and 2) faculty development to promote curriculum development and organizational change.

Faculty Development to Promote Teaching Excellence

Teach the Cognitive Base

As stated at the outset, role modeling and the implicit teaching of professionalism are no longer sufficient. We need to equip our teachers with the cognitive base underlying professionalism as well as a common language, so that they will be able to communicate their vision and understanding of the attributes of professionalism (as outlined in Chapter 1). In line with this thinking, faculty development efforts should include the definition of professionalism, its historical roots, the relationship between professionalism and the ever-changing social contract between medicine and society, and the obligations necessary to sustain professional status.[1,40] Teachers also need to develop a common understanding of the attributes of professionalism and the behaviors expected of a professional. This is essential, as diverse definitions exist, and teachers often see professionalism as a vague concept lacking a cognitive base. Faculty development programs should therefore provide teachers with operational definitions that can be taught and evaluated. Appendix B outlines the core attributes of professionalism that we have used to guide teaching and learning in our setting. It is offered as an example to guide the work of others in this field.

Translate Content into Practice

To be effective, the attributes of professionalism must be taught and *demonstrated* in the clinical setting. Accordingly, clinicians need to translate the core content into practice and see its applicability and relevance. In our own setting, we chose to promote the latter by defining professionalism and its attributes, using case examples (outlined in Appendix C), and asking faculty members to complete action plans following a faculty development workshop in order to ensure implementation.[8] We also provided our teachers with a written matrix (included in Appendix D) to help guide their teaching practices.

Start with a Focus on Teaching

The need to focus on *teaching* professionalism arises from several factors. Virtually every accrediting, licensing, and certifying body requires that professional behaviors in students and residents be evaluated.[41–43] However, if professionalism is to be evaluated, it must first be taught. Based on our own experience in this area,[8,9] we believe strongly that a focus on *teaching* professionalism is less threatening to health care professionals than a focus on *being* professional. We would therefore encourage others to start with a focus on teaching, and with time, take a more careful look at the professional behaviors of their colleagues. This challenge is also addressed in Chapter 15 on continuing professional development.

Facilitate Experiential Learning and Promote Self-Reflection

Reflection "in action" and "on action" has recently been identified as central to the teaching and learning of professionalism.[44] Faculty development activities must therefore include activities that promote self-reflection, awareness, and change. If we believe that professional identity arises from "a long-term combination of experiences and reflection on experience"[45] and that our students require both experience and reflection in order for learning to occur, then we must model these strategies when working with our faculty members. The literature on reflection[46–49] has grown significantly in recent years and has highlighted the importance of a safe environment, peer support, and mentorship in promoting "mindfulness." These attributes must also characterize a robust faculty development initiative.

Faculty Development to Promote Curriculum Development and Organizational Change

Faculty development programs should not be designed or delivered in isolation from other factors such as institutional support, organizational goals and priorities, resources for program planning, or individual needs and expectations.[18] At the same time, they can also serve as useful instruments in the process of change.[9] Faculty development can help to build consensus, generate support and enthusiasm, and implement a change initiative; it can also help to change the culture within the institution by altering the formal, informal, and hidden curriculum. For example, the "informal" curriculum consists of unscripted, unplanned, and highly interpersonal forms of teaching and learning that take place between faculty and students.[16] Students and residents are always learning from faculty members, be it in elevators, corridors, or social settings, and faculty development activities must address these informal interactions.

Lanphear and Cardiff[50] have described the role that faculty development can play in supporting curriculum change. A well-known model for "leading change" can also serve as a useful framework for promoting organizational reform. Kotter[51,52] has outlined a series of eight steps that can lead to transformational change in a variety of settings. In our experience,[9] these steps can be applied effectively when trying to promote curricular or organizational change. They include the following:

- Establish a sense of urgency – establishing urgency demands that the sources of complacency be removed or minimized in order for change to occur.
- Form a powerful guiding coalition – because major change is so difficult to accomplish, a powerful team is required to implement and sustain the process.
- Create a vision – vision clarifies the direction of the change and helps to both motivate and align key players.
- Communicate the vision – those involved in the change must have a common understanding of its goals and direction.
- Empower others to act on the vision – change requires the efforts of many.
- Generate short-term wins – short-term wins help to promote change by fine-tuning the vision, reinforcing the efforts taken, and building momentum.
- Consolidate gains and produce more change – it is essential to consolidate gains and sometimes produce "more change" as resistance to change can undermine early success.
- Anchor new approaches in the culture – new approaches must be institutionalized in the culture to assure transformation.

Table 9.1 illustrates how we have been able to use Kotter's model in analyzing a change initiative in our context.

A CASE STUDY

In our own setting, we have been involved in the design and delivery of faculty development for the teaching and learning of professionalism for over ten years. In this section, we will briefly describe the process that we used to promote consensus and buy-in as well as some of the outcomes that arose from our faculty development initiatives. At the same time, we must highlight that our faculty development program is still a "work in progress" as our activities continue to evolve in response to student and faculty needs.

Process

When we first began our work in this area, we had expected some resistance to the concept of professionalism and its core attributes, as a consensus on its

Table 9.1. Using Kotter's framework to analyze change[9]

Steps in "leading change"[51,52]	Faculty development initiatives	Impact on the faculty and the undergraduate curriculum
Create a sense of urgency	Medical education rounds on professionalism	Highlighted to the faculty the increasing importance of professionalism in medical education
Form a powerful guiding coalition	"Think tank" on teaching professionalism	Established an informal "interest group" on professionalism and contributed to enhanced visibility within the faculty
Create a vision	Invitational workshop on teaching professionalism	Resulted in the creation of a cohort of small-group teachers knowledgeable in this emerging domain; led to a set of general recommendations regarding the teaching of professionalism
Communicate the vision	Faculty-wide workshop on teaching professionalism	Contributed to the dissemination of the vision throughout the academic community (e.g., via hospital-based grand rounds, small-group sessions on professionalism in the undergraduate curriculum, peer-reviewed articles)
Empower others to act on the vision	Departmental workshops on teaching professionalism	Resulted in a detailed report submitted to the associate dean, which led to the establishment of working groups on professionalism, healing, and evaluation.
Generate short-term wins	"Think tank" on evaluating professionalism; faculty-wide workshop on evaluating the physician as healer and professional; faculty-wide workshop on teaching communication skills	Resulted in the development and piloting of a specific tool to evaluate professionalism (i.e., the P-MEX)[59]; led to the adoption of a particular model to teach communication skills; helped to catalyze the creation of a task force mandated to renew the curriculum based on the concept of physicianship
Consolidate gains and produce more change	Faculty retreat on curricular renewal	In partnership with the curriculum committee, this retreat led to a formal endorsement of the physicianship curriculum
Anchor new approaches in the culture	Faculty development workshops for the Osler fellows	Enables the ongoing preparation and "renewal" of faculty members involved in the implementation and delivery of the physicianship curriculum

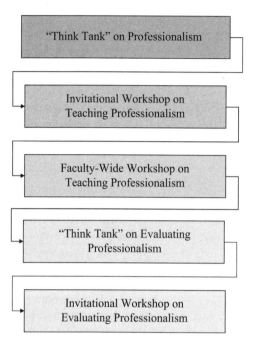

Figure 9.1. The faculty development process at McGill University.[8]

importance, values, and definitions had not been established. We therefore chose a systematic approach, consisting of "think tanks" and workshops as key educational methods, to promote buy-in. Both methods allowed participants to explore their values and beliefs, acquire core content and skills, and begin to take "ownership" of this content area.

The following steps (outlined in Figure 9.1) were used in the development of our faculty development initiative, which has been described previously.[8] We hope that some of our "lessons learned" will be helpful to others interested in mounting faculty development programs in this area.

"Think Tank" on Teaching Professionalism

To initiate a discussion about teaching professionalism, the dean of our medical school invited twenty-five educational leaders to a half-day session, to highlight the importance of professionalism, to develop consensus, and to discuss outreach to faculty members. The participants included the dean, the associate deans for undergraduate and postgraduate medical education, members of the Faculty Development Team, key departmental chairs, program directors at the undergraduate and postgraduate levels, and local content experts. The "think tank" started with a brief overview of the core content of professionalism and proceeded to examine how professionalism was being taught at all levels of the curriculum. At the end of the session, a plan for a faculty development workshop had been developed. Other outcomes included a consensus on the importance of teaching profession-alism, a review of how professionalism was being taught, and agreement on content. Most importantly, however, this "think tank" was fundamental to the success of our faculty development endeavor, and it has served as a model for curricular development in other areas.

Invitational Workshop on Teaching Professionalism

Following the "think tank," all departmental chairs and undergraduate and postgraduate program directors were invited by the dean to a half-day work-shop on *The Teaching of Professionalism*. This workshop was limited to thirty-five participants so that we could "test" the working definitions of the attributes of professionalism, examine the strengths and weaknesses of diverse teaching methods, and receive immediate feedback. The workshop was organized into three parts: the "core content" of professionalism, per-sonal views and beliefs, and strategies for teaching. Appendix B presents the definition of professionalism's core attributes that were refined by the group members. Participants were also asked to discuss a number of case vignettes (based on real clinical or classroom encounters and described in Appendix C), to identify attributes of professionalism and to match available teaching methods to the different attributes. The workshop concluded with the com-pletion of an action plan for each department. By the end of the workshop, we had broadened consensus regarding the importance of professionalism and its core content, and developed a plan for a faculty-wide workshop. We had also prepared a cohort of small-group facilitators for future workshops and teaching sessions, and outlined a series of recommendations regarding the teaching of professionalism that would be presented to the undergraduate and postgraduate curriculum committees. Two key messages emerged from this workshop: 1) the importance of *role modeling* and 2) the need to make the teaching of professionalism *explicit*.

Faculty-Wide Workshop on Teaching Professionalism

Following the invitational workshop, a faculty-wide workshop welcomed sixty-five participants, representing all major specialties. The workshop's goals were to highlight the importance of teaching professionalism in the faculty of medicine and to improve the teaching of this content area by trans-mitting core content, discussing key teaching strategies, and developing an action plan for each department. A written matrix, designed to facilitate the "matching" of methods to attributes, was developed to guide the discussion and highlight the value of examining the strengths and limitations of diverse approaches (see Appendix D). The outcome of this workshop was increased buy-in among the faculty members, new content experts, and an array of educational resources that could be used for teaching purposes at both the undergraduate and the postgraduate level.

"Think Tank" on Evaluating Professionalism

We realized at the outset that, for teaching to be successful, professionalism would need to be evaluated in a more systematic way. Although aspects of professionalism were being assessed on in-training evaluations, improvement was needed. We therefore held another "think tank" with twenty educational leaders and content experts, to examine methods for evaluating professionalism and to develop the content and method of a workshop in this area. We also realized that the attributes of a physician as professional and healer had to be integrated in order for evaluations to be comprehensive. Accordingly, definitions of healing attributes were developed and agreed upon (e.g., caring and compassion, openness and insight, presence). The outcome of this session was a detailed plan for a faculty-wide workshop.

Faculty-wide Workshop on Evaluating the Physician as Healer and Professional

The goal of this workshop, which welcomed ninety-five faculty members, was to develop methods for evaluating professionalism at the undergraduate and postgraduate level. To accomplish this objective, we examined different approaches to evaluating professionalism,[53–56] assessed the benefits and limitations of different evaluation methods (e.g., global rating scales, portfolios, critical incidents), and defined specific, measurable behaviors for each attribute. The latter was done to highlight the importance of behavior specificity and identify a bank of behaviors that could be used in the development of assessment tools. Matrices were also used to guide the generation of behaviors, the matching of methods to behaviors, and the feasibility of the different assessment approaches. By the end of the workshop, we had developed consensus on the need to improve our evaluation of professionalism, identified behaviors that demonstrated the attributes, and developed a series of recommendations that were presented to the faculty of medicine (e.g., each attribute must be evaluated on a regular basis).

Our experience in designing faculty development activities for teaching and evaluating professionalism highlighted the value of the following lessons:

- Define core content and develop a "common language"
- Provide conceptual frameworks to guide thinking and learning
- Enable experiential learning and promote application to personal settings
- Work to promote buy-in

- Emphasize the "teaching" of the competency
- Build on participants' strengths
- Incorporate follow-up tasks and activities

We also saw the benefit of using situated learning, which is based upon the notion that knowledge is *contextually situated* and fundamentally influenced by the *activity, context*, and *culture* in which it is used,[57] as an educational framework for our work in this area.

Faculty Development Outcomes

In our own setting, our faculty development program played a major role in promoting change at the undergraduate and postgraduate level.[9] Some of these changes have included renewal of our undergraduate curriculum to include an emphasis on the physician as healer and professional,[58] increased teaching of this core competency to residents and faculty members, a renewed focus on the evaluation of professionalism among students and residents and validation of an instrument to assess professionalism,[59] and faculty development programs in other areas (e.g., interprofessional education and practice) based on the model used in teaching and learning professionalism.

CONCLUSIONS

In summary, faculty development is a critical component in the teaching and learning of professionalism. As we move forward in this area, we should strive to:

- Bring about change at the *individual* and the *organizational* level.
- Target diverse stakeholders and ensure that there is agreement on the definitions, attributes, and behaviors of professionalism.
- Ensure that faculty development takes place in a variety of settings, using diverse formats and educational strategies.
- Incorporate appropriate educational frameworks and principles of effective instructional design.
- Evaluate the impact of all activities to ensure that predetermined goals and objectives are being met.

As we have stated previously, faculty development can help to build consensus, generate support and enthusiasm, and implement a change initiative. Faculty development can also help to prepare teachers for their multiple roles and change the culture within the institution by altering the formal, informal, and hidden curriculum. The true test of faculty development, how-ever, is in the improvement of teaching and learning for students across the educational continuum, and ultimately, patient care.

REFERENCES

1. Cruess, RL, Cruess, SR. Teaching medicine as a profession in the service of healing. *Acad Med.* 1997;72(11):941–52.
2. Cruess, SR, Cruess, RL. Professionalism must be taught. *BMJ.* 1997;315(7123): 1674–7.
3. Gordon, J. Fostering students' personal and professional development in medicine: a new framework for PPD. *Med Educ.* 2003;37(4):341–9.
4. Coulehan, J. Today's professionalism: engaging the mind but not the heart. *Acad Med.* 2005;80(10):892–8.
5. Ludmerer, KM. Instilling professionalism in medical education. *JAMA.* 1999; 282(9):881–2.
6. Wear, D, Bickel, J. *Educating for Professionalism: Creating a Culture of Human-ism in Medical Education.* Iowa City (IA): University of Iowa Press; 2000.
7. Whitcomb, ME. Professionalism in medicine. *Acad Med.* 2007;82(11):1009.
8. Steinert, Y, Cruess, S, Cruess, R, Snell, L. Faculty development for teaching and evaluating professionalism: from programme design to curriculum change. *Med Educ.* 2005;39(2):127–36.
9. Steinert, Y, Cruess, RL, Cruess, SR, Boudreau, JD, Fuks, A. Faculty development as an instrument of change: a case study on teaching professionalism. *Acad Med.* 2007;82(11):1057–64.
10. Centra, JA. Types of faculty development programs. *J Higher Educ.* 1978; 49(2):151–62.
11. Bland, C, Schmitz, C, Stritter, F, Henry, R, Aluise, J. *Successful Faculty in Academic Medicine.* New York: Springer-Verlag; 1990.
12. Sheets, KJ, Schwenk, TL. Faculty development for family medicine educators: an agenda for future activities. *Teach Learn Med.* 1990;2:141–8.
13. Steinert, Y. Faculty development in the new millennium: key challenges and future directions. *Med Teach.* 2000;22(1):44–50.
14. Steinert, Y. Learning together to teach together: interprofessional education and faculty development. *J Interprof Care.* 2005;19(2 Suppl. 1):60–75.
15. Wilkerson, L, Irby, DM. Strategies for improving teaching practices: a compre-hensive approach to faculty development. *Acad Med.* 1998;73(4):387–96.
16. Hafferty, FW. Beyond curriculum reform: confronting medicine's hidden curric-ulum. *Acad Med.* 1998;73(4):403–7.
17. McLellan, H. *Situated Learning Perspectives.* Englewood Cliffs (NJ): Educational Technology Publications; 1996.
18. Steinert, Y. Staff development. In Dent, JA, Harden, RM, editors. *A Practical Guide for Medical Teachers.* Edinburgh (UK): Churchill Livingstone; 2005.
19. Rubeck, RF, Witzke, DB. Faculty development: a field of dreams. *Acad Med.* 1998;73(9 Suppl.):S32–7.

20. Grant, J. Learning needs assessment: assessing the need. *BMJ.* 2002;324(7330):156–9.

21. Lockyer, J. Needs assessment: lessons learned. *J Contin Educ Health Prof.* 1998; 18(3):190–2.

22. McLeod, P, Steinert, Y, Nasmith, L, Conochie, L. Faculty development in Canadian medical schools: a 10-year update. *CMAJ.* 1997;156(10):1419–23.

23. Steinert, Y, Mann, K, Centeno, A, Dolmans, D, Spencer, J, Gelula, M, Prideaux, D. A systematic review of faculty development initiatives designed to improve teaching effectiveness in medical education: BEME guide no. 8. *Med Teach.* 2006;28(6):497–526.

24. Ulian, J, Stritter, F. Faculty development in medical education with implications for continuing medical education. *J Contin Educ Health Prof.* 1996;16:181–90.

25. Steinert, Y, Nasmith, L, McLeod, PJ, Conochie, L. A teaching scholars program to develop leaders in medical education. *Acad Med.* 2003;78(2):142–9.

26. Steinert, Y, McLeod, P. From novice to informed educator: the teaching scholars program for educators in the health sciences. *Acad Med.* 2006; 81(11):969–74.

27. Flynn, SP, Bedinghaus, J, Snyder, C, Hekelman, F. Peer coaching in clinical teaching: a case report. *Educ Res Methods.* 1994;26(9):569–70.

28. Sekerka, LE, Chao, J. Peer coaching as a technique to foster professional development in clinical ambulatory settings. *J Contin Educ Health Prof.* 2003;23(1):30–7.

29. Schön, DA. *Educating the Reflective Practitioner: Toward a New Design for Teaching and Learning in the Professions.* San Francisco (CA): Jossey-Bass; 1987.

30. Westberg, J, Whitman, N. Resource materials for faculty development. *Fam Med.* 1997;29(4):275–9.

31. Beasley, BW, Kallail, KJ, Walling, AD, Davis, N, Hudson, L. Maximizing the use of a web-based teaching skills curriculum for community-based volunteer faculty. *J Contin Educ Health Prof.* 2001;21(3):158–61.

32. Knowles, MS. *The Modern Practice of Adult Education: From Pedagogy to Andragogy.* New York: Cambridge Books; 1988.

33. Kaufman, DM, Mann, K, Jennett, PA. *Teaching and Learning in Medical Education: How Theory Can Inform Practice.* Edinburgh (UK): Association for the Study of Medical Education; 2000.

34. DeWitt, TG, Goldberg, RL, Roberts, KB. Developing community faculty: principles, practice, and evaluation. *Am J Dis Child.* 1993;147(1):49–53.

35. Langlois, JP, Thach, SB. Bringing faculty development to community preceptors. *Acad Med.* 2003;78(2):150–5.

36. Stufflebeam, DL. Alternative approaches to educational evaluation. In Popham WJ, editor. *Evaluation in Education: Current Applications.* Berkley (CA): McCutchan Publishing; 1974.

37. Popham, WJ. *Educational Evaluation.* Boston (MA): Allyn and Bacon; 1993.

38. Wholey, IS, Hatry, HP, Newcomer, KE. *Handbook of Practical Program Evaluation.* San Francisco (CA): Jossey-Bass; 1994.

39. Kirkpatrick, DL. *Evaluating Training Programs: The Four Levels.* San Francisco (CA): Berrett-Koehler Publishers; 1997.

40. Swick, HM. Towards a normative definition of professionalism. *Acad Med.* 2000;75(6):612–6.

41. American Board of Internal Medicine (ABIM). *Project Professionalism*(revised). Philadelphia (PA): American Board of Internal Medicine; 1999 [cited November 27, 2007]. Available from: www.abimfoundation.org/professional.html.

42. American Association of Medical Colleges (AAMC). *Learning Objectives for Medical Student Education: Guidelines for Medical Schools*. Washington (DC): American Association of Medical Colleges; 1998.

43. Royal College of Physicians and Surgeons of Canada. CanMEDS 2000 project – skills for the new millennium: report of the societal needs working group. 2005 [cited November 27, 2007]. Royal College of Physicians and Surgeons [24 screens]. Available from: http://rcpsc.medical.org/canmeds/CanMEDS_e.pdf.

44. Cruess, RL, Cruess, SR. Teaching professionalism: general principles. *Med Teach*. 2006;28(3):205–8.

45. Hilton, SR, Slotnick, HB. Proto-professionalism: how professionalization occurs across the continuum of medical education. *Med Educ*. 2005;39(1):58–65.

46. Epstein, RM. Mindful practice. *JAMA*. 1999;282(9):833–9.

47. Novak, DH, Epstein, RM, Paulsen, RH. Toward creating physician-healers: fostering medical students' self-awareness, personal growth, and well-being. *Acad Med*. 1999; 74(5):516–20.

48. Maudsley, G, Strivens, J. Promoting professional knowledge, experiential learning, and critical thinking for medical students. *Med Educ*. 2000;34(7):535–44.

49. Mamede, S, Schmidt, HG. The structure of reflective practice in medicine. *Med Educ*. 2004;38(12):1302–8.

50. Lanphear, JH, Cardiff, RD. Faculty development: an essential consideration in curriculum change. *Arch Pathol Lab Med*. 1987;111:487–91.

51. Kotter, JP. Leading change: why transformation efforts fail. *Harv Bus Rev*. 1995;73:59–67.

52. Kotter, JP. *Leading Change*. Boston (MA): Harvard Business School Press; 1996.

53. Arnold, L. Assessing professional behaviors: yesterday, today, and tomorrow. *Acad Med*. 2002:77(6);502–15.

54. Ginsburg, S, Regehr, G, Hatala, R, McNaughton, N, Frohna, A, Hodges, B, Lingard, L, Stern, D. Context, conflict, and resolution: a new conceptual framework for evaluating professionalism. *Acad Med*. 2000;75(10 Suppl.):S6–11.

55. Papadakis, MA, Osborn, EH, Cooke, M, Healy, K. A strategy for the detection and evaluation of unprofessional behavior in medical students. *Acad Med*. 1999; 74(9):980–90.

56. Van Luijk, SJ, Smeets, JG, Smits, J, Wolfhagen, I, Perquin, ML. Assessing professional behaviour and the role of academic advice at the Maastricht Medical School. *Med Teach*. 2000;22(2):168–77.

57. Brown, JS, Collins, A, Duguid, S. Situated cognition and the culture of learning. *Educ Res*. 1989;18(1):32–42.

58. Boudreau, D, Cassell, E, Fuks, A. A healing curriculum. *Med Educ*. 2007;41(12):1193–201.

59. Cruess, R, McIlroy, JH, Cruess, S, Ginsburg, S, Steinert, Y. The professionalism mini-evaluation exercise: a preliminary investigation. *Acad Med*. 2006; 81(10 Suppl.):S74–8.

10 The Relationship between Teaching Professionalism and Licensing and Accrediting Bodies

Sir Donald Irvine, C.B.E., M.D., F.R.C.G.P., F. Med.Sci.

INTRODUCTION

The essential character of a profession is that its members have specialized knowledge and skills, which the public will wish to use.[1] Medical regulation in its various forms – licensure, certification, and accreditation in particular – is therefore the means through which the state makes sure that the public is served by doctors who are well trained and completely up to date, and who are therefore competent, show sound judgment, are ethical, and are capable of making and sustaining good relationships with patients.[2] In some countries, for example, the United States and British Commonwealth, the state has delegated part of its responsibility to organizations within the medical profession through the principle of self-regulation. By definition self-regulation is therefore a privilege granted by the state that has to be earned and constantly justified. It is not the right that some doctors think it is.[3–5]

Medical professionalism has been defined as a set of values, behaviors, and relationships that underpins the trust the public has in doctors.[6] Professional regulation, which is founded on the values and standards of practice of the day, may therefore be seen as a formal expression of doctors' professionalism and the basis for the profession's "social contract" with the public.[7] Medical education is the principal (but not the only) means whereby such values and standards are taught, learnt, digested, internalized, and continuously refreshed at all stages in a doctor's career.[8] This is why, from the earliest days of the modern medical profession, the relationship between medical education and medical regulation has been so fundamental.

The basic instrument of regulation is licensure. Licensing authorities are statutory bodies entrusted by legislatures to ensure that only people they consider to be properly qualified are allowed to practice medicine. So a license to practice is restrictive – one cannot practice without it. Licenses are granted to new entrants who reach the standard required by the authority and may be restricted or withdrawn altogether from those who do not sub-sequently maintain that standard. The licensing authorities may be national, like the General Medical Council (GMC) in the United Kingdom, or they may be regional where the jurisdiction rests in a state or province as in the United States and Australia, and in Canada, respectively. They implement their statutory functions by maintaining registers or lists of practitioners whom they have licensed to practice.

Certification, which may or may not be statutory, marks the satisfactory completion of specialist training and training for family practice. Specialty-specific professional bodies such as specialty boards and Royal Colleges decide the standards needed for practice in their respective fields and the training necessary to achieve those standards. These specialty-specific standards complement the generic standards needed for licensure. Historically, certification has been indicative, that is to say highly desirable but not – like licensure – absolutely restrictive. So, for example, it is still possible to practice as a general practitioner or specialist in the United States while not being board certified. Employers, insurers, and others may link financial incentives and penalties, and eligibility for institutional practicing privileges, to certification but there is no automatic bar to practice without it. However, the tendency is toward making certification more restrictive by establishing a linkage with licensure – as happens now in Canada and is to be implemented shortly in the United Kingdom.

Accreditation is the process whereby designated authorities approve the educational experience and standards of training offered by educational institutions.[9] The US Accreditation Council for Graduate Medical Education (ACGME), which accredits postgraduate training, and the Education Committee of the General Medical Council, which accredits basic medical education in UK medical schools, are examples. There are usually close formal and informal relationships between teachers (academics) and the accrediting authorities because it is teachers who deliver the educational experience needed for licensure and certification.

Public policy on professional regulation is broadly informed by the public's expectations and experiences of doctors. Klein put his finger on the nub of the relationship between public policy and professional regulation when he said, "The aim of public policy is to make the medical profession collectively more accountable for its performance. The aim of professional self-regulation is to make individual practitioners more accountable to their peers. Control over the medical profession collectively is a complement to – not a substitute for – control by the medical profession of its members. The precise balance between the two will depend on the extent to which the medical profession demonstrates that it can be trusted to deliver its part of the bargain."[10]

These, then, are the basic principles that inform the culture and governance of the medical profession. Every doctor must understand them and know how they relate to their professional duties and responsibilities as individuals and collectively as members of the profession. For teachers, students, and trainees, understanding begins by putting the principles into the context of the public's expectations and experiences of doctors and the medical profession today, so that there can be in no doubt about what patients regard as truly patient-centered care.

What the People Say

The public believe that everyone should have a "good" doctor. Patients do not knowingly choose a "bad" doctor or even one who they think is just "not good enough."[2] They expect the regulators, educators, and, where appropriate, employers to deliver good doctors on their behalf to make sure they stay that way and to act to protect them when doctors do not.

Patients' Ideas of a Good Doctor

For patients and their relatives, a good doctor is one whom they feel they can trust without having to think about it.[11] They equate "goodness" with integrity, safety, up-to-date medical knowledge and diagnostic skill, and an ability to form a good relationship with them. For them, good doctors are clinically expert yet know their limitations. They are honest, interested in them, listen to them, will put themselves out for them, are kind, courteous, considerate, empathetic, respectful, and caring. These attributes matter because patients know their doctors' advice and decisions can affect the outcome of their illness – even make the difference between life and death, or between enjoying a speedy recovery and suffering serious disability.[2,12]

We can all put our own personal gloss on this vignette but there is ample evidence from recent patient surveys and focus groups to show that it is essentially accurate (e.g., Chisholm et al.[13] and Coulter[14]). For example, in 2006, the Picker Institute[15] reported the results of surveys it organized in eight European countries (the Czech Republic, Denmark, Italy, The Netherlands, Poland, Spain, Switzerland, and the United Kingdom), to find out what patients and relatives thought about the qualities they looked for in intensive care doctors. What mattered most were medical skill and experience, particularly clinical knowledge, decisiveness in decision making, and the ability to act calmly in a crisis. Almost equally important was the ability to exchange information, to communicate effectively, and to deal sensitively with anxious patients and relatives.

Similarly, a systematic review of 19 studies on patients' priorities in general practice ranked "humaneness" in 86 percent of studies, "competence/accuracy" in 64 percent, "patient involvement in decisions" in 63 percent, and "time for care" in 60 percent.[16] In another study of patients attending the Mayo clinic, the researchers identified seven ideal physician behaviors: according to these patients, good physicians are confident, empathetic, humane, personal, forthright, respectful, and thorough.[17] And of course the public today wants doctors to involve them, to the extent that they decide appropriate, in decisions about their care.[18,19]

Patients' Experiences of Doctors

In general terms, it seems that patients' experience of their doctors matches their expectations, which is why so many doctors enjoy a high level of personal patient satisfaction and trust in many countries.[20] That is good news. However, the medical profession's historical tolerance of poor practice is becoming less acceptable to the public (see below), and professional institutions therefore trusted less. This may be because the public is becoming more aware of the evidence of wide variations in doctors' performance.

This variation is well illustrated in the cluster of behaviors that fall loosely under the headings of communication and professionalism. In a recent study – the latest in a series over several years – the Commonwealth Fund has compared patient experience in five countries, the United Kingdom, Australia, Canada, New Zealand, and the United States.[21] Box 10.1 shows five examples – doctor-patient communication, involving patients in treatment decisions, giving clear goals and a treatment plan, explaining medication side effects, and giving patients access to their records. Most patients have a positive experience. However, a sizable minority of patients – significant in terms of the millions of people in a population who may be affected – do not experience such care. The size of this minority may help to explain the background buzz of discontent one often hears about doctors' attitudes and communication skills.

Public Expectations of Professional Regulation

In 2005, the UK government commissioned a major study of attitudes to medical regulation and revalidation among the general public and doctors.[20] The first striking finding was that three fifths of people surveyed knew nothing about the assessment of doctors. For them the inner workings of licensure and certification were a closed book, taken on blind trust. Nevertheless, when asked, respondents had clear ideas about what aspects of a doctor's practice are important to them, and which should therefore be assessed throughout a doctor's career. Nine in ten UK citizens want their doctors to demonstrate

Box 10.1. Patients' experiences of five measures of doctor's professionalism in five countries

A: Doctor always/usually involves patient in treatment decisions

B: Doctor gives clear goals and treatment plan

C: Doctor explains medication side effects

D: Patient can access medical records

E: Doctor–patient communication

regularly that they have good clinical knowledge and technical skills and, equally, competence in the interpersonal aspects of care. About half want these checks done annually.

In Ontario, Canada, a 2006 survey of members of the public and doctors showed that 93 percent of lay people and 52 percent of doctors said there must be regular competence checks to maintain licensure.[22] Similarly, 85 percent of lay people and 44 percent of doctors thought that doctors must receive formal feedback from their colleagues and other health professionals, while 84 percent of lay people and 42 percent of doctors thought the same about feedback from patients about their communications. The situation in the United States is similar, with a strong public (but not medical) preference for mandatory knowledge testing as part of recertification.[23]

Three things need to be emphasized when teaching about professionalism. First the public think of doctors' professionalism holistically, and not simply as the narrower humanistic/ethical subset favored by many medical regulators and educators today. Second, despite the high levels of trust in the profession, people nevertheless want to be sure that their doctors are up to the mark. This is why the overwhelming majority of the public think that doctors must be regularly tested throughout their active professional lives through some process of revalidation. The clear implication is that doctors who fail must quickly remedy the problem or lose their unrestricted license to practice. Third, and by contrast, doctors are much more divided about the necessity for and especially the rigor of any revalidation process. Some think that the very idea of revalidation demeans their professionalism, whereas other doctors and the public think it would enhance it. Today these conflicted expectations represent a huge challenge for professional leaders and teachers not least because they are themselves divided but it was not always so.

Evolving Ideas about Professionalism and Professional Regulation

Most people tend to use the generic word "professional" to describe a combination of strongly positive qualities and attributes including high technical performance, integrity, conscientiousness, commitment, dependability, selflessness in putting the interests of others first (altruism), and general excellence. In medicine, earlier interpretations of professionalism were based on the possession of an exclusive body of knowledge held and accessed only by doctors, on physician autonomy, and on implicit values and standards of practice and education that were determined almost exclusively by doctors themselves.[4,5] So it is not surprising that doctors liked this concept of professionalism – it carried with it connotations of trustworthiness, high public esteem, self-worth, self-control, and self-respect. It made them feel good.

This doctors' view of professionalism was taken for granted in the nineteenth century and most of the last century – a long time. It was the received wisdom among the leaders of the medical schools, postgraduate organizations, colleges, professional associations, and regulatory bodies, and was the culture that was passed on to new generations of doctors.[24] The public willingly accepted this perspective of doctors' duties and responsibilities, not least because they could see the benefits for themselves that were flowing from the burgeoning new medical science and technology. Doctors, it seemed, could be trusted, individually and collectively, to make sure that patients were always served by good doctors who belonged to a profession that put the public interest first. Hence, the public's relatively uninformed and understandably uncritical endorsement of self-regulation during that period despite dissenting voices critical of the profession's tolerance of cases of incompetent or simply poor practice.[5,24]

But within the last quarter century, this traditional view of medical professionalism has attracted serious criticism inside and outside the profession. In particular, it became clear that the energetic pursuit of scientific knowledge and skills, especially in academia, had reduced the attention given to the ethical and human dimensions of medical practice with detrimental effects on the quality of patients' experience.[4,12,25] More generally, patients wanted to take charge of their own lives as evidenced through the rapidly evolving consumer, women's rights, and civil rights movements in the Western world. These movements were the spearhead of a societal change that emphasized the rights and entitlements of the individual, and thus eschewed paternalism, passive deference, and therefore patients' resigned tolerance of poor practice.

In this climate embarrassing, well-publicized medical disasters in the United Kingdom raised new questions about patient safety, in particular whether the collective profession had the stomach to deal effectively with poorly performing doctors or whether it would continue to give doctors rather than patients the benefit of the doubt.[11,26,27] The public were in no doubt. While patients' trust in individual doctors remained strong where their personal experience was good, the hitherto unquestioning trust of medical regulation began to be replaced by assertive questioning coupled with a demand for better protection from poorly performing doctors, more public involvement in regulation, more accountability, concrete evidence of consistency of doctors' lifetime competence and performance, and less self-interested protectiveness.[11,25,26] In future, trust in the collective profession must be evidence based and founded on a "patient-centered" culture of medical practice and a system of professional regulation and medical education that put patients unequivocally first.

For doctors the choice was clear. They could accept the validity of the public's criticisms of their professionalism with good grace, adapt their ideas of professionalism to meet society's new expectations, and so rebuild the relationship of trust both parties want. Or they could reject or ignore the criticisms, or give a grudging, minimalist response, in which event the inevitable consequence would be continuing loss of status and perceived trustworthiness as doctors' wide discretionary clinical and professional privileges were further eroded or even replaced by managerial control.

In the event the profession has inclined to favor the former and so in several countries today is in the process of making a system-wide transition from the old to a "new professionalism."[5,24] The essential elements are described below. The change is coming about largely because of informal alliances between reforming doctors – many of them leading teachers – and progressive patients' organizations who together have sought to push things forward.[24] Even so the process of change has proved to be far more difficult, slow, and emotionally charged than many doctors are prepared to admit. Old habits die hard and medicine is socially still an inward looking, conservative profession.[25] The present generation of medical students and new doctors, who are the future, must be active in promoting and supporting needed change. It is in their interests to help create and maintain a relationship with society founded on trust.

New Professionalism, New Professional Regulation

So what does the profession have to do to rebuild trust? To answer this it is essential to go back to the public's starting point. As we have seen, when people become ill they expect to be under the care of a fully trained specialist or family practitioner. So their focus is entirely on an "established" doctor. They expect this doctor to have a good standard of up-to-date knowledge and skill, and "professional" behavior, however long he or she has been qualified. They assume that the regulatory and medical educational systems, and employers, are focused on their doctor to make sure this happens. The public's assumptions are perfectly logical and valid.

These assumptions are not, however, borne out by the facts. Historically, and even today, the mindset and main edifice of both medical regulation and education are geared primarily to the selection and preparation of new entrants – making students into doctors and then doctors into specialists. The profession has taken this important phase of preparation very seriously, which is why by and large it has been thorough, rigorous, and effective. This high order of educational and regulatory professionalism contrasts sharply with the permissive, arbitrary, "do-as-you-please" individualism and dare one say amateurism that has characterized the collective approach to the continuing professional development and the maintenance of professional standards among career doctors. Until very recently, the profession has been content to rely on doctors' personal conscience as the main guarantor of their continuing professionalism rather than to take the collective responsibility for individual physician performance that Klein[10] wrote about. Now the price of public trust is that the profession takes this responsibility equally seriously.

And indeed this is beginning to happen, as the professionalism of the career doctor moves toward the center of the frame. The change in focus sounds deceptively simple. In fact, as doctors are now discovering, it will have profound consequences for the medical mindset and culture, the governance of the profession particularly at the workplace, the practicing and learning environment, the design of regulatory and educational institutions and processes, and for relationships with other health professions as well as the public.

Modernized medical regulation is one result of this change of focus. The new model is founded on values, standards, and competencies that can form the basis for doctors' fitness to practice, a fitness they are expected to demonstrate regularly throughout their active professional lives.[2,28] In this model, regulation and education assume a new significance because together they become the primary instruments for internalizing and embedding the standards in the professional culture and in the minds and actions of individual doctors. The model embodies the principles of accountability, transparency, and partnership with the public. It is proactive rather than reactive. It requires attention to the assessment of performance as well as of competence. Licensure and certification are no longer seen as stand-alone processes but rather as very important elements in a wider framework of continuous quality improvement and quality assurance at doctors' places of work.

Professional Standards

Professional standards are at the heart of the new professionalism and consequently must be an integral part of all teaching programs. New thinking about values and standards, and the duties and responsibilities of doctors, began to emerge in the early 1990s from within the profession itself. The main driving force was the realization among some professional leaders that relying on an implicit understanding of what a good doctor is was no longer sufficient as the basis for regulation and education, and for communicating effectively with the public. Indeed, it was proving difficult for doctors to communicate and secure agreement among themselves about some pretty fundamental matters, far less given a coherent explanation of their professionalism to the outside world. Communication, relationships with patients, attitudes to teamworking, and standards of performance are examples of hot topics at the time. A vehicle for setting out common ground had to be found.

The initiative began independently around the same time in the United States, the United Kingdom, and Canada. A consortium led by the American Board of Internal Medicine Foundation wrote a Physicians Charter to provide a basis for the renewal of professionalism.[29] The GMC started work on a statement setting out the duties and responsibilities of doctors in the United Kingdom in the booklet Good Medical Practice.[30] It planned from the outset to use this for regulatory purposes, starting with its management of fitness to practice cases. And the Royal College of Physicians and Surgeons of Canada created their CanMEDS document around the competencies for training in patient-centered practice.[31]

In 1999, the ACGME defined six general competencies for use in graduate medical education. These are medical knowledge, patient care, interpersonal and communication skills, professionalism, practice-based learning and improvement, and systems-based practice. These competencies have been adopted subsequently across US medicine and form the basis for the maintenance of certification under the auspices of the American Board of Medical Specialities. In 2005, the US Federation of State Medical Boards initiated an informal National Alliance for Physician Competence to promote effective medical regulation. It has taken up the work begun by the National Board of Medical Examiners and other organizations in the United States to create an American version of Good Medical Practice. The Alliance believes that a unified code can provide a new foundation for education, licensure, and certification for American medicine. The Alliance also plans to develop a consensus on the data needed to provide evidence of meeting the standards of Good Medical Practice United States [32] throughout the career of a doctor.

Meanwhile, in Britain the Department of Health (DoH) in 2006 described a professional code of practice for doctors as a set of clear, unambiguous, and, where possible, assessable set of standards that relate closely to the work of a doctor.[28] A code should be capable of being operationalized if it was to be of any practical use.[2,28] It should thus provide the vehicle for making sure that doctors know what is and is not expected of them. It should provide a benchmark by which patients can test their expectations and judge their experiences, and should ensure that all those who contract with doctors have a shared understanding. It should provide greater transparency for patients, public, and employers.

The latest edition of Good Medical Practice, also published in 2006, provides some sixty generic standards.[30] It is underpinned by careful research on patients' expectations of doctors.[33] It meets the DoH criteria. It provides the framework for the assembly of specialty-specific standards now being undertaken by the Royal Colleges. It is now the benchmark against which UK doctors' fitness to practice is assessed and judged when complaints are made against them, is the basis for medical curricula in all stages of medical education, provides a framework for the new NHS appraisal scheme, and will be the generic template for revalidation.[28]

Revalidation

Revalidation is the process through which doctors demonstrate regularly that they are fit to practice in their chosen field. A recent study of twenty-four countries in the Western world has shown that at present none have a completely satisfactory set of arrangements for revalidation.[34] The systems are usually partial, based on varying degrees of rigor, and so inevitably leave sections of the population still at risk from poor performance.

In the United Kingdom, there is to be a two-strand model based on relicensure by the GMC and complementary recertification by the Royal Colleges. Assessment will be against the generic standards described above.[28] Relicensure will be every five years and will involve satisfactory participation in annual National Health Service appraisal at the workplace, informed by standardized multisourced feedback. Recertification, also five yearly, will use assessment tools calibrated against specialty standards.

The American experience with recertification provides a reasonably robust working model.[35] The American Board of Medical Specialities has agreed a common framework for professional development and assessment based on the ACGME competencies. The development of assessment methods is greatly helped by the fact that there are organizations like the National Board of Medical Examiners and the specialty boards who specialize in medical assessment. A recent review offers good evidence that recertification improves the quality of doctors' practice.[36] However, this optimistic picture needs qualification. Estimates of US doctors who are not recertified range from 8 to 15 percent with some estimates rising to 25 percent (Richard Hawkins, personal communication). Physicians whose current competency status is unknown therefore look after large absolute numbers of people in the United States.

New Professionalism, New Learning, and Teaching

The new regulatory requirements provide a huge opportunity and challenge for medical education. By its nature regulation is directive. Doctors know all too well that it can feel heavy handed and oppressive particularly if it appears to be being done to them without their wholehearted agreement. That makes meaningful compliance difficult to secure. The task for the educators is to help all members of the profession work through the standards while reflecting on their own practice, to promote understanding and a depth of commitment that goes beyond a superficial nod in the direction of changed behavior. It is about doctors taking ownership, of making their professionalism part of their identity.[37]

A great deal of progress has already been made on the teaching of professionalism and on the development of suitable assessment methods. The burgeoning literature in the past ten years on the subject is testament to this activity. However, much of the attention has focused on raising the profile of professionalism through redesigned curricula and innovative teaching and assessment methods.[38,39] The hidden curriculum, particularly the impact of role modeling, of the learning environment, and of the professionalism of clinical teachers themselves as doctors, is much more difficult and complex.[38] How common it is today to attend meetings of enthusiasts where the hidden curriculum is fully recognized and talked about yet is accompanied by a sense of hopelessness about how to take things forward beyond the efforts of individual enthusiasts.

This brings me straight to the point. If the educational system is to respond adequately to the challenge of public expectation and the new regulation, and to serve doctors well, it will need a comparable mindset and general systems change. What this means in practice is that the quality of the practice of clinical teachers has to move center stage. In medical education, so heavily dependent as it is on experiential learning, the teachers are the gold in the bank. Everyone knows that their influence, by deed as much as by word, is critical. The change will not happen unless and until the high command of medicine requires that it shall be so, and sets about national implementation as though it were running a military campaign. It needs the regulators (including the accrediting agencies) and the colleges to set the direction but they cannot do the job on the ground. That will fall to the university medical schools and to the various postgraduate organizations, which between them manage medical education in the field. They are the organizations that need to take the responsibility, singly and collectively, for making this happen.

Making change on this scale will be daunting and will take time. But it can be done. For example, in the 1970s, in UK general practice, determined doctors set about achieving such a national transformation against a background of some lamentable practice. They used the new vocational training as the vehicle for introducing a standard setting system for clinical teachers that put feedback on their performance and formative professional development at the forefront. Within five years, there were fine examples of practice and teaching of a very high order coupled with high morale, across the country.

The doctors involved saw that they could achieve a higher level of professionalism and at the same time find the whole experience enjoyable and rewarding. Self-esteem and self-respect are powerful motivators. It was all about leadership and hearts and minds.[2,40]

CONCLUSIONS

Medical regulation and medical education are inextricably entwined. The new professionalism, grounded firmly on the public's expectations of doctors, is fundamental to the safety and well-being of patients and the health of the medical profession. It requires the regulatory and educational institutions of medicine, and medical leaders and teachers, to work closely together to make sure that doctors and students always put the interests of patients first. That is the only way for the profession to maintain public trust in future.

REFERENCES

1. Secretary of State for Social Services. Report of the Committee of Inquiry into the regulation of the medical profession. Chairman Dr A W Merrison. Cmnd 6018. London: HMSO; 1975.
2. Irvine, DH. Everyone is entitled to a good doctor. Abridged version of the 30th William Osler lecture delivered at McGill University, Montreal, 2006. *MJA*. 2007;186(5):256–61.
3. Irvine, D. The performance of doctors. I: Professionalism and self-regulation in a changing world. *BMJ*. 1997;314(7094):1613–5.
4. Freidson, E. *Professionalism Reborn: Theory, Prophecy, Policy*. Cambridge: Polity Press; 1994.
5. Stacey, M. *Regulating British Medicine: The General Medical Council*. Chichester (UK): Wiley; 1992.
6. Royal College of Physicians of London. Doctors in society: medical professionalism in a changing world. Report of working party on medical professionalism. London: Royal College of Physicians; 2005.
7. Cruess, SR. Professionalism and medicine's social contract with society. *Clin Ortho Relat Res*. 2006;449:170–6.
8. Cruess, RL, Cruess, SR, Johnston, SE. Professionalism: an ideal to be sustained. *Lancet*. 2000;356(9224):156–9.
9. Lynch, D, Leach, DC, Surdyk, PM. Assessing professionalism for accreditation. In Stern, DT, editor. *Measuring Medical Professionalism*. New York: Oxford University Press; 2006: 265–80.
10. Klein, R. *Regulating the Medical Profession: Doctors and the Public Interest. Healthcare 1997/1998*. London: Kings Fund; 1998.
11. The Shipman Inquiry. *Safeguarding Patients: Lessons from the Past, Proposals for the Future*. Chairman Dame Janet Smith. London: Stationery Office; 2004.

12. Gerteis, M, Edgman-Levitian, S, Daley, J, Delbanco, T L. *Through the Patient's Eyes: Understanding and Promoting Patient Care.* San Francisco: Jossey-Bass; 1993.

13. Chisholm, A, Cairncross, L, Askham, J. *Setting Standards: The Views of Members of the Public and Doctors on the Standards of Care and Practice They Expect of Doctors.* Oxford: Picker Institute Europe; 2006 [cited May 22, 2006]. Available from: www.pickereurope.org/Filestore/Publications/Setting_Standards_with_ISBN_web.pdf.

14. Coulter, A. What do patients and the public want from primary care? *BMJ.* 2005;331:1199–201.

15. Hasman, A, Graham, C, Reeves, R, Askham, J. *What Do Patients and Relatives See as Key Competencies for Intensive Care Doctors?* Oxford: Picker Institute Europe; 2006 [cited May 22, 2006]. Available from: www.pickereurope.org/Filestore/Publications/CobatriceFull_report_with_isbn_web_(2).pdf.

16. Wensing, M, Jung, HP, Mainz, J, Olesen, F, Grol, R. A systematic review of the literature on patient priorities for general practice care. Part 1: Description of the research domain. *Soc Sci Med.* 1998;47:1573–88.

17. Bendapudi, NM, Berry, LL, Frey, KA, Parish, JT, Rayburn, WL. Patients' perspectives on ideal physician behaviours. *Mayo Clin Proc.* 2006;81:338–44.

18. Ellins, J, Coulter, A. *How Engaged Are People in Their Health Care?* Findings of a national telephone survey. London: The Health Foundation; 2005 [cited May 22, 2006]. Available from: www.pickereurope.org/Filestore/Publications/Patient-Activation-Survey.pdf.

19. Coulter, A, Ellins, J. *Patient-Focused Interventions: A Review of the Evidence.* London: The Health Foundation; 2006 [cited May 22, 2006]. Available from: www.pickereurope.org/Filestore/Publications/QEI_Review_AB.pdf.

20. IPSOS-MORI. *Attitudes to Revalidation and Regulation of Doctors.* London: Department of Health; 2005 [cited November 27, 2007]. Available from: www.ipsos-mori.com/polls/2005/pdf/doh.pdf.

21. Coulter, A. *Engaging Patients in Their Healthcare: How Is the UK Doing Relative to Other Countries?* Oxford: Picker Institute Europe; 2006 [cited May 22, 2006]. Available from: www.pickereurope.org/Filestore/Publications/Six_country_study_with_ISBN_web.pdf.

22. College of Physicians and Surgeons of Ontario. Revalidation consultation summary. April 7, 2006 [cited May 22, 2006]. Available from: www.cpso.on.ca/Whats_New/RevalConsultApr06.pdf

23. The Gallup Organisation for the American Board of Internal Medicine. *Awareness of and Attitudes towards Board/Certification of Physicians.* Princeton (NJ): The Gallup Organisation; 2003.

24. Irvine, DH. *The Doctors' Tale: Professionalism and Public Trust.* Oxford: Radcliffe Medical Press; 2003.

25. Irvine, D. A short history of the General Medical Council. *Med Educ.* 2006;40:202–11.

26. Bristol Royal Infirmary Inquiry. Learning from Bristol: the report of the public inquiry into children's heart surgery at the Bristol Royal Infirmary 1984–1995. *Chairman Sir Ian Kennedy.* London: Stationery Office; 2001.

27. Institute of Medicine. *Crossing the Quality Chasm*. Washington (DC): Institute of Medicine; 2001.

28. Donaldson, L. *Chief Medical Officer. Good Doctors, Safer Patients*. London: Department of Health; 2006.

29. American Board of Internal Medicine Foundation. *Physicians' Charter*. Philadelphia: American Board of Internal Medicine Foundation; 2004.

30. General Medical Council. *Good Medical Practice*. 4th ed. London: General Medical Council; 2006 [cited June 5, 2007]. Available from: www.gmcuk.org/guidance/good_medical_practice/GMC_GMP.pdf.

31. Royal College of Physicians and Surgeons of Canada. CanMEDS 2000 project. Ottawa: RCPSC; 1996. http://rcpsc.medical.org/canmeds/index.php (Accessed June 5, 2007).

32. National Alliance for Physician Competence. Good medical practice-USA. Version 0.1 August 15, 2007. National Alliance for Physician Competence; 2006 [cited November 27, 2007]. Available from: www.gmpusa.org.

33. Chisholm, A, Askham, J. *A Review of Professional Codes and Standards for Doctors in UK, USA and Canada*. Oxford: Picker Institute Europe 2006 [cited June 5, 2007]. Available from: www.pickereurope.org/Filestore/Publications/PCP_codes_with_ISBN_for_web.pdf.

34. Allsop, J, Jones, K. Quality assurance in medical regulation in an international context. University of Lincoln; 2005 [cited November 27, 2007]. Available from: www.lincoln.ac.uk/policystudies/Research/docs/CMOReport.pdf.

35. Lipner, RS, Bylsma, WH, Arnold, GK, Fortna, GS, Tooker, J, Cassel, CK. Who is maintaining in certification in internal medicine — and why? A national survey 10 years after initial certification. *Ann Intern Med*. 2006;144:29–37.

36. Sutherland, K, Leatherman, S. Does certification improve medical standards? *BMJ*. 2006;333:439–41.

37. Hafferty, F. Measuring professionalism: a commentary. In Stern, DT, editor. *Measuring Medical Professionalism*. Oxford (UK): Oxford University Press; 2006:281–302.

38. Cruess, RL. Teaching professionalism: theory, principles, and practices. *Clin Orthop Relat Res*. 2006;449:177–85.

39. Cohen, JJ. Professionalism in medical education, an American perspective: from evidence to accountability. *Med Educ*. 2006;40(7):607–17.

40. Coulehan, J. Today's professionalism: engaging the mind but not the heart. *Acad Med*. 2005;80(10):892–8.

11 Educating the Public about Professionalism: From Rhetoric to Reality

Jordan J. Cohen, M.D., and Linda L. Blank

Professionalism has become something of a contemporary preoccupation. The public's persistent worry about professionals, often somewhat misleadingly described as concern about professional "ethics," is in fact a suspicion that professionals have broken faith with the public. Frequently, especially in popular journalism, the accusation is that professionals have abandoned the public; they have become self-protective and aloof from the significance of what they do.[1]

INTRODUCTION: FRAMING THE ISSUE

This book is devoted to the teaching and learning of medical professionalism. As is true of virtually all discussions of medical professionalism, its principal focus is on what individual physicians and the professional bodies composing organized medicine can and must do to sustain medical professionalism. So too was the focus of the physician *Charter,* which has been hailed appropriately as a milestone in the profession's efforts to fulfill its contract with society.[2,3] The *Charter* called on physicians to affirm three principles underlying professionalism – the primacy of patient interest, patient autonomy, and social justice – and laid out ten categories of responsibilities for physicians to discharge in actualizing those principles.

Clearly, the need for physicians, both individually and collectively, to understand the nature of professionalism, to exemplify the attributes and behaviors required to manifest professionalism, and to appreciate the contemporary threats to professionalism's continued survival cannot be overestimated. But its critical importance notwithstanding, such inwardly directed emphasis leaves unexamined the public's stake in medical professionalism and the role the public must play to ensure that it continues to obtain the benefits of professionalism. The value of educating the public about professionalism – and how we might go about doing so – is the focus of this chapter.

The Public's Stake in Medical Professionalism

Maintaining health and combating disease are among the most fundamental needs of any society. From the beginning of recorded history, all societies have vested much of the responsibility for addressing these needs in "healers," individuals with special knowledge and experience who were entrusted with (or assumed) the duty of forestalling ill health, treating the sick, and advancing community well-being.

As scientific knowledge and technologies evolved, the "healer" class became more empowered. The gap between the knowledge and skills of its members and that of the public widened significantly.[4,5] As a consequence, it became increasingly important to ensure that those in possession of specialized knowledge (e.g., physicians) used their expertise primarily in the interest of patients and the public, and not in pursuit of self-interest. Three methods have emerged for providing this critical assurance: 1) reliance on government supervision, the "regulatory" model; 2) reliance on market forces, the "commercial" model; and 3) reliance on a social contract, the "professionalism" model.[1,6]

The *regulatory* model assumes that a central, usually governmental authority can formulate standards of physician behavior and that conformity to those standards can be achieved through laws and regulations. The *commercial* model assumes that informed consumers operating in a competitive environment can exert discipline on physicians through their purchasing choices. The *professionalism* model assumes that neither government supervision nor the commercial market can anticipate the myriad opportunities physicians have for using their special expertise to advance their own interests over those of their patients and the public. Rather, this model assumes that the public's and patients' interests can be fully served only if physicians are committed to act on their own volition to subordinate their self-interest.

In today's developed countries, with their increasingly complex and costly health care systems, none of the three models has proven sufficient by itself to meet society's needs. Virtually every country has found that some combination of government oversight and free market conditions is necessary to gain the unique advantages of a well-functioning profession governed by a social contract.

The need for appropriate regulation and a measure of market discipline notwithstanding a health care system in which physicians are committed to the tenets of professionalism, and choose as a matter of principle to subordinate their self-interest to their patients' welfare, provide individual patients and the public at large with the greatest assurance of safe, effective, and compassionate care. No regulatory scheme or marketplace arrangement has the potential to provide comparable assurance of high quality, ethically sound health care. It is for this reason that the public has an abiding interest in seeing that professionalism prevails and that physicians remain dutiful to their professional responsibilities.

The Public's Role in Sustaining Professionalism

Many, if not most, of today's physicians practice in settings that thwart their ability to fully comply with their responsibilities to patients. Many of the impediments they face are so deeply imbedded in the structure of all health care systems that they are beyond the control of physicians, whether acting alone or collectively. Indeed, only those in a position to effect system-wide changes on behalf of the public (e.g., elected officials, ministers of heath) can eliminate these structural impediments. For example, neither individual physicians nor the medical profession as a whole can guarantee universal access to care, establish the information technology infrastructure and legal arrangements needed to support patient safety efforts and enable robust quality improvement activities, provide the financial and policy conditions necessary for effective medical education and research, create a financing scheme for the health care system that supports evidence-based decision making and discourages waste or fully safeguard patients and the public from the damaging effects of conflicts of interest.

Consequently, if the public is to continue to enjoy the unique benefits that medical professionalism can offer, it is not enough for physicians to understand the nature of professionalism and to be held accountable for meeting their professional responsibilities in the real world of medical practice. It is equally important for the public to understand their stake in medical professionalism and their essential role in eradicating the structural barriers impeding the profession's ability to fulfill its obligations.

EDUCATING THE PUBLIC ABOUT PROFESSIONALISM

The first issue to address here is what "public" is to be educated? As defined in *The Oxford Dictionary*, the "public" refers to "Ordinary people in general, the community; a section of the community with a shared interest or activity." Even more problematic, some argue that, "there is no such thing as 'the public',[rather] there are a hundred small segments of the public described as some general, assumed but unexamined, taken-for-granted notion . . . a vision grounded on fragmentary, anecdotal, estimated, guessed, projected or imagined evidence."[7] The ill-defined nature of "the public" notwithstanding, it is clear from the countless public opinion polls and patient satisfaction surveys about physicians' performance that concern about the profession of medicine is widespread among the general population.

It is not so clear, however, how to channel that concern into constructive activities in defense of medical professionalism. The key public audience to be made more aware of the value of medical professionalism, as noted above, is the policymaking community – elected officials, secretaries and ministers of health, legislative analysts, and others. These are the individuals who are in a position to address the existing barriers that frustrate individual physicians in their efforts to adhere to the tenets of professionalism. Unfortunately, the messages to be conveyed to policymakers can be easily misconstrued as being self-serving and, hence, easily rejected. Appeals by physicians – or by professional organizations on their behalf – to restructure the payment system, to invest in information systems, to modify professional liability laws, or to extend health insurance coverage to everyone are all examples of reforms that are needed to promote patient welfare and foster professionalism, but that can appear to the wary policymaker as attempts to promote narrow self-interest.

To overcome their natural wariness and prompt policymakers to implement the needed reforms will likely require efforts beyond those that can be mounted by the profession alone. Engaging patients and potential patients (i.e., the public) in a functional alliance with the medical profession would appear to offer the best hope.[8]

IN PREPARATION FOR EDUCATING THE PUBLIC

Before crafting effective strategies for educating the public, a better understanding of what the public presently perceives about medical professionalism would be advantageous. Toward this end, the Picker Institute Europe launched a comprehensive research program in 2004 that was designed to assess public expectations of doctors and the health care system for the purpose of establishing effective health policy and quality improvement programs in the United Kingdom and other European countries.[9] The institute's research entailed extensive surveys of members of the public and of physicians, and results of the three-year effort are scheduled for dissemination in late 2008. The US-based Picker Institute also has developed survey instruments to assess what patients desire and value from physicians and the health care system.[10] The Kaiser Family Foundation[11] and its Health08 Web site[12] offer yet another source of public polling data and analyses of health care issues.

These and similar initiatives are models of effective means whereby public awareness of the current state of medical professionalism could be assessed

Table 11.1. Strategies for educating the public

Harnessing the mini-med school
Engaging hospital-based programs
Utilizing professional and lay publications
Empowering public voices inside the profession
Enlisting professional organizations

and the public's understanding of their stake in preserving professionalism could be probed.

SPECIFIC STRATEGIES FOR EDUCATING THE PUBLIC

No single strategy is likely to suffice to educate the public about their stake in preserving medical professionalism. Rather, a variety of approaches will almost certainly be required to generate a functional alliance between the public and the medical profession sufficiently robust to convince policymakers to address the existing barriers that impede physicians' ability to adhere to their responsibilities as professionals. Among the reforms the envisioned alliance might effectively advocate are the following:[8]

- Ensure that all members of society have access to a basic set of preventive and medical services
- Provide the infrastructure necessary to foster improvement in the quality and safety of health care services
- Construct and maintain a medical liability system that encourages wide dissemination of lessons learned from medical errors
- Align payment systems with professional values and performance
- Provide adequate support for the education and training of physicians
- Provide adequate support for medical and health sciences research
- Recognize and minimize opportunities for conflicts of interests

These reforms could well be used as curricular elements for specific educational strategies designed to improve the public's understanding of professionalism.

Harnessing the Mini-Med School

The Mini-Med School concept was developed by John J. Cohen, M.D., Ph.D., in 1989 as a means to enhance the relationship between medical schools and their local communities. Mini-Med School curricula typically comprise a series of thematic lectures spread over several weeks during which faculty engage interested members of the public in open discussion of topics of interest. Since its inauguration at the University of Colorado Health Sciences Center, the Mini-Med School movement has expanded rapidly with sessions now held in at least thirty-four states and three countries under the sponsorship of over seventy medical schools, universities, research institutions, and hospitals.[13] Some 75,000 people attend one or more of these programs annually.

The Mini-Med School format would appear to be ideally suited for the purpose of examining components of medical professionalism from the public perspective. Mini-Med faculty lectures or expert panels could center on several professional responsibilities that could promote the desired medical-societal alliance; examples include:

- What does it take to educate and train a competent, caring doctor in the twenty-first century?
- Does the public have an advocacy role in garnering support (governmental/other) for pre- and postdoctoral medical education and for medical and health sciences research?
- How can the public and the profession partner to ensure that all members of society have access to basic preventive and medical services?
- Who should determine what services are essential?
- How can the public and the profession work together to convince policy-makers to fulfill this fundamental responsibility?

Engaging Hospital-Based Programs

Community hospitals have historically provided programs at which the public and the profession have opportunities to discuss matters of mutual interest. As with Mini-Med Schools, these programs are tailor made for addressing topics in professionalism. An existing example is the Institute of Medicine & Humanities, a joint program of St. Patrick Hospital and Health Sciences Center and the University of Montana, Missoula.[14] The purpose of the institute is to explore the interface between the humanities and medicine in order to better understand the human dimensions of health care. Formal programs (four Monday evenings for two to three hours) featuring panel discussions and an open conversational forum are scheduled twice yearly and integrate participants from the medical center, university, and community at large. A typical topic might be the roles of the public and the profession in recognizing and minimizing opportunities for conflicts of interest in health care delivery.

Utilizing Professional and Lay Publications

For well over a decade, the multiple challenges facing the health care systems in the United States, Canada, and other countries have been headlined in prominent medical journals, in international, national, and local news media, and increasingly in political and financial blogs. Although an erosion of medical professionalism is clearly among those challenges, it has received much less prominence – certainly in the popular media – than have more visible challenges (e.g., cost escalation, lack of universal health insurance, lapses in patient safety, uneven quality, health care disparities). With some notable exceptions, few voices have been raised within public ear shot about the dangers lurking should professionalism continue to erode.[15–17]

Medical journals have an important role to play but can only do so much by way of public education. Newspapers and other lay publications are obviously better positioned to take on this responsibility but need more dogged encouragement by individual physicians and the professional organizations that represent them. A concerted campaign to pepper local newspapers with op-ed pieces and letters to the editor should be considered. Petitions to appear on National Public Radio, National Public Television, and other cable networks should be filed. Utilizing existing or newly created blogs is yet another possible strategy by which to reach a wider public.

Empowering Public Voices Inside the Profession

Myriad organizations within medicine have governing boards and/or advisory groups that include prominent members of the public. Such individuals are especially well positioned to be conduits of information and aspiration on behalf of the profession to the larger public. Much could be gained directly and indirectly by engaging governing and advisory bodies of hospitals, academic medical centers, research institutes, specialty societies, professional associations, certifying boards, and the like in candid discussions about the challenges that physicians face in sustaining their commitment to professionalism.

Enlisting Professional Organizations

Physician-based professional associations and societies could greatly assist the public education effort by utilizing their national meetings and other venues to showcase and discuss civic professionalism.[18] By impressing on their membership, the need for a public/profession partnership to preserve professionalism and by energizing their membership to communicate with their patients and with their social networks, a grassroots effort toward needed reforms might be ignited.[18–21]

SUMMARY

The importance of educating medical students, residents, and practitioners about the critical role of professionalism in maintaining public trust in the profession cannot be overestimated. Ensuring that future and current members of the profession understand and remain committed to their multiple responsibilities in service to professionalism is a key objective of all medical educators. No single lesson is more fundamental for the good physician to learn than the need to subordinate self-interest in adhering to the primacy of patients' interest.

Many aspects of contemporary medical practice, however, pose substantial barriers to the full expression of professionalism, barriers that are simply beyond the control of individual physicians, and even of the profession as a whole. Convincing policymakers to implement reforms that can overcome these barriers will require a strong alliance between the profession and the public. Crafting that alliance, in turn, will require a public that is better informed about its stake in maintaining medical professionalism, a stake that derives from the realization that physicians acting on their own volition to maintain the primacy of patients' interest affords the public unique protections from the vicissitudes of twenty-first century medicine.

Educating the public about their stake in medical professionalism is a tall order and requires much more than rhetoric. It will require the reality and rigor of multiple strategies implemented over a long time and the concerted effort of the entire profession.

REFERENCES

1. Sullivan, WM. *Work and Integrity: The Crisis and Promise of Professionalism in America.* 2nd ed. San Francisco: Jossey Bass; 2005.
2. ABIM Foundation, ACP-ASIM Foundation, European Federation of Internal Medicine. Medical professionalism in the new millennium: a physician charter. *Ann Intern Med.* 2002;136:243–246.
3. Medical Professionalism Project. Medical professionalism in the new millennium: physicians' charter. *Lancet.* 2002;359:530–532.
4. Starr, P. *The Social Transformation of American Medicine.* New York: Basic Books; 1982.
5. Krause, E. *Death of the Guilds: Professions, States and the Advance of Capitalism, 1930 to the Present.* New Haven: Yale University Press; 1996.

6. Freidson, E. *Professionalism: The Third Logic.* Chicago: University of Chicago Press; 2001.

7. Smelser, NJ. Constituency perspectives: patients and the public. ABIM Summer Conference Report. Philadelphia: American Board of Internal Medicine; 1997.

8. Cohen, JJ, Cruess, S, Davidson, C. Alliance between society and medicine: the public's stake in medical professionalism. *JAMA.* 2007;298:670–673.

9. www.pickereurope.org. <accessed April 23, 2008>

10. www.pickerinstitute.org. <accessed April 23, 2008>

11. www.kff.org. <accessed April 23, 2008>

12. www.health08.org. <accessed April 23, 2008>

13. www.science.education.nih.gov/home2.nsf/index.htm. <accessed April 23, 2008>

14. www.saintpatrick.org. <see Education and Research for Institute of Medicine and Humanities, accessed April 23, 2008>

15. Relman, AS. Medical professionalism in a commercialized health care market. *JAMA.* 2007;298:2668–2670.

16. Sox, HC. Medical professionalism and the parable of the craft guilds. *Ann Intern Med.* 2007;147:809–810.

17. Sox, HC. The ethical foundations of professionalism: a sociologic history. *Chest.* 2007;131:1532–1540.

18. Gruen, RL, Pearson, SD, Brennan, TA. Physician-citizens – public roles and professional obligations. *JAMA.* 2004;291:94–98.

19. Gruen, RL, Blumenthal, D, Campbell, EC. Public roles of US physicians: community participation, political involvement and collective advocacy. *JAMA.* 2006;296:2467–2475.

20. Sullivan, W, Benner, P. Challenges to professionalism: work integrity and the call to renew and strengthen the social contract of the professions. *Am J Crit Care.* 2005;14:78–84.

21. Larson, EB. Physicians should be civic professionals, not just knowledge workers. *Am J Med.* 2007;120:1005–1009.

PART FOUR

Practice: Case Studies in Teaching
Professionalism across the Continuum

12 Teaching Professionalism in a Traditional or Organ-Based Curriculum

Erika Goldstein, M.D.

INTRODUCTION

Defining and understanding professionalism in medicine is a challenging undertaking. Translating that definition and understanding into the complex world of medical education is even more challenging. My goal in this chapter is to describe how these challenges are addressed in the setting of a traditional, or organ-based, medical school curriculum at the University of Washington School of Medicine (UWSOM).

Well into the UWSOM faculty's work on introducing medical professionalism into the curriculum, we became aware of the debate among medical education experts working in the field of professionalism between those who emphasize a didactic approach focusing on definitions and a specific knowledge base and those who emphasize narrative and experiential learning.[1–3] Interestingly, through our work in developing and implementing a curriculum on professionalism, we have found it necessary to intertwine these two approaches as we attempt to create a successful curriculum. The theoretical debates between the two schools of thought both helped us to understand what we were already doing and to become more deliberate as we moved the professionalism curriculum forward. A merging of these two threads appears to be consistent with the direction this debate is taking for others as well.[4]

Another interesting aspect of the complex undertaking involved in teaching medical professionalism became apparent in the course of our work. We learned that it is important to focus on an "aspirational" approach to professionalism in teaching this material. That approach means that, regardless of level of training or practice, we are all – students, trainees, teachers – involved in, and must work continuously toward honing, refining, and enhancing our medical professionalism. To expect perfection or to pinpoint the needs or shortcomings of any specific level of training or professional activity runs the risk of alienation; conversely, an inclusive, aspirational approach introduces commonality and acknowledges that professionalism is difficult for everybody yet is critical as a goal. Thus, we took the approach of focusing on "continuous professional improvement" within our teaching and stated approach and thereby moved beyond undergraduate medical education and graduate medical education into the area of reinvigorating medical professionalism throughout our institutional culture.[5]

UWSOM STRUCTURE

The UWSOM curriculum is organized into a traditional sequence of two years of preclinical training followed by two years of clinical training. The first year consists of discipline-based, basic science courses, and the second year consists of organ system courses. The third year comprises six basic clerkships, each of which is six weeks in length (with the exception of internal medicine, which is twelve weeks). The fourth year includes several required four-week clerkships (neurology, emergency medicine, surgical subspecialties, and chronic care) as well as two- and four-week elective rotations, culminating in a capstone course at the end of the fourth year that focuses on preparing students for internship.

The two preclinical Introduction to Clinical Medicine courses, ICM I in year one and ICM II in year two, run continuously throughout the first two years and focus on training students in basic clinical skills and professionalism. In addition, a single-quarter problem-based learning (PBL) course within the second year attempts to integrate some of the basic science material in organ system courses taught at the same time. Standardized patients (SPs) are used in both the first and the second year ICM curriculum for teaching purposes, both in developing general interviewing skills and in specific content areas (e.g., alcohol and substance use history, sexual history, and working with interpreters). All students participate in formative and summative objective structured clinical examinations (OSCE) at the end of second year and again at the beginning of fourth year.

Two unique features of the UWSOM have widespread implications for our curriculum and for our training in professionalism. First, the UWSOM is the only medical school in the five-state region of Washington, Wyoming, Alaska, Montana, and Idaho (WWAMI) and serves as the regional medical school for all these states. The primary component of the WWAMI program consists of offering the first-year curriculum at five different state university sites. Approximately 100 students complete their first year in Seattle, Washington; 16 Wyoming resident students complete their first year in Laramie, Wyoming; 20 Alaska resident students in Anchorage, Alaska; 20 Montana resident students in Bozeman, Montana; and 20 Idaho resident students and 20 additional

Washington resident students complete their first year at a combined site in two border cities several miles apart in Moscow, Idaho, and Pullman, Washington. In addition, all students can complete a portion of their third- and fourth-year clerkships in training sites across the five-state region.[6] There is considerable variation in the number of clerkships that individual students complete at WWAMI sites; some students complete most of their clerkships at regional sites and some complete most in Seattle. In addition, through the WWAMI Rural Integrated Training Experience Program, 10–12 students with strong interest in rural primary care have the opportunity to complete some of their required clerkships early in the third year and then spend five months in a single rural community with a family medicine preceptor where they complete the remainder of their core clerkships in an integrated fashion.

The second unique feature of the UWSOM is its "Colleges Program."[7,8] This program, which began with the entering class of 2001, started with thirty faculty members who are divided into five Colleges, with six faculty in each College. One of the faculty in each College serves as the College head. Each College faculty member mentors a cadre of 24–30 students spread across the four years of the student curriculum. Upon matriculation, each student is assigned to a College and, within that College, to a faculty member. That faculty member serves as the student's mentor throughout his/her tenure at the UWSOM. In addition, the ICM II course in the second year is taught by College faculty members. This involves weekly bedside teaching sessions with the mentors' six second-year students, as well as classroom teaching from the entire College faculty and others.

The emphasis in the ICM II course is on teaching and honing advanced skills in medical interviewing and physical examination, written documentation, oral case presentations, clinical reasoning, and professionalism and ethics. In the course of the year, each student performs a comprehensive history and physical examination on six patients in the presence of and under the guidance of the College mentor. The students then present the patients they interviewed and examined to their small group at the bedside and also complete a write-up on their patient. The write-up is submitted to the students' electronic learning portfolio and is reviewed, with extensive feedback, by their mentors. College faculty also provide mentoring for students outside of the hospital experience through classroom experiences, College-specific activities, peer advising sessions, individual mentoring sessions, and small-group social gatherings throughout the year. After second year is completed, College faculty continue to support and mentor their students throughout the third and fourth years of the curriculum by means of email contact, telephone calls, individual counseling and advising sessions, peer advising, and all-College meetings and social gatherings.[7]

The College faculty are responsible for collaborating with other faculty throughout the medical school to create and deliver a four-year integrated curriculum in clinical skills and professionalism. Our approach is to teach these skills in a "spiral development" fashion, introducing many of the skills in the first-year ICM course and then adding increasing complexity as the students move through the four years of training.[9] Through this iterative process, topics initially introduced early in the first year are revisited later in first year and then in second, third, and fourth years with increasing complex but developmentally appropriate goals for learning. We are working toward developing specific "benchmarks" for each level of training in each competency area – interviewing, physical exam (broken down into specific organ system exams), medical documentation, oral case presentations, and clinical reasoning – in addition to professionalism and ethics. The College faculty are responsible for developing and delivering that curriculum in the ICM II course and work with other faculty in developing other curricular elements.

TEACHING PROFESSIONALISM

Preclinical Curriculum

Training in professionalism begins at the first-year student orientation with several group exercises that focus on the professional development of physicians. One session, for example, involves sharing with students the definition of professionalism and its specific elements that have been adopted at the UWSOM. The definition of professionalism we have adopted is that put forth by Arnold and Stern: "Professionalism is demonstrated through a foundation of clinical competence, communication skills, and ethical understanding, upon which is built the aspirations to and wise application of the principles of professionalism."[10] We further delineate seven specific professional values that the College faculty have defined more specifically: The professional values that we have identified to seek to live out and demonstrate to others include:

1. Altruism
2. Honor and integrity
3. Caring, compassion, and communication
4. Respect
5. Responsibility and accountability
6. Excellence and scholarship
7. Leadership

A second session involves analyzing the meaning of each line of the Hippocratic Oath (at our medical school we use a slightly modified version of the Geneva version of the Hippocratic Oath). In this exercise, students work in small groups to discuss their assigned line from the oath in terms of what it means for physicians, for medical students, and for the public at large. The students then present a summary of their small-group discussion to the entire group. In another exercise, students, working in small groups, draw a composite picture of the "ideal physician." They then present their drawing to the large group, explaining the significance of the various aspects of their drawing.

ICM I

Once the formal curriculum begins, much of the teaching about professionalism in the first year is within the ICM I course. This includes didactic components, reflections on experiences in both large- and small-group settings, and patient interviews. Each student also completes at least one quarter- or semester-long preceptorship in first year, working with a clinician in his/her practice setting for one morning a week. Students shadow the physician during patient clinic visits and/or hospital rounds, and the preceptor provides informal instruction. These activities occur both in Seattle and at the various WWAMI first-year sites, with some site-based variation.

A central goal of the ICM I course is to introduce students to the medical interview. Students begin interviewing hospitalized patients in their second week of school, initially obtaining the social history and adding additional aspects of the complete medical database over the course of the year. A major focus in ICM I is teaching students patient-centered interviewing. We start with a focus on the patient's illness experience and then, over the course of the first quarter or semester, show how the patient's illness narrative is gathered by the interviewer and transformed into the medical story of the history of present illness, or HPI. We emphasize to the students the importance of remaining mindful of the patient's narrative and experience even as they must reshape it into a medical narrative.

All of the teaching of patient-centered medical interviewing and doctor-patient communication is infused with elements related to professionalism, which are addressed explicitly within lecture presentations as well as small-group discussions. For example, after teaching basic interviewing skills and after the students have conducted several interviews on their own, we hold a large-group session on "difficult questions." In this session, we emphasize 1) the importance of sensitivity to and respect for those areas that the patient might find difficult yet which we do not and 2) the importance of understanding our own discomfort with certain areas and learning to address these areas in a way that is caring and respectful of patient's values and needs in a nonjudgmental fashion.

In addition to teaching interviewing, a number of other topics related to medical professionalism are introduced in the ICM I course. These include discussions of medical ethics, diversity (both among patients and among colleagues), continuity of care and what that means for patients and physicians, asking "difficult questions" (described above), dealing with difficult interview situations, dealing with controversial topics in which there appear to be values differences between physicians and patients or between physician colleagues, the patient's view of their experience of interactions with physicians and with the health care system, and the role of the physician's personal affective responses in the care of patients. These sessions each has readings and specifically articulated goals.

A number of these topics are presented through role-plays and large-group discussions followed by small-group discussions. This format is used for dealing with controversial topics and for understanding the role of the physicians' affective responses. Other topics, such as patients' experiences of the health care system, are presented with panel discussions or patient interviews. For other sessions, such as the session on diversity in health care, students present their own reflective writing, followed by discussion. Important elements of professionalism are interwoven into the topic presentations, such as interviewing patients about alcohol and substance use, care of patients with disabilities, care of sexual minorities, and cross-cultural medicine.

Students also meet weekly in small groups with the same two faculty leaders throughout the year to discuss issues that arise in their interviews and preceptorship experiences, as well as material covered in the large-group lectures (and at the smaller first-year WWAMI sites, with the entire group, which is small in size). In addition, students are asked to read several essays in association with their preceptorship and to complete three written reflections that focus on a continuity curriculum. One is based on their preceptor's thoughts about continuity; the second focuses on a discussion with a patient concerning his/her experience of continuity; and the third is a self-reflection of their own or a family member's experience of continuity of care.

Self-reflection and its role in professional development and practice for physicians is a theme throughout ICM I and II. The topic of continuity is the students' first explicit reflection "assignment." The students also write reflections on a visit to a skilled nursing facility in their first year. Other written reflections related to self-care, balance, and burnout may be added to the first-year curriculum in the future.

ICM II

Since all students spend their second year in Seattle, the ICM II course brings all the students together for a common experience. The ICM II course is taught by the College faculty. The continuation of the course, as in first year, focuses on development of clinical skills and professionalism.

The year begins with a discussion of two elements of professionalism. One is the set of expectations the College faculty have for student behavior and performance in the ICM II course. The second is the UWSOM definition of professionalism and its specific components. These are presented to the students in the form of benchmarks for professionalism (clear statements about what the students are expected to master). Course expectations and the professionalism benchmarks are presented in the first small-group session of the second year when each small group of six students and their faculty mentor meets for the first time. The College faculty worked together as a group to develop an approach to presenting the introductory material on both these elements of professionalism.

For the College faculty, there is a clear connection between ICM course expectations and the professionalism benchmarks. Over time, however, we have learned the importance of separating the two and addressing them somewhat differently in order to avoid student perception of a rule-based approach to professionalism that is delivered by those who "have it" to those who don't. ICM course expectations for professional behavior include punctuality, respect for patients and colleagues, confidentiality, and appropriate dress. The professionalism benchmarks are somewhat more complex and include definitions of the seven domains of professionalism adopted by the UWSOM, and examples of what these look like in operational terms for medical students in the preclinical curriculum. The professionalism benchmarks can be found on the UWSOM Colleges Web site (http://courses.washington.edu/colleges).

Benchmarks for ethics are presented separately to students. These benchmarks include a core ethical knowledge base and an approach to ethical problem solving that is introduced in a large lecture format. After the lecture, students participate in an ethics exercise formally analyzing an ethics "case" from their own experiences and discussing the cases in small groups.

Didactic sessions in large-group settings throughout the second year include presentations, physician and patient panels, and discussions concurrent with small-group discussions and self-reflections shared with mentors and with colleagues. Large-group sessions cover a number of topics, including the challenge of maintaining balance and clarity of values throughout training and practice, uncertainty and mistakes in medicine, and caring for patients with life-threatening and terminal illness. Students prepare written reflections related to the topic for each session, sharing their reflections with their mentor through electronic portfolios and also discussing them within the small-group setting.

Much of the teaching of professionalism in ICM II occurs interactively within weekly morning teaching sessions in hospitals. As described above, the groups of six students with their College mentor work at the bedside, learning and practicing clinical skills (history taking, physical exam, oral case presentation, clinical reasoning). At the bedside, students have many opportunities to experience and learn about professionalism issues in "real time" through their own experiences with patients, observing patients interact with their mentors, and observing fellow students, other faculty, residents, students, nurses, and staff interact with patients and family members. Patients share powerful stories with students and small groups, including what it means to cope with serious illness or face a terminal diagnosis, challenges in dealing with the medical system, and issues of poverty, homelessness, and/or mental illness. These situations provide excellent opportunities for discussion of professionalism issues in the context of real-life experience. Every bedside interaction ends with the mentor asking the patient to tell the small group of students "what makes a good doctor?" These are often very moving moments and are undoubtedly among the most powerful learning experiences in professionalism that the students experience up to that point in their training.

Professionalism Working Group

The Colleges have a number of "working groups" that address specific areas of student development and teaching, such as mentoring, clinical reasoning, physical examination. The teaching of professionalism in the second year, and, more broadly, throughout the undergraduate curriculum, has been coordinated by the Colleges' professionalism working group. This working group, composed of College faculty and other faculty involved in ethics and professionalism at our institution, is one of the most active of the College faculty working groups.

In the first several years of the College curriculum, the professionalism working group addressed an interesting challenge to professionalism that may resonate with faculty at other schools: the challenge of second-year medical students' negative reaction to "the P-word" (referring to the use of the word "professionalism"). Initially, it appeared that our approach to professionalism was too far removed from the students' experience. This growing understanding resulted from student responses and comments on end-of-year surveys and exit interviews completed for evaluation purposes.

Professionalism, or the "P-word," was perceived as consisting of self-evident platitudes about physician behavior that were thought by the students to be too vague and obvious to be of any meaning. When faculty became aware of these reactions among students, they worked to bring professionalism closer to the lives of students and talk about what constitutes professional behavior for medical students. In the process, we perhaps swung the pendulum too far to the other direction. Students began to perceive the professionalism curriculum as a series of rules that we (the faculty), who "had" professionalism, were imparting to them (the students), who did not "have it."

In response to the students' negative reactions to both approaches, the professionalism working group convened a "student advisory group," consisting of first- and second-year students in leadership roles at the medical school with an interest in professionalism. During discussion sessions, these students indicated that they learned best from the stories that preceptors and faculty mentors share with them concerning the faculty's own clinical experiences. The students recommended that the working group gather stories from the College faculty about challenges they had experienced to their own professionalism. As a result of this set of recommendations from students, each College mentor was asked to provide two brief clinical stories, or vignettes, to the working group that were meaningful to them in terms of experiences relevant to professionalism with patients, both positive or negative, successes and failures. The resulting sixty short vignettes written by College faculty were edited to remove identifying information and then were shared with the student advisory group. These vignettes range from one sentence to several paragraphs in length. They cover experiences that faculty had as residents, as attending physicians, and in their practices, and include experiences with both patients and colleagues.

When the students were asked to select the best of these vignettes for use in teaching sessions, they suggested that the faculty should share *all* of the stories – that all of the stories were meaningful and helpful. These vignettes have since become the basis for several small-group teaching sessions throughout the year between mentors and their small groups.

The strong reaction to the P-word seems to be waning somewhat, perhaps as a result of the fact that we have shared with students our own challenges with professionalism. Discussion and reflection on these challenges let students know that the faculty are remarkably similar to students in facing ongoing professionalism challenges. We have previously described this process in more detail and with specific examples.[11] Despite some improvement in student responses to this curriculum, we recognize that we still have a long way to go. This process of creating a curriculum, assessing the students' response, re-examining the curriculum and its goals with student input, revising the curriculum, and reassessing the students' response is an early example of the "continuous professionalism improvement" approach described above.[5]

At the end of second year, students complete a series of formative and summative OSCEs, one of which is a professionalism case. Students also participate in a "transition to the clerkships" series after their second-year classes are completed. This series addresses several professionalism topics, including professional boundaries, physician burnout and impairment, medicine and the law, and working in the health care team. The second year ends with a "clinical transition ceremony." During this formal ceremony, emphasizing the professional transition and attended by families, friends, and other teachers, students receive white coats from their mentors.

Clinical Curriculum

Working on professionalism in the clinical curriculum remains one of the faculty's greatest challenges. In past years, students had the opportunity to participate in "ward ethics" sessions during selected third-year clerkships.[12] These sessions involved bringing students on their medicine or surgery rotations together with one or two faculty facilitators who were not involved in their current clerkship for a discussion of professional and ethical challenges they observed or experienced. These sessions varied widely in the number of participants and topics covered. We hope to re-institute these sessions with some modifications in the near future.

College faculty have also been working actively with directors of the required clerkships in third and fourth year to move the developmental clinical skills and professionalism curriculum into clinical training in a consistent manner. Each required clerkship director is paired with a College faculty liaison from the same clinical department with whom to work. For the past three years, combined clerkship and College liaison faculty have met once or twice a year for day-long retreats. During the retreats, clerkship directors and selected faculty work with College liaison faculty on a variety of areas related to advancing the developmental curriculum and assessing student performance. Each clerkship has created a "mini-CEX" for teaching and assessing a specific clinical skill. A similar model is being developed for "professionalism CEXs" but has not yet been enacted. The overall long-term goal is to have each basic clerkship identify one or more specific areas of professionalism appropriate to their specialty for which they will create a set of benchmark expectations, with a curriculum and a mini-CEX appropriate to the content. It is hoped that each of these will include a topic and assignment for a written reflection that can be shared with College mentors as they follow their students through clinical training.

Other areas of collaborative work between clerkship directors and Colleges faculty have included developing standards for assessing professionalism and developing professionalism OSCE cases for the OSCEs that students are required to complete at the start of their fourth year. The intent is to base these stations on the professionalism benchmarks and curriculum being created and taught within the clerkships. Professionalism topics are also continuously developed and revised for the capstone course that students participate in at the end of their fourth year immediately prior to graduation.

In addition to the activities described above, the College professionalism working group has been working with the clerkship directors on all these areas. To facilitate this dialogue, the working group has developed a grid for the seven domains of professionalism across the developmental continuum of undergraduate training. This document has been a source of ongoing dialogue and has been refined as work continues with the clerkship faculty to integrate training in these areas into the clinical curriculum and as we continue work in the preclinical curriculum.

Overarching Curriculum Components

While a major component of College activities occur in the context of teaching ICM II in the second-year curriculum, mentors continue to serve in a supporting and coaching role throughout their students' medical education. They provide critical academic and professional support to students and are an important resource as students encounter challenging personal and professional issues. Further opportunities to enhance contact around these issues are being developed through dialogue and reflection exercises in all four years of the curriculum.

OSCEs in second year and fourth year are central to teaching and evaluation of students. OSCE cases include material from the professionalism curriculum and we continue to work at improving the connection between the professionalism benchmarks and curriculum that supports it and the evaluation of students' mastery of that content. Similarly, we continue to work on integrating the professionalism curriculum into the major "transitions" in undergraduate medical education: the transition to clinical training at the end of the second year and the transition to residency training at the end of the fourth year in the capstone course.

Other Components

The College's professionalism working group has evolved from a group that focuses strictly on the ICM professionalism curriculum to one that plays an active role in integrating professionalism across the four-year undergraduate medical education curriculum. The group uses the same model of "spiral development" that we use in integrating all our clinical skills training throughout our medical school curriculum. In addition, the professionalism working group actively collaborates with our graduate medical education programs and links the work in the undergraduate curriculum to residency training. They have also begun to play an increasingly important role in faculty development related to teaching and modeling professionalism.

Another component of work in the area of professionalism is in an initiative launched by a group of College faculty and staff that focuses on "patients as teachers." This initiative involves eliciting feedback from patients about our ICM I and II programs and curricula, as well as providing opportunities for patients to give feedback to individual students. One of the initiative's intentions is to empower patients to understand their important role as teachers of medical students and to help students understand the role that patients play in teaching and guiding them. This process has been extremely beneficial in providing information regarding professional development from a very important constituency.

The area of feedback and evaluation on professional development has been an ongoing challenge. Our work in defining developmental benchmarks has been very helpful in creating feedback and evaluation tools for our first- and second-year ICM courses. Work is ongoing in developing uniform feedback and evaluation for students regarding professionalism in the clinical clerkships. In addition, a system of "professionalism incident reporting" is being planned across the four-year curriculum to provide opportunities for faculty, staff, and peers to formally document breaches of professionalism independent of other aspects of academic performance. We also hope to implement a mechanism soon for giving students opportunities to provide feedback on both instances of exemplary professionalism and breaches of professional behavior they observe and experience among residents, faculty, and staff throughout their training.

All professionalism training takes place within the overarching environment and culture of our institution as a whole. Our institution-wide continuous professionalism improvement efforts provide an important backdrop for our efforts within undergraduate medical education. The lessons we have learned have been and will continue to be of use to those broader efforts. In turn, the institution-wide emphasis on professionalism helps our efforts within undergraduate education by sending a very important message to students that professionalism is an ongoing aspirational goal for all physicians at all levels of training and practice. The ultimate goal is that students not have one set of expectations, while residents, faculty, and staff have a different set of expectations.

Lessons Learned

The primary lessons we have learned in teaching professionalism in an undergraduate curriculum thus far have been threefold. The first is the importance of weaving the teaching of professionalism throughout the curriculum in a developmental fashion that incorporates didactic components, with definitions and explicit skills training, and opportunities for experiential learning and reflection.

The second lesson is the importance of providing examples of professionalism for students that include both situations that are immediate to the students' level of training – what does it mean to be professional as a first-year student, a second-year student, a clinical student – and situations that will be meaningful and important in residency and in practice beyond. Using only examples from the former can leave the students feeling that these are "trivial" and not connected to the important questions they will be facing. Using only examples from the latter may make the students feel that the issues of professionalism are not of concern to them now and that the issues are only important "later" when they are in practice.

Finally, we have learned the importance of placing all of this within the broader cultural context of the institution as a whole. Inherent in this lesson is the importance of faculty development in continuing to teach professionalism throughout undergraduate medical education. This means explicitly addressing the existence and influence of the "hidden curriculum" and including residents and fellows in faculty development. It also means speaking explicitly about the aspirational nature of efforts to improve the culture of professionalism in our institution as a whole.

In many very clear ways, the efforts and energy spent teaching professionalism in undergraduate medical education at our institution have been a driving force behind these broader efforts at an institutional level. The undergraduate professionalism curriculum and approach is meaningless without an institution-wide focus, and vice versa.

REFERENCES

1. Huddle, TS; Accreditation Council for Graduate Medical Education (ACGME). Viewpoint: teaching professionalism: is medical morality a competency? *Acad Med*. 2005;80(10):885–91.
2. Coulehan, J. Viewpoint: today's professionalism: engaging the mind but not the heart. *Acad Med*. 2005;80(10):892–8.
3. Cruess, RL, Cruess, SR. Teaching medicine as a profession in the service of healing. *Acad Med*. 1997;72(11):941–52.

4. Cruess, RL, Cruess, SR. Teaching professionalism: general principles. *Med Teach*. 2006;28(3):205–8.

5. Fryer-Edwards, K, Van Eaton, E, Goldstein, EA, Kimball, HR, Veith, RC, Pellegrini, CA, Ramsey, PG. Overcoming institutional challenges through continuous professionalism improvement. *Acad Med*, 2007;82:1073–1078.

6. Ramsey, PG, Coombs, JB, Hunt, DD, Marshall, SG, Wenrich, MD. From concept to culture: the WWAMI program at the University of Washington School of Medicine. *Acad Med*. 2001;76(8):765–75.

7. Goldstein, EA, Maclaren, CF, Smith, S, Mengert, TJ, Maestas, RR, Foy, HM, Wenrich, MD, Ramsey, PG. Promoting fundamental clinical skills: a competency-based college approach at the University of Washington. *Acad Med*. 2005;80(5):423–33.

8. Whipple, ME, Barlow, CB, Smith, S, Goldstein, EA. Early introduction of clinical skills improves medical student comfort at the start of third-year clerkships. *Acad Med*. 2006;81(10 Suppl.):S40–3.

9. Harden, RM, Stamper, N. What is a spiral curriculum?. *Med Teacher*. 1999; 21(2):141–3.

10. Arnold, L, Stern, DT. "What is medical professionalism?" In Stern, DT, editor. *Measuring Medical Professionalism*. New York, NY: Oxford University Press;2006; page 19.

11. Goldstein, EA, Maestas, RR, Fryer-Edwards, K, Wenrich, MD, Amies-Oelschlager, AM, Baernstein, A, Kimball, HR. Professionalism in medical education: an institutional challenge. *Acad Med*. 2006;81(10):871–6.

12. Fryer-Edwards, K, Wilkins, MD, Baernstein, A, Braddock, CH. Bringing ethics education to the clinical years: ward ethics sessions at the University of Washington. *Acad Med*. 2006;81(7):626–31.

13 Learning Professionalism in a Problem-Based Curriculum

Gillian Maudsley, M.B.Ch.B., M.P.H. (dist.), M.Ed. (dist.), M.D., and Rev. David C.M. Taylor, B.Sc., M.Ed., Ph.D.

"There is responsibility now. What happens in the next five years will shape my attitude to medicine. Before there was little need for memory to last longer than the end of an exam – this is no longer true."

"Learning to be a doctor may not be just an academic challenge but also a social challenge where other important skills, such as communication skills must be mastered."

"– no one to tell you what to do.
a lot of pressure to get things right
it's not just a question of learning material for marks but you have to know the material, understand and be able to apply it. Tests more than just knowledge but strength of character and communication skills."

> Year 1 Liverpool medical students (1999 entrants) describing how
> they think that "learning to be a doctor" might differ from their
> experience as a learner at school/college[1]

BACKGROUND

Medical students are likely to perceive many pressures to develop their professional persona. A few examples illustrated above are:

- Learning for the purposes of being the best possible doctor (rather than merely to survive the next examination);
- Learning beyond mere recall of bioscience facts;
- Becoming socially adept for medicine;
- Developing appropriate attitudes;
- Taking responsibility for own learning and practice;

We thank the students who have contributed, over the years of this curriculum, their ideas, and efforts to the educational research and to the routine in-curriculum evaluations that have informed this overview.

- Knowing how to "get things right"; and
- Building "a strong character."

Curricula whose philosophical focus is on learning rather than teaching do still need to provide very clear signposting, triggers, and opportunities to learn how to assume a well-measured medical mantle. The longstanding Liverpool undergraduate medical curriculum underwent a comprehensive transformation to a problem-based curriculum in 1996, underpinned by a wholesale shift in educational philosophy, design, and implementation. This included a more systematic and explicit approach to promoting professionalism. Over a decade later, it is timely to reflect on how this aspiration has fared. This is especially so with the concept of medical "professionalism" (and whether it is "caught or taught") regularly featuring prominently[2] in medical education debate, such that different expressions of its core attributes[3] abound.

The formal notions of professionalism underpinning the 1996 Liverpool redesign echoed General Medical Council requirements about being self-critical, good as a team player, ethically instinctive, responsive to change in a constructive way, and committed to advancing the art and science of medical practice and to lifelong learning. The General Medical Council's "Duties of a Doctor" have remained in the forefront since the outset,[4] and the ethical principles for guiding clinical decision making were made explicit,[5,6] with an ethicist now leading the ethics input to PBL (problem-based learning) scenarios and assessments.

The best laid plans are, however, vulnerable to the vagaries of changing policy priorities, drifting implementation, and, inevitably, the hidden curriculum, that is, "customs, rituals, and taken-for-granted aspects"[7(p404)] that influence what students learn in formal and informal settings. This includes the informal curriculum conveyed by interpersonal communication,[8] that is, by word of mouth from peers and staff in the "corridors" of learning and clinical practice rather than the "classrooms" or "clinic."

In its "moral and symbolic transformation of a lay person …,"[9(p135)] professionalization will convey a particular version of "how to be a good doctor."[10(p205)] Indeed, each student will undergo an individual professionalization journey, overlapping closely with the journeys of peers in the same curriculum. How medical students conceptualize professional practice could also be viewed by borrowing Cornwell's concepts of health beliefs, where people present "public accounts" (the socially approved versions of reality) and "private accounts" (the individual versions of reality that arise from personal experience).[11]

In a problem-based curriculum, the reliance on subtle triggers and conducive conditions (rather than on heavy contact time, formal "instruction," and structure) would suggest greater opportunities for diversity of experience and, in particular, greater reliance on the informal curriculum. Given that "part of the potency of the hidden curriculum is that it is unwritten and largely un-discussed,"[12(p58)] if a problem-based philosophy is working well, it should be focusing on what is being *learnt* rather than taught[8] and on challenging assumptions via small-group discussion. While recognizing that attempts to formalize the informal can be counterproductive, educators should be able to facilitate an incremental uncovering of key "hidden" assumptions about medical professionalism throughout the problem-based curriculum.

This chapter sets out to reflect on how students learn professionalism ("professional quality, character, or conduct"[13]) in a problem-based curriculum, how it is assessed, and lessons learnt from its implementation, with reference to local research evidence.

THE CONTEXT

The context within which students socialize into the professional role conveys official cues about the key features of good medical practice and unofficial cues about alternative and complementary norms. The way in which professionalism is assumed will relate to characteristics of the curriculum, its participants, and the political, policy, and practice setting. In the Liverpool five-year curriculum, well over three quarters of entrants are eighteen to twenty-one years and entering directly from school, which has particular implications for induction into active learning in higher education. Plans for the "problem-based" system adopted from 1996 incorporated and informed responses to the General Medical Council recommendations of the time,[14,15] resulting in key features that supported progressive acquisition of professionalism.

Using a problem-based system meant a "problem-first" learning philosophy.[16] This included problem-based learning as the main way of acquiring the knowledge base, that is, relying heavily on self-directed generation of learning objectives from "problem" scenarios, typically studied in three 2-hour sessions per fortnight, facilitated by a tutor. This focused on "LIVER-pool" goals[17] (rooted in Maastricht's Seven Steps[18]):

- *L*ook for phenomena requiring explanation
- *I*nvestigate prior knowledge and experience
- *V*olunteer shared learning objectives
- *E*xplain the essence of the case scenario
- *R*eflect and evaluate.

In this system, PBL was only one of the core elements, but other activities had to complement and not distract from the self-motivated learning ethos.

Such features supported the professional requirements of, for example, self-motivation, small-group work, collaborating, rehearsing lifelong learning skills, critically analyzing evidence and decision making, acknowledging uncertainty and limits in their understanding, coping with changing knowledge and context, viewing staff as facilitators, managing their own time in sessions, and self-evaluating progress. Personal development was also promoted in challenging and defending assumptions uncovered in group discussion (and in developing a professional identity in a group).

Integrating core knowledge into four curriculum themes gave a more applied and holistic approach:

- Structure and function in health and disease (S&F)
- Individuals, groups, and society (IGS)
- Population perspective (PP)
- Professional and personal development (PPD)

This used horizontal integration (between subjects) and vertical integration (revisiting concepts throughout, and blurring the conventional preclinical/clinical divide), intended to trigger discussion of the themes in all scenarios in all PBL sessions in Years 1–4, and facilitating a more community-orientated approach to medical practice. This feature supported the professional requirements of, for example, considering psychosocial, population, and ethicolegal dimensions of a clinical scenario, while having the care of the "patient" as the main focus. This feature also encouraged consideration of bioscientific principles underpinning that care, and trying straightforward ways of explaining core concepts across all themes complemented these.

Having a spiral core curriculum design encouraged progression in learning by revisiting key concepts in progressively greater breadth, depth, and application. This feature supported the professional requirement of, for example, developing a good standard of practice and care founded on a solid base of core knowledge and skills.

Having professional and personal development as one of these themes (Box 13.1) (including a history of medicine strand[19]) underlined very clearly its importance, with a formal requirement for students to discuss and reflect upon professional issues regularly, from the outset, guided by triggers in the scenarios (Box 13.2).

These features supported the professional requirements of, for example, applying ethical principles to common clinical presentations and personal development, and learning lessons for contemporary professional practice from earlier practices.

Box 13.1. Liverpool MBChB curriculum: professional and personal development theme framework (2007/08)

1. **How do the *General Medical Council's Duties of a Doctor*[4] relate to this scenario/situation and the doctor's role?**

Are there specific issues related to the doctor's approach to being able to[4]:

- "Make the care of your patient your first concern
- Protect and promote the health of patients and the public
- Provide a good standard of practice and care
  - Keep your professional knowledge and skills up to date
  - Recognise and work within the limits of your competence
  - Work with colleagues in the ways that best serve patients' interests
- Treat patients as individuals and respect their dignity
  - Treat patients politely and considerately
  - Respect patients' right to confidentiality
- Work in partnership with patients
  - Listen to patients and respond to their concerns and preferences
  - Give patients the information they want or need in a way they can understand
  - Respect patients' right to reach decisions with you about their treatment and care
  - Support patients in caring for themselves to improve and maintain their health
- Be honest and open and act with integrity
  - Act without delay if you have good reason to believe that you or a colleague may be putting patients at risk
  - Never discriminate unfairly against patients or colleagues
  - Never abuse your patients' trust in you or the public's trust in the profession.

You are personally accountable for your professional practice and must always be prepared to justify your decisions and actions."

2. **What legal issues and requirements relate to this scenario/situation for the doctor, other health professionals, and other people involved?**

3. i) Which ethical *issues*/moral dilemmas are relevant for the doctor, other health professionals, and other people involved in this scenario/situation?
   ii) Are the four principles identified by Beauchamp and Childress (respect for autonomy, beneficence, non-maleficence, and justice) relevant to this scenario, and if so how are they relevant?[5]

4. i) How does this scenario/situation illustrate the history of increasing professionalization of medicine, and the changing role of medicine in health care?
   ii) What historical context/examples might help you explain in this scenario/situation why a contemporary aspect of, for example:
   - ... public or political expectation ...
   - ... health or social service organization ...
   - ... professional practice or professional knowledge base ...
   has developed as it has done?

5. **What personal beliefs/assumptions might affect how well you understand this scenario/situation, and what personal development do you need?**

Box 13.2. Liverpool MBChB curriculum: examples of professional and personal development theme triggers extracted from four of the PBL (problem-based learning) scenarios* studied by year 1 medical students in their first semester (with permission)

A Raging Thirst

"... The [general practitioner], Dr. Ray Cornwall, refers Mrs Buckingham to the diabetes clinic. A diabetes nurse specialist reviews her weight and gives her a diet-sheet about protein, fat, carbohydrate, and vitamins. [In the back of her mind, when giving the advice, the nurse specialist is implicitly balancing beneficence with non-maleficence, treating them as *prima facie* (not absolute) principles.] ..." [This triggers learning about team-roles and about two ethical principles.]

A Wheezy Adolescent

"... Later, the practice nurse, Nurse Alwen Archer, discusses with Dr Allison the problems of managing anxious patients with chronic disease in the community. With the ethical principle of 'justice' uppermost in his mind, he leaves for a [primary care trust] meeting about distributing the limited local funds for respiratory health services fairly – he is ruminating about whether 'need', 'social contribution', or 'the free-market' would really sort any of this out ..." [This triggers learning about another ethical principle, and about how society or the profession might prioritize when allocating resources.]

Cold Feet

"... [Dr Patel] also knows that Mr Todd has the right to – *respect for private and family life, home and correspondence* – as enshrined in Article 8 of the Human Rights Act (1998), and that it is therefore up to Mr Todd whether he attends the vascular referral appointment ..."

"... Dr Lee says, "How can you know whether a reported association with smoking is 'causal' in those two broad study designs? It's not like anatomy knowledge is it? Think what they must have known 400 years ago! ..." [This triggers learning about human rights legislation and about lessons from history about the nature of knowledge ...]

Sudden Onset of Weakness

"[Mr Webster said] ..."I know the hospital is always busy after Friday night pub 'closing time', but Meg was very embarrassed at being examined in the corridor, which felt like an invasion of privacy ..."

"... Bearing in mind the importance of patient confidentiality, Dr Kumar asks Mrs Webster if he can discuss her details with Social Services." [This triggers learning about the issue of privacy versus confidentiality.]

* The scenarios are each about 350–550 words and usually focused on one individual's symptoms, signs, and personal situation/feelings, with reference to local community context, etc., and to key members of the health care services and their actions/reactions.

Reducing "factual overload" included making whole-year plenary sessions noncompulsory and much less frequent than in a lecture-based curriculum. This freed up more curriculum time and space for self-directed study and a more discriminating use of this medium by staff and students alike. Remaining plenaries allowed some structure and an opportunity to set context, convey less accessible or very recent material, or allow good speakers to convey the enthusiasm driving their own practice or research. This feature supported the professional requirements of, for example, time management, self-motivation, taking responsibility to keep up-to-date, and developing a professional identity with peers.

Early, incremental, and sustained clinical context and contact complemented the core themes. This comprised the clinical context of scenarios and the practicalities of early and ongoing compulsory clinical[20] and communication skills[21] training. Clinical placements had nearly one third of time in community general practice (to reinforce the more community-orientated approach to medicine). These features supported the professional requirements of, for example, being competent to provide a good standard of practice and care, critical analyzing evidence in context,[22] and being able to justify the personal knowledge and skills base in terms of future clinical practice.

Recognizing the key role of assessment in driving learning led to a more efficient use of assessments, having fewer of them, and coordinating them centrally. The focus was on "minimum-level competence" for clinically relevant material across all four curriculum themes and clinical/communication skills. Year 5 assessment (by an incremental portfolio of evidence) reinforced this using a clinical governance framework,[23,*] to consolidate such strands as risk management, clinical effectiveness, information management, and good communication/teamworking. The National Health Service (NHS) has used a clinical governance framework for a decade, whereby all staff are accountable for improving service quality in the pursuit of excellence. These features of assessment supported the professional requirement of, for example, a recurrent focus on issues in the Professional and Personal Development theme, such that a poor performance on this theme could not be compensated by good clinical/communication skills or Structure and Function performance.

Managing the curriculum centrally (culminating in a School of Medical Education to do this), rather than from individual subject disciplines, allowed a more coordinated approach to curriculum design and assessment. This was intended to reduce redundant overlap, and supported the professional requirement of, for example, taking a more integrated and patient-focused approach to medicine rather than thinking in subject-focused compartments.

---

* "A framework through which NHS organisations are accountable for continuously improving the quality of their services and safeguarding high standards of care by creating an environment in which excellence in clinical care will flourish."[23]

In summary, opportunities for learning professionalism were embedded in the curriculum design. Under the problem-based philosophy, PBL scenarios encouraged students to deliberate regularly about professionally relevant issues.

OPPORTUNITIES FOR LEARNING PROFESSIONALISM

Besides embodying them in one of four core themes integral to the content and process of PBL, the formal curriculum provides opportunities for learning professionalism via documented curriculum outcomes in the student handbook, a public declaration at induction, and the self-reflection, self-assessment, and peer-review activities that are integral to the curriculum design.

Pellegrino highlighted that there are two sides to being a member of a profession.[24] On the one hand, it involves accepting the need to acquire a panoply of knowledge, skills, and attitudes as the esoteric basis for admission. On the other hand, becoming a professional also involves a public declaration to use this esoteric knowledge to benefit others without fear or favor.

On Day 1 now, the students encounter the Royal College of Physicians (RCP) definition of medical professionalism[25]:

> Medical professionalism signifies a set of values, behaviours, and relationships that underpins the trust the public has in doctors.[25(p14)]

. . . and its further description:

> Medicine is a vocation in which a doctor's knowledge, clinical skills, and judgement are put in the service of protecting and restoring human well-being. This purpose is realised through a partnership between patient and doctor, one based on mutual respect, individual responsibility, and appropriate accountability.
>
> In their day-to-day practice, doctors are committed to:
>
> - integrity
> - compassion
> - altruism
> - continuous improvement
> - excellence
> - working in partnership with members of the wider healthcare team.

These values, which underpin the science and practice of medicine, form the basis for a moral contract between the medical profession and society. Each party has a duty to work to strengthen the system of healthcare on which our collective human dignity depends.[25(p14,15)]

It is noteworthy that the RCP considered and excluded the concepts of "mastery, autonomy, privilege, and self-regulation," the last of these for not being of itself a core professional value or behavior but a collective action to govern the profession.

Documented curriculum outcomes focus on Duties of a Doctor,[4] plus:

- Attending satisfactorily, and being punctual, reliable, honest, respectful, courteous, and well presented
- Recognizing the impact of own health on own ability to undertake medical practice, and respond appropriately
- Agreeing to take the "Declaration of Geneva"[26]
- Working in teams in an interdisciplinary setting
- Tolerating uncertainty in professional practice, and demonstrating leadership as appropriate
- Being committed to advancing the science and art of medical practice for the benefit of patients, the population, the profession, and personal development.

One of the rites of passage for a newly qualified doctor (or in Liverpool any of the graduating health professionals) is the public assent to the Hippocratic Oath. In the United Kingdom, it has often, appropriately, been made at the point of admission to the profession (defined as being graduation), but other possibilities include the first entry to the clinical arena (such as in a "white coat" ceremony[27]). The idea in Liverpool was to ensure that the expectations of a health care professional were made explicit from the outset, so students assent to the Declaration of Geneva (the contemporary World Medical Association equivalent of the Hippocratic Oath) on their first day. Those privileged to observe the occasion have noted that the students start the declaration as a matter of speaking by rote. As they grasp the enormity of their promise, the atmosphere in the lecture theatre changes palpably.

This early public assent serves two purposes. Firstly, it serves as a rite of passage, and starts to form professional identity. Other curricula might regard induction to the mysteries of the dissecting room as another important rite of passage. This rite has a different emphasis in Liverpool, where students use human anatomy resource and clinical skills resource laboratories to learn anatomy from prosected specimens and models and alongside clinical skills,[28] rather than undertaking compulsory dissection practice. PBL scenarios and other experiences also trigger complementary discussions about ethicolegal issues in the use of human tissue. In this curriculum, students also have a rolling introduction to clinical practice, with Year 1 students undertaking preliminary community-based activities with general practitioners, a "baby clinic," and a family with children. There is no clear-cut point at which to assume a "white coat identity," and this would also seem incongruous when there is such an emphasis on retaining strong community orientation in all settings. Secondly, the declaration focuses students' attention on related outcomes of the curriculum, which echo the professional Duties of a Doctor declared, in principle and via the law, by the General Medical Council.[4]

Reflection about own and group learning and performance are integral to PBL sessions, although some students and staff might struggle with this activity[29] without a clear rationale and the requisite skills. Examples of formative self-assessment opportunities are:

- A formal exercise where, each semester, the tutor and the student each complete a proforma about the student's performance in PBL sessions, and then meet to discuss these, which supports aspects of professionalism such as reflection, group participation, communication, and critical thinking;
- Self-marking some short-answer responses (against the official marks schedule) from formative written assessments, as a required part of the assessment process, which supports aspects of professionalism such as self-awareness and probity.

Alongside academic contact, students complete a reflective portfolio of online documents related to personal development planning, which obliges them to reflect upon their experiences. The students are required to email extracts to their personal tutors (who have a mentoring/pastoral role) and their PBL tutors (who know about their academic abilities and group performance):

- In Year 1, they learn the skills of reflection, through discussing relatively unthreatening situations such as their reasons for choosing medicine, adjusting to university life, and their formative assessment results.
- In Years 2 and 4, a series of questions directs them to consider events that they have experienced on their clinical placements.
- In Year 3, there is a specific exercise where the students must reflect upon an example of either good or bad professional practice that they have observed.

Over time, the curriculum design has been refined, and has taken account of the 2003 update of the General Medical Council recommendations,[30] redoubling efforts to promote attitudes, behavior, and qualities suitable for a good doctor with responsibilities to patients, colleagues, and society generally. There are continuing efforts to recognize that the hidden curriculum can also confound the intended implementations and the intended outcomes related to professionalism, despite systematic attempts to uncover and tackle the more negative aspects.

In summary, besides four core themes integral to the content and process of PBL, the formal curriculum provides opportunities for learning professionalism via documented curriculum outcomes in the student handbook, a public declaration at induction, the self-reflection, self-assessment, and peer-review activities integral to the curriculum design, and culminating in another public declaration at graduation.

ASSESSING PROFESSIONALISM AND FITNESS FOR PRACTICE

In the scheme of assessment, for each summative assessment there is a formative assessment some months previously, giving a dress rehearsal and learning feedback opportunity (including about aspects of the professional and personal development theme). Attention to formative assessment systems, clear messages about expected levels of achievement, and interventions aimed at fostering "healthy" approaches to studying should reduce the stress of unrealistic expectations.[31]

For Years 1–4, written assessments of knowledge, understanding, and critical analysis for clinical practice are based on the student learning activities triggered for all themes by all PBL scenarios, such that some aspect of professionalism will appear in each. This could include professional behavior, ethical dilemmas, ingrained assumptions to be challenged, legal interpretations, interprofessional relationships, or lessons from a historical perspective. Each PBL group reports its learning objectives electronically to a year-group "virtual learning environment," generating a shared resource, which also informs the contents of the formative and summative examinations. Assessments also require competence in clinical and communication skills such that, if retaking a year, students must also retake these assessments, even if previously attained, to demonstrate that they have maintained competence. These assessments include various elements of professional demeanor and behavior.

There are other examples of summative assessment including some aspect of professionalism, for example:

- There is a summative self- and peer-assessment opportunity as part of the Year 3 "critical thinking" submission (a study proposal).[32] For this, a student provides anonymous formal comments on two of their peers' study design proposals, and incorporates into their own study design proposal the comments of two of their peers and responds formally to these.

- Year 5 differs in its assessment process, which comprises the "professional education and training appraisal," culminating in the submission of a portfolio of evidence, rather than assessments under examination conditions. The five 7-week placements (each finished by a reflective Week 8) are aligned more with students' forthcoming preregistration house officer (PRHO) (intern) year, now called foundation year (FY) 1. At the start of each placement, students complete a proforma with their educational supervisor indicating their intended learning outcomes under a number of domains (including professional behavior and communication), and how they will demonstrate attaining these. Students are assessed summatively against their statements during and at the end of the placement. Two of the placements each require a written report on either a current clinical guideline or a clinical dilemma, the latter choice being likely to require review of professional practice and ethical dimensions. In addition to portfolio material supplied by the student, other members of the health care team (including other health care professionals) are involved in assessing the student's professional behavior in all the placements. It is particularly important that this behavior occurs and is assessed in the clinical environment given Klass' observation that competence, including here competence in professionalism, demands a match between the behavior of the would-be doctor and the patient's expectations.[33]

An ongoing dilemma is the difficulty in assessing professionalism given the lack of explicit criteria, which is particularly important if an element of peer assessment (in Year 3) or assessment by other members of the health care team (in Year 5) is to be included.

Local research in progress is attempting to identify an appropriate set of criteria for the cognitive elements of professionalism, researching different groups of students' perceptions of the defining characteristics. So far, this research has shown that Liverpool students and recent graduates (FY1 doctors) regard technical knowledge and competence as being important. As the student progresses through the curriculum, elements concerning interpersonal skills become increasingly more important, until shortly after graduation when personal qualities, such as honesty and integrity, are seen as the most important elements describing professionalism.[34]

How "fitness for practice" procedures address professionalism is a contentious issue, but recent guidance from the General Medical Council and Medical Schools Council is helping to clarify responsibilities.[35] Following a change in the law in the United Kingdom, the General Medical Council will now, before granting provisional registration, consider each medical graduate's formal declaration about his/her fitness for practice. Medical schools should address behavior that undermines a "student's ability to continue on a medical course, or their fitness to practise as a doctor after graduation."[35(p24)] Medical schools are trying to pre-empt future difficulties, for example, by identifying where a full FY1 performance could not realistically be achieved, even with appropriate support (or, as a separate, albeit related issue, with reasonable adjustment for disabilities). Liverpool has clear fitness for practice mechanisms when there are concerns about a student's suitability for professional practice on the grounds of health or conduct (such as personal integrity, group relationships, attitudes, or attendance). Engaging in illicit drug misuse, drug dealing, or recurrent intoxication would trigger these mechanisms, and students must also report, in confidence, concerns about other students misusing drugs or alcohol, all of which complies with the General Medical Council guidance.

A "yellow card" system for student support allows for a "concern form" to be written where staff or students are concerned about some aspect of a student's behavior. Support can be triggered by a minor matter that turns out to link to a series of other reported behaviors causing concern from various parts of the curriculum. The report might come from the staff with whom a student is in contact (sometimes because the student has raised the issue first), or worried peers, and the student is aware of the contents of the report. Potentially, this system has crucial implications for professional practice. It encourages students' personal accountability for disclosing problems in their own or colleagues' practice, if there are potential implications for safe clinical practice. Mostly, an interview between the student and a senior member of faculty is sufficient to help start addressing the issue. Furthermore, the school reserves the right to refer a student to its own school clinical psychology service, or to the health services in an adjoining region with which it has reciprocal arrangements. Wherever possible, the emphasis is developmental rather than punitive.

In summary, the formal student assessment framework is designed to highlight the professional knowledge, attitudes, and behavior that the curriculum intends to promote, and fitness for practice issues are addressed in related processes.

CURRICULUM EVALUATION AND IMPLEMENTATION ISSUES FOR PROMOTING PROFESSIONALISM IN A PROBLEM-BASED CURRICULUM

Evaluating success in these attempts to promote professionalism is an ongoing activity. There was early evidence that students perceived that they were better prepared for independent learning than were their predecessors in the conventional curriculum.[36] An interview study of the educational supervisors of the first cohort of graduates found that they considered them to be better prepared for preregistration house year than their predecessors, and very aware of their own limitations and when to ask for help.[37] A study of the graduates themselves found them to feel well prepared for the practicalities of house year,[38] although within both studies there were conflicting perceptions about whether the core knowledge base was sufficient or not. More recently, Liverpool graduates in local PRHO posts were more likely than those graduating elsewhere to report feeling prepared by medical school for using critical appraisal skills,[39] which are crucial in developing a professional approach.[40]

Ongoing evaluation of the PBL "modules" (plenaries, resources, PBL sessions) and other curriculum elements have informed improvements in implementation but have not necessarily focused on the four-theme design. Indeed, evaluation theory would suggest that outcome evaluation should concentrate on distinctive aspects of curriculum design, such that integrated curriculum themes, for example, should be very prominent in student assessment *and* curriculum evaluation.[41] The strategy for what and how to evaluate is under review. From a professionalism perspective, it is timely that Mattick and Bligh have, for example, proposed that ethics input to British undergraduate medical curricula should now be reviewed against an established national consensus statement.[42,43] Curriculum evaluation fatigue is, however, a danger in curricula undergoing much innovation, and the first cohort of students through the Liverpool curriculum felt, for example, that they had been asked to contribute to too much curriculum evaluation.[38]

Other local research has given glimpses into the realities of the students' professionalization experience. When prompted to reflect on problems in PBL from the tutoring perspective, junior students' main thwarted expectation was of good intervention, particularly if tutors contributed excessively.[29] The hidden curriculum revealed by a few students suggested the problems caused if tutors undermined PBL "rules."[29] Nonreflective role models and interference from the informal curriculum of personal interactions with disgruntled staff may well encourage socialization into low expectations of PBL sessions, tutors, and by inference professionalism. Inconsistencies in implementation and "philosophical drift" remain constant threats to the success of the problem-based system.

It was also clear from local research that it was unrealistic to expect junior students' appreciation of the full implications of professionalism.[44] Using nine emergent themes from researching their descriptions a "good doctor" at entry to medical school, and then replaying these themes for them and their successors (and prospective medical students) to rank, showed a good doctor as a "compassionate, patient-focused carer" and "listening, informative communicator" more than an "exemplary, responsible professional." Their views generally corresponded with the three "Cs" that patients are purported to value most: communication, caring, and competence.[45] It cannot be assumed, however, that the students were forsaking professionalism but merely de-emphasizing it when ranking a closed system of themes, or tussling with its import early in their professionalization journey.

Students' continuing exposure to professionalism concepts as learning opportunities under an assessed core curriculum theme was clearly necessary but not sufficient to raise its profile. Working with the learners' notions of professionalism, in this way, and exploring what curriculum aspects are effective in promoting appropriate behaviors, rather than just focusing on what is assessed (or abstract notions about attitudes), are important avenues for continuing work.[46]

Concerning staff development, the introduction of a problem-based curriculum meant a need for a change of staff mindset and much effort to prepare staff to be PBL tutors,[47] and maintaining a critical mass of suitable tutors is an ongoing challenge. Although there is a consensus in medicine that professionalism is "a good thing,"[25] it is evident that many colleagues regard it as something that can be absorbed. The value of staff development – in both formal and informal settings – is to encourage such colleagues that professionalism is something that they can and should model, and also can be assessed formally and explicitly. Steinert *et al.*'s reports about staff development related specifically to promoting professionalism (including how to view this through a change management framework) are rare in the literature.[48,49]

Those becoming PBL tutors found the experience a challenge, whether due to the facilitation skills and restraint required or due to the breadth of content to be facilitated,[50,51] and there is evidence that, as with such curricula elsewhere, reflective role models cannot be assumed.[29] There may be pockets of unabashed, intransigent, nonreflection alongside pockets of enthusiastic, enlightened, critical reflection, yet the conflict between these can prevent curriculum complacency and stimulate more robust evidence- and theory-based approaches.

One side product of the summative written examination papers being subject to an Angoff[52] standard setting panel of six to twelve staff is that this gives an opportunity for them to experience what it feels like to be confronted with questions, for example, about ethical issues and professional practice. A greater insight into students' perceived misconceptions can then be used to advocate for specific refinements in the curriculum or to inform personal changes in education practice regarding professionalism. Including aspects of professionalism in all elements of the curriculum reaps benefits for staff as well as students.

Another example comes from a longitudinal study that started before the introduction of the problem-based curriculum.[53] Using a variety of techniques, students have been asked to identify the attributes of a good personal tutor. These overlap very closely with the expectations required of the students themselves in assenting to the Declaration of Geneva. This has proved an invaluable aid in informing the staff development scheme.

In summary, running a problem-based system has the constant challenge of showing success to students, staff, and other stakeholders, and there is a danger of overevaluation. Staff development also remains a big challenge, as there are issues with staff recruitment and reward for key tasks, and the required role models for professionalism cannot be assumed.

LESSONS LEARNED

Over a decade on from the problem-based transformation of this curriculum, there are clear strengths and weaknesses in the way that the curriculum develops the students' professionalism.

*A **strength*** of the system described is learning about professionalism in context and constantly being challenged to develop an appropriate professional persona within a planned, supportive framework. Sustained contact with PBL tutors can act as an extra safety net for pastoral care,[54] for example, as problems get detected earlier. The need for professional self-awareness is unavoidable in this system.

*A **weakness*** is that some people will perceive that, unless they are "being told" or "telling" others what it takes to be a good doctor, "it" cannot possibly work. Indeed, tolerating the uncertainties surrounding changing professional practice and contexts is another aspect of professionalism. It is also difficult to maintain continuity, appropriate progression, and consistent learning opportunities for professional and personal development, let alone organizational memory for the overall philosophy (and the rationale for why things should be done in certain ways). The dangers are that staff and students might become very formulaic in carrying out particular activities (short-circuiting the elements for which, despite controversy,[55] there is generally strong evidence of benefit[56–59]), that the power of role models might be undervalued, and that educational research might not receive appropriate attention within an institution generally.

In terms of lessons learnt, the key to success seems to be congruence. When Liverpool introduced a student-focused, problem-based, integrated curriculum, it was important to give a clear message, and ensure that all elements of the curriculum worked together to support the overall curriculum goals, which were made explicit at each stage of development. Similarly, the emphasis on the importance of professionalism was integral to this endeavor, and is therefore made explicit from the first day in medical school and the formal curriculum supports this. Challenges remain in uncovering and tackling the hidden curriculum elements that potentially short-circuit self-directed learning[60] or squash aspirations to a better version of professionalism than can sometimes confront students in their everyday curriculum experience. Research needs to continue exploring some of the "private accounts"[11] of how things are for students rather than how the school assumes them to be. There are many variables in the Liverpool problem-based system[61] that should promote key aspects of professionalism, if implemented properly.

In terms of developments and future directions, the School of Medical Education bid successfully for a £4.5 million Centre of Excellence in Teaching & Learning (CETL) specializing in professionalism in undergraduate medical education, which was launched in 2006. The CETL's remit focuses on developing sound ways of assessing students' professional attitudes and behavior (and promoting their learning), developing early career guidance to help them develop professional career plans, and developing criteria by which excellence in clinical educators can be identified and rewarded. It is intended that this will include hidden curriculum issues, as well as overt characteristics of educators, and the problematic notion of role models spans both. The CETL will help develop and embed mechanisms for supporting and assessing professionalism, and the intention is to emphasize that professionalism is something that should develop throughout a career.

When Liverpool students assent to the Declaration of Geneva at their graduation, they use the same form of words that they used on their first day – the difference is that, when they say it on their last day of medical school, they are in a position to make an informed choice, and should be suitably prepared to take their place in their chosen profession.

REFERENCES

1. Maudsley, G. Medical students' expectations and experience as learners in a problem-based curriculum: a 'mixed methods' research approach. [Doctor of Medicine (MD) thesis, Public Health/Medical Education]. The University of Liverpool: Liverpool, 2005.
2. Bligh, J. Professionalism. *Med Educ.* 2005; 39(1): 2005.
3. Jha, V, Bekker, HL, Duffy, SRG, Roberts, TE. Perceptions of professionalism in medicine: a qualitative study. *Med Educ.* 2006; 40(10): 1027–1036.

4. General Medical Council. *Good Medical Practice*. London: General Medical Council, 2006.

5. Beauchamp, TL, Childress, JF. *Principles of Biomedical Ethics*. Oxford: Oxford University Press, 2001.

6. Lloyd-Jones, G, Ellershaw, J, Wilkinson, S, Bligh, JG. The use of multidisciplinary consensus groups in the planning phase of an integrated problem-based curriculum. *Med Educ.* 1998; 32(3): 278–282.

7. Hafferty, FW. Beyond curriculum reform: confronting medicine's hidden curriculum. *Acad Med.* 1998; 73(4): 403–407.

8. Hundert, EM, Hafferty, F, Christakis, D. Characteristics of the informal curriculum and trainees' ethical choices. *Acad Med.* 1996; 71(6): 624–633.

9. Haas, J, Shaffir, W. Ritual evaluation of competence—the hidden curriculum of professionalization in an innovative medical school program. *Work and Occupations* 1982; 9(2): 131–154.

10. Cribb, A, Bignold, S. Towards the reflexive medical school: the hidden curriculum and medical education research. *Studies in Higher Education* 1999; 24(2): 195–209.

11. Cornwell, J. *Hard-Earned Lives: Accounts of Health and Illness from East London*. London: Tavistock, 1984.

12. Fryer-Edwards, K. Addressing the hidden curriculum in scientific research. *The Am J. Bioethics* 2002; 2(4): 58–59.

13. *Oxford English Dictionary*. [2nd edition with updates] June 2007. Last available May 3, 2008 from: http://dictionary.oed.com.

14. General Medical Council. *Tomorrow's Doctors: Recommendations on Undergraduate Med Educ.*. London: General Medical Council, 1993.

15. Bligh, J. Identifying the core curriculum—the Liverpool approach. *Med Teach.* 1995; 17(4): 383–390.

16. Maudsley, G. Do we all mean the same thing by "problem-based learning?"—a review of the concepts and a formulation of the ground rules. *Acad Med.* 1999; 74(2): 178–185.

17. Maudsley, G. Roles and responsibilities of the problem based learning tutor in the undergraduate medical curriculum. *BMJ* 1999; 318(7184): 657–661.

18. Schmidt, HG. Problem-based learning: rationale and description. *Med Educ.* 1983; 17(1), 11–16.

19. Sheard, S. Developing history of medicine in the University of Liverpool medical curriculum 1995–2005. *Med Educ.* 2006; 40(10): 1045–1052.

20. Bradley, P, Bligh, J. One year's experience with a clinical skills resource centre. *Med Educ.* 1999; 33(2): 114–120.

21. Humphris, GM, Kaney, S. Assessing the development of communication skills in undergraduate medical students. *Med Educ.* 2001; 35(3): 225–231.

22. Bradley, P, Humphris, G. Assessing the ability of medical students to apply evidence in practice: the potential of the OSCE. *Med Educ.* 1999; 33(11): 815–817.

23. Scally, G, Donaldson, LJ. Looking forward: Clinical governance and the drive for quality improvement in the new NHS in England. *BMJ* 1998; 317: 61–65.

24. Pellegrino, ED. Professionalism, profession and the virtues of the good physician. *Mt. Sinai J. Med.* 2002; 69(6): 378–384.

25. Royal College of Physicians. *Doctors in Society: Medical Professionalism in a Changing World.* Report of a Working Party of the Royal College of Physicians of London. London: RCP, 2005.

26. World Medical Association. *Declaration of Geneva* (last amended 2006). Ferney-Voltaire: World Medical Association, 2006 version: [page on the Internet]. Last available May 3, 2008 from: www.wma.net/e/policy/c8.htm.

27. Wear, D. On white coats and professional development: the formal and the hidden curricula. *Ann Int. Med.* 1998; 129(9):734–737.

28. Dangerfield, P, Bradley, P, Gibbs, T. Learning gross anatomy in a clinical skills course. *Clin Anat.* 2000; 13(6): 444–447.

29. Maudsley, G, Williams, EMI, Taylor, DCM. Problem-based learning at the receiving end: a 'mixed methods' study of junior medical students'. *Advances in Health Sciences Education* 2007 ['Online First': DOI 10.1007/s10459-006-9056-9]

30. General Medical Council. *Tomorrow's Doctors: Recommendations on Undergraduate Med Educ..* London: General Medical Council, 2003.

31. Humphris, G, Kaney, S. The encouragement of 'perfect' health professionals. *Med Educ.* 1998; 32(5): 452–455.

32. Platt, MJ, Alfirevic, Z, McLaughlin, PJ. The 'Critical Thinking Module'—a grant proposal simulation exercise. *Med Educ.* 2000; 34(11): 951–952.

33. Klass, D. A performance-based conception of competence is changing the regulation of physicians' professional behavior. *Acad Med.* 2007; 82(6): 529–535.

34. Taylor, DCM, Royles, B, Sayle, E. The student view of professionalism changes as they progress through an undergraduate medical course. [Abstract] Parallel session presentation at "Association for the Study of Med Educ. (ASME) Annual Scientific Meeting" ASME scientific meeting 2007; Keele University, September 11–13, 2007.

35. General Medical Council and Medical Schools Council. *Medical Students: Professional Behaviour and Fitness to Practise.* London: General Medical Council and Medical Schools Council, 2007.

36. Bligh, J, Lloyd-Jones, G, Smith, G. Early effects of a new problem-based clinically oriented curriculum on students' perceptions of teaching. *Med Educ.* 2000; 34(6): 487–489.

37. Watmough, S, Taylor, D, Garden, A. Educational supervisors evaluate the preparedness of graduates from a reformed UK curriculum to work as pre-registration house officers (PRHOs): a qualitative study. *Med Educ.* 2006; 40(10): 995–1001.

38. Watmough, S, Garden, A, Taylor, D. Pre-registration house officers' views on studying under a reformed medical curriculum in the UK. *Med Educ.* 2006; 40(9): 893–899.

39. Doran, T, Maudsley, G, Zakhour, HD. Time to think? Questionnaire survey of pre-registration house officers' experiences of critical appraisal in the Mersey Deanery. *Med Educ.* 2007; 41(5): 487–494.

40. Maudsley, G, Strivens, J. Promoting professional knowledge, experiential learning and critical thinking for medical students. *Med Educ.* 2000; 34(7): 535–544.

41. Maudsley, G. What issues are raised by evaluating problem-based undergraduate medical curricula? Making healthy connections across the literature. *J. Eval in Clin Practice* 2001; 7(3): 311–324.

42. Mattick, K, Bligh, J. Undergraduate ethics teaching: revisiting the consensus statement. *Med Educ.* 2006; 40(4): 329–332.

43. Anonymous. Consensus statement by teachers of medical ethics and law in UK medical schools. Teaching medical ethics and law within medical education: a model for the UK core curriculum. *J. Med Ethic* 1998; 24(3): 188–92.

44. Maudsley, G, Williams, EMI, Taylor, DCM. Junior medical students' notions of a 'good doctor' and related expectations: a mixed methods study. *Med Educ.* 2007; 41(5): 476–486.

45. Martin, S. What is a good doctor? Patient perspective. *Am J. Obs Gyn.* 1998; 178(4): 752–754.

46. Ginsburg, S, Stern, D. The professionalism movement: behaviors are the key to progress. *Am J. Bioethics* 2004; 4(2): 14–15.

47. Evans, PA, Taylor, DCM. Staff development of tutor skills for problem-based learning. *Med Educ.* 1996; 30(5): 365–366.

48. Steinert, Y, Cruess, S, Cruess, R, Snell, L. Faculty development for teaching and evaluating professionalism: from programme design to curriculum change. *Med Educ.* 2005; 39(2):127–136.

49. Steinert, Y, Cruess, RL, Cruess, SR, Boudreau, JD, Fuks, A. Faculty development as an instrument of change: a case study on teaching professionalism. *Acad Med.* 2007; 82(11): 1057–1064.

50. Maudsley, G. Making sense of trying not to teach: an interview study of tutors' ideas of problem-based learning. *Acad Med.* 2002; 77(2): 162–172.

51. Maudsley, G. The limits of tutors' 'comfort zones' with four integrated knowledge themes in a problem-based undergraduate medical curriculum (Interview study). *Med Educ.* 2003; 37(5): 417–423.

52. Fowell, S, Fewtrell, R, McLaughlin, PJ. Estimating the minimum number of judges required for test-centred standard setting on written assessments. Do discussion and iteration have an influence? *Adv Health Sci Educ.* 2008; 13(1): 11–24. [2006 'Online First': DOI 10.1007/s10459-006-9027-1]

53. Taylor, D. What students want from their pastoral care system. In: *Adv Med Educ.* Scherpbier, AJJA, van der Vleuten, CPM, Rethans, JJ, van der, Steeg (editors). Dordrecht: Kluwer Academic Publishers, 1997: 803–804.

54. Taylor, D. Personal development. *Med Educ.* 1997; 31(Suppl. 1: Conference proceedings on: The transition from medical student to medical practitioner. Cambridge, July 16–18, 1997): 15–16.

55. Norman, GR, Schmidt, HG. Effectiveness of problem-based learning curricula: theory, practice and paper darts. *Med Educ.* 2000; 34(9): 721–728.

56. Norman, GR, Schmidt, HG. The psychological basis of problem-based learning: a review of the evidence. *Acad Med.* 1992; 67(9): 557–565.

57. Albanese, MA, Mitchell, S. Problem-based learning: a review of literature on its outcomes and implementation issues. *Acad Med.* 1993; 68(1): 52–81.

58. Vernon, DTA, Blake, RL. Does problem-based learning work? A meta-analysis of evaluative research. *Acad Med.* 1993; 68(7): 550–563.

59. Berkson, L. Problem-based learning: have the expectations been met? *Acad Med.* 1993; 68(10 Suppl.): S79–S88.

60. Lloyd-Jones, G, Hak, T. Self-directed learning and student pragmatism. *Adv Health Sci Educ.* 2004; 9(1): 61–73.

61. Dangerfield, P, Dornan, T, Engel, C, Maudsley, G, Naqvi, J, Powis, D, Sefton, A. *A Whole System Approach to Problem-Based Learning in Dental, Medical and Veterinary Sciences—A Guide to Important Variables.* Manchester: The Centre for Excellence in Enquiry Based Learning (CEEBL); a Centre of Excellence in Teaching & Learning (CETL); University of Manchester, 2007: [on the Internet]. Last available May 3, 2008 from: www.campus.manchester.ac.uk/ceebl/resources/resourcepacks/pblsystemapproach_v1.pdf.

14 Teaching Professionalism and Fostering Professional Values during Residency: The McGill Experience

Linda Snell, M.D., M.H.P.E., F.R.C.P.C., F.A.C.P.

Learning how to be a professional is a vital part of residency training. Although professional socialization starts in medical school, professional attitudes and behaviors are internalized during residency as the resident learns medicine over a period of years of supervised practice. Providing illustrations from McGill University, this chapter will present a model of how professionalism can be taught and evaluated at the postgraduate or residency level and address lessons learned.

THE CONTEXT

Professionalism is a standard for accreditation of postgraduate programs in most Western countries, as found, for example, in the CanMEDS roles for specialty residencies in Canada, and the Accreditation Council for Graduate Medical Education's competencies in the United States.[1,2] Other countries use documents such as the General Medical Council's "Good Medical Practice" in the United Kingdom or the Charter on Professionalism to outline appropriate professional behaviors for all physicians.[3,4] As such, the curricular content for a residency program is broadly outlined, and there is an expectation that residents' professional behaviors will be assessed. National residency accrediting bodies usually include a general definition of "professionalism" in their standards. As well, these bodies usually describe elements of professionalism, including concepts relating to professional attributes and humanistic behaviors, professional relationships (e.g., the social contract), the organizational and legal aspects of professionalism (e.g., profession-led regulation), ethical principles and practice, sensitivity to diversity, and physician health and sustainable practice.

In Canada, both the Royal College of Physicians and Surgeons and the College of Family Physicians have mandated all residency programs to teach and evaluate professionalism. It is also assessed on national final residency examinations. Similarly, a number of Specialty Boards in the United States (e.g., the American Board of Paediatrics[5]) request that residency program directors assess and document professionalism prior to board certification. However, little guidance to implementation is provided, with few details of curricular content, teaching strategies, or evaluation methods.[6,7] The residency program director or curriculum planner is thus left to translate the general descriptions into goals and objectives, and to design learning methods and assessment processes that will be effective for their specialty and for the level of the resident. This frequently must be done in the context of little buy-in or understanding by faculty members, or within the constraints of a hidden curriculum that subverts these efforts.

TRANSLATING CONCEPTS INTO EDUCATIONAL PRACTICE: A FRAMEWORK

At McGill University, we have been guided by a number of beliefs and principles, which have provided a framework for the teaching of professionalism at the residency level. As outlined elsewhere in this volume, we believe that there is a need to teach the cognitive base of professionalism,[8] which will give a structure for all learners and will provide a common vocabulary for teachers and residents to discuss professional issues in the workplace. Just as there is a scientific knowledge base that a resident applies to their clinical practice of medicine, there is a base of knowledge about professionalism that can be applied to their professional practice, and this must be explicitly taught. There are also skills important to certain aspects of professionalism; we feel that these can be taught. We also feel that the residents must have multiple opportunities to apply these concepts of professionalism in their practice, and to internalize them into attitudes that are expressed in professional behaviors. The latter process is fostered by learning methods such as experiential learning, role modeling, and reflection. As the cognitive base and the latter teaching strategies are often new to most faculty members, faculty development is essential. Finally, as evaluation drives learning,[9] we feel that professional behaviors and knowledge of the concepts must be assessed, both formatively and summatively. This must be done with strong institutional support and a positive learning environment. Table 14.1 shows these essential elements, with some examples of learning activities for professionalism currently provided at our university.

We have introduced a Postgraduate Core Competencies Program (PCCP), with a mandate for faculty-wide oversight of educational activities for all core competencies (i.e., CanMEDS roles and Family Medicine competencies). At a cross-disciplinary level, this program assists the residency program directors by defining resident's educational needs (content, format, level)

Table 14.1. Essential elements (with examples) for learning professionalism at the resident level

	Faculty-wide	Program/ specialty	Individual learner
Learning the cognitive base of professionalism			
Academic half-day on professionalism	+		
Principles of ethics: lectures, half-days	+	+	
Risk management, self regulation, medicolegal issues	+	+	
Principles of teaching	+	+	
Physician health and sustainable practice: Resident Wellness Day	+		
Learning the skills of professionalism			
Ethics-associated communication skills: teaching OSCE		+	
Advanced communication skills		+	+
Teaching skills	+	+	
Teamwork	+	+	
Time management	+	+	
Conflict resolution	+	+	
Mentorship – how to select a mentor	+		
Developing professional attitudes and fostering professional behaviors: transferring learning into practice			
Experiential learning			+
Role modeling			+
Guided reflection			+
Mentorship		+	+
Portfolios		+	
Changing the learning environment	+	+	
Evaluating professionalism			
Cognitive base: written examinations	+		
Individual residents: P-MEX		+	
End of rotation and composite in-training assessments	+		
Evaluation of portfolios		+	
Specialty examinations: OSCE stations	+		
Faculty development			
Contribution to a definition that is understood by faculty members and for which there is buy-in by teachers	+		
Development of an institutional approach to teaching and evaluation of professionalism, and dissemination with workshops	+		

Table 14.1. Continued

	Faculty-wide	Program/ specialty	Individual learner
Program directors' retreat on teaching core competencies (includes professionalism)	+		
Program directors' retreat on evaluating core competencies (includes professionalism)	+		
Guidelines for teaching and resource lists (e.g., ethics)		+	
Workshop and other activities on role modeling	+		
Workshop and other activities on reflection	+		
Royal College of Physicians and Surgeons of Canada train-the-trainer module for professionalism	+		

in the area of core competencies, providing resources, implementing activities, and developing a cohort of motivated and skilled faculty. The PCCP is part of the Faculty of Medicine Postgraduate section, and as such, links with all residency programs. Members of the PCCP planning group include content experts, program directors, residents, and faculty developers. The PCCP educational activities complement and supplement the formal and informal learning that occurs at the department level and for individual residents. In specific content areas such as ethics education, the PCCP has developed guidelines that are used by the residency program directors; these include suggested learning strategies and print and Internet resources. The "Professionalism for Residents" half-day was the first offering of the PCCP, and educational activities for other competencies have been modeled on this.

EXAMPLES OF EDUCATIONAL ACTIVITIES FOR RESIDENTS FOR LEARNING PROFESSIONALISM AT MCGILL UNIVERSITY

Learning the Cognitive Base

At our institution, we have instituted a number of educational activities to help residents learn about the cognitive base of professionalism. We require an annual half-day on professionalism for all second-year residents in all specialties. A number of other large-group cross-specialty activities also address elements of professionalism. Residents also participate in discipline-based (department-specific) activities such as Grand Rounds, freestanding lectures, retreats, and didactic presentations at departmental resident half-days. Details of these will be described below.

Academic Half-Day on Professionalism

Our annual faculty-wide cross-specialty mandatory half-day on "Professionalism for Residents" is aimed at second-year residents. This level was chosen because by this time the residents have, for the most part, adapted to their program, improved their communications skills, and are "clinically comfortable." They are able to reflect on the behaviors of themselves, their teachers, and their colleagues. As well, this fits with the other educational activities of the PCCP, which offers level-specific activities in other core competencies (e.g., communication skills in first year, teaching, leadership, and management in the senior years). As in many medical schools, expertise in professionalism was limited to a few individuals, and we felt it would be more efficient to provide the didactic part of a program to larger numbers of residents, rather than asking these few experts to lecture to smaller numbers in over fifty residency programs. We have given this program to approximately 140 residents a year since 2001.

Our goals are that by the end of the half-day, the resident will be able to define professionalism, identify the attributes of professionalism in clinical contexts, describe the social contract between physicians and society, and discuss how it applies to residents, and apply this information to their current and future professional and clinical settings. As the program evolved and many residents had been exposed to the topic as medical students, we added another learning objective: to describe how codes of ethics and the Charter on Professionalism fit into the resident's role as a professional.

The four-hour program begins with a plenary lecture given by experts in the topic. This presentation identifies major issues, key concepts, and definitions; describes core attributes of professionalism; and outlines the social contract (the cognitive base is described in Chapter 1). The definition used was agreed upon by faculty members for use in teaching professionalism at all levels.[10] The program has evolved over the years. There is now more lecture time devoted to the social contract. In some years, a vignette with questions is provided before the lecture to raise awareness and motivate residents as well as to "situate" the topic in the residents' context. As many McGill undergraduate medical students go on to undertake a residency at McGill, they have already been exposed to the material. Consequently, in recent years we have given a separate, more advanced lecture to the McGill graduates, while maintaining a more basic one for those who did their undergraduate education elsewhere.

The lecture is immediately followed by 2.5-hour small-group sessions for groups of eight to ten residents from diverse training programs. The purpose of the small-group session is to allow the residents an opportunity to apply the content to their own context, using a discussion of case vignettes, focused questions, and guided reflection. The vignettes, based on real events, were specifically geared to the resident context, in many specialty areas. This allows the learning to be collaborative, and "situated" in the residents' own context, as mentioned in Chapter 2 in this volume. We chose cases that exemplified both the positive and the negative aspects of professionalism, and vignettes were developed with input from residents. Sample vignettes are provided in Appendix C. The residents use the vignettes and a worksheet[7] (Appendix E) to identify the attributes and elements of professionalism raised by each case, and then discuss their approaches to the issues. The small-group session has evolved over time, with additional discussion questions on the social contract and codes of ethics added (Appendix F).

The small-group facilitators consist of a faculty member and senior resident working together. The faculty members have all attended faculty development sessions on teaching professionalism[10] and they are skilled in leading small-group discussions and promoting reflection. The fourth-, fifth-, and sixth-year residents have all attended the half-day as second-year learners. As well, a training session is given to all facilitators several weeks prior to the session, and they are provided with a group leader guide (Appendix G). We found that the combination of senior resident and faculty member was very effective; the faculty provided experience and teaching expertise, and the senior residents were easily able to translate the concepts into the participants' contexts.

The half-day is evaluated by the residents using a post-session questionnaire consisting of open-ended questions, ratings using a Likert scale, and a retrospective pre-post analysis (Appendix H). By using multiple methods, we hoped to assess participant satisfaction and whether there was improved knowledge and the ability to apply it. The residents found the content of the half-day very relevant and thought that the discussion of vignettes helped them apply concepts. They appreciated the interaction with others in different disciplines. As shown in Figure 14.1, the retrospective pre-post analysis showed significant increase in self-perceptions of knowledge about professionalism and in the ability to apply it in clinical contexts.

Resident knowledge about professionalism has been assessed before and after the session using case vignettes asking them to identify the attributes of professionalism that apply to the case. Before the session, the residents had an understanding of general concepts, had tacit knowledge of professionalism,

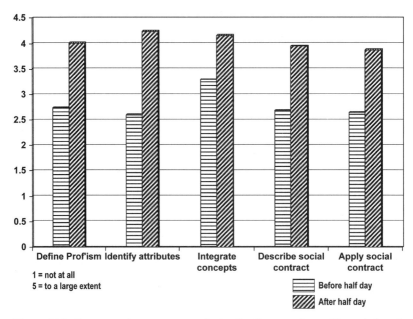

Figure 14.1. Retrospective pre-post analysis of self-perceptions of knowledge about professionalism and ability to apply it.

and could provide rich narrative descriptions of the professional issues in the vignettes. Following the session, the residents were more likely to use a common framework for approach to cases, to recognize issues described in the cases as "professional," and to use correct terminology.

The small-group facilitators also evaluate the half-day. They have provided useful suggestions to improve vignettes (number, type, and media) and have made valuable comments that have improved the program over time. They endorse the combination of senior resident and faculty member as effective. They consider pre-course training sessions essential. Both faculty and senior resident facilitators felt that their own knowledge and skills improved as a result of leading the group discussion and that they would apply the concepts in their own teaching practice. Almost all commented on the need to complement the formal teaching with other methods to promote integration of the cognitive base into the residents' practices.

Other Large-Group Learning Activities to Teach the Cognitive Base

Several elements of the professional role not addressed directly in the above-mentioned half-day are described in the CanMEDS document[1]: physician health and sustainable practice, peer review, disclosure of adverse events and errors, and bioethical theories and principles. A number of large-group activities at our institution address these. These are a combination of interactive presentations and workshops.

At McGill, ethics has been taught separately from, and in parallel to, the professionalism program, primarily at the departmental (specialty) level. Faculty-wide didactic presentations addressing the cognitive base of ethics are provided by ethics experts. Most clinical teachers have a basic knowledge of ethical principles and can help residents to apply these in the clinical context. As well, clinical ethicists are consulted about ethical issues in the resident's patients and contribute to the residents' experiential learning by helping the residents to analyze the ethical and legal aspects of a clinical situation.

Presentations from the national malpractice organization deal with risk management, medical error, teamwork responsibilities, and other medicolegal aspects of practice. The ability to teach well is considered a part of professionalism by many authors as teaching fosters and develops respect for fellow learners and the team.[11] Improving residents' skills as educators and enhancing their role as a teacher is considered part of developing the residents' professionalism.[5] Our resident-as-teacher program combines large-group presentations on the principles and theory of teaching with skill-building sessions. An annual "Resident Wellness Day" open to all residents of any level or discipline provides resources and presentations to help residents cope with stress, and improve their physical, psychological, and financial wellness and work-life balance. Professionalism concepts addressed on this day include recognizing and managing unprofessional behaviors, advocacy, and choosing a mentor.

Learning the Skills of Professionalism

As well as a cognitive base, there are specific skills that can assist residents develop professional behaviors. A number of skill-building activities are provided at a program or faculty-wide level. These activities have varied formats, all of which facilitate the acquisition of skills. Workshops including group discussion and role-play are used for developing teamwork, conflict resolution, and time management skills. A series of hands-on modules with practice sessions and microteaching are used to improve teaching skills. Advanced communication skills and practical ethics are taught at our simulation centre using standardized patients in scenarios in which the residents practice and get feedback.

Developing Professional Attitudes and Fostering Professional Behaviors: Transferring Learning into Practice

A helpful element is ensuring that learning objectives include expectations of professional behaviors and characteristics. An example of the goals and objectives about professionalism in the internal medicine program is shown in Table 14.2.

The residents receive these annually with a recommendation that they be reviewed at the beginning of each rotation.

Experiential Learning: Role Modeling, Guided Reflection, and Mentorship

Developing professional attitudes and encouraging professional behaviors is more difficult than increasing knowledge about professionalism. As mentioned elsewhere in this volume, one must address the informal and hidden curriculum as well as the formal curriculum.[8] Using case studies and vignettes may start the resident thinking about professionalism in their own practice. However, much of the learning about professionalism occurs "on the job" in the clinical context, by observing positive and negative professional behaviors, by working with role models (faculty, peers, and other health professionals), by practice with feedback, and by informal discussions with colleagues.[12] The learning methods used must recognize the dual role of the resident as "apprentice learner" and practitioner, and should use the residents' rapidly expanding experience in the clinical setting, as described in Chapter 2 in this volume. As young physicians proceed through two to seven years of residency and are progressively socialized into the profession, they are given graded responsibility and independence. During this evolution, their ability to self-reflect and to apply the cognitive base of professionalism increases as they internalize attitudes and behaviors, as diagrammed in Figure 14.2.

We use a number of learning strategies to ensure that the residents' knowledge of professionalism is truly internalized and expressed in professional behaviors. These primarily rely on explicit role modeling and guided self-reflection.[13,14] Clinical teachers are encouraged to specifically address issues of professionalism that arise in the patient care setting and to promote reflection in a safe environment. The residents' experience of concrete professional behaviors (e.g., punctuality, accurate charting, truth telling, self-regulation, similar to those described by other authors[6]) is accompanied by open discussion and contemplation of professional issues, using a vocabulary and framework that both the teachers and learners share. Some programs are starting to use learning portfolios to guide reflection about professional issues. Learning professionalism thus becomes an active rather than a passive experience.[12]

The Learning Environment

Clearly, one cannot expect residents to develop as good professionals if the learning environment does not explicitly exhibit models of excellence at all

Table 14.2. Sample curriculum for professionalism for internal medicine residents

Internal medicine goals and objectives: professional role

The curriculum is structured to occur through teaching sessions, academic half-days (e.g., on professionalism and medicolegal issues), and through the patient care context.

Regular evaluation of a resident's knowledge skill and attitudes in this domain is part of the monthly evaluation for each clinical rotation.

As a result, the resident will be able to deliver quality care with integrity, honesty, and compassion.

The resident will exhibit appropriate personal and interpersonal behaviors.

The resident will practice medicine ethically, consistent with the obligations of a physician.

The resident's knowledge, attitudes, and skills in this content will show appropriate evolution over training, with mastery of more advanced attitudes and skills in being a professional as the resident's clinical training progresses.

Ethics curriculum

The ethics curriculum is structured to occur through regular teaching sessions with clinical ethicists, in the patient care context through the recognition and application of basic ethical principles, and in the context of academic half-days.

Regular evaluation of a resident's knowledge skill and attitudes in this domain is part of the monthly evaluation for each clinical rotation.

The resident will demonstrate knowledge of common ethical issues encountered in practice, including consent, capacity, substitute decision making, confidentiality, truth telling, conflicts, boundary issues, end-of-life decisions, resource allocation, professionalism, and medicolegal issues.

The resident will appreciate the ethical dimensions of medical decision making.

The resident will appreciate the professional, legal, and ethical codes to which physicians are bound; and will recognize and know how to address unprofessional behaviors in clinical practice.

The resident will be able to analyze the ethical and legal dimensions of a clinical situation; to communicate with colleagues, families, and patients about these issues; and to recognize and deal with conflicts.

The resident's knowledge, attitudes, and skills in this content will show appropriate evolution over training, with appropriate mastery of more advanced concepts in clinical ethics as the resident's clinical training progresses.

From: McGill University Faculty of Medicine Internal Medicine Residency Learning Objectives, 2007.

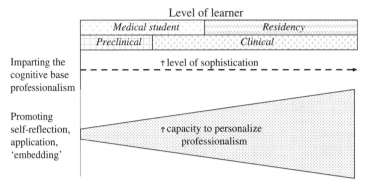

Figure 14.2. Developmental stages in learning professionalism.

levels.[15,16] The "hidden curriculum," as described elsewhere in this volume, is addressed in a number of ways specific to the residency level.

In many programs, the role of the resident as professional is addressed in the interview associated with the residency selection process. In pediatrics, for example, candidates are asked to describe role models and their influence on the resident, to discuss the "larger meaning of professionalism" (e.g., "what does it mean to you to be a professional, beyond being a good person"), and to analyze their own experiences with lapses in professionalism that they have observed.

In some disciplines, residents have participated in departmental retreats about professionalism alongside their faculty mentors and have contributed to the discussion of professional behaviors relevant to the specialty.

Many programs require residents to also rate their attending teachers on the professional role. For example, in internal medicine, the evaluation form has two items: "the attending staff role modeled and promoted the values of the highest levels of integrity and honesty," and "the attending staff role modeled and promoted the values of compassion and empathy in clinical encounters with patients and families." In pediatrics, the residents rate these two items, and as well assess their attending staff "sensitivity and respect for diversity," recognition of own limitations, and application of the principles of ethics to clinical situations. Thus, professional behaviors are explicitly discussed and encouraged in both teachers and learners.[6]

Evaluation

Another helpful means to ensure that professionalism is learned is to formally evaluate it on every clinical rotation,[17] using explicit behaviors as

Table 14.3. Professionalism evaluation items on in-training assessment forms

Criterion	Description
Integrity and honesty	Judges whether the trainee is dependable, reliable, honest, and forthright in all information and facts.
Sensitivity and respect for diversity	Judges whether the trainee is able to understand and be sensitive to issues related to age, gender, cultures, and ethnicity.
Responsible and self-disciplined	Judges whether the trainee adequately accepts professional responsibilities, placing the needs of the patients before the trainee's own; ensuring that the trainee or his/her replacement are at all times available to the patient. The trainee is punctual and respects local regulations relating to the performance of his/her duties.
Communicates with patients	With compassion and empathy
Recognition of own limitations, seeking advice when needed	Judges that the trainee is able to self-assess his/her limits of competence, and is able to seek and give assistance when necessary.
Understands the principles of ethics, applied to clinical situations	Judges the trainee's understanding of the principles and practice of biomedical ethics as it relates to the specialty. The trainee practices in an ethically responsible manner.

From: McGill University Faculty of Medicine Postgraduate In-Training Evaluation Form, 2008.

outcome measures.[5,6] This is done using monthly in-training assessment forms used by all residency programs and on the biannual composite assessments. Ratings of the professional role are done in six categories: "integrity and honesty"; "sensitivity and respect for diversity"; "responsibility and self-discipline"; "communicates with compassion and empathy"; "recognizes own limitations, seeks help when needed"; "understands ethical principles and applies them to clinical situations." These are described in more detail in Table 14.3.

We have also attempted to assess individual residents' professional behaviors using the Professionalism Mini-Evaluation Exercise described elsewhere in this volume. The P-MEX assesses twenty-one observable professional behaviors during a brief real clinical encounter and has shown good construct validity.[18] However, we have not had complete acceptance of or buy-in to this means of evaluation at the resident level by either the residents or their teachers.

Knowledge about professionalism must be assessed specifically, and not indirectly through the evaluation of other competencies.[19] The Canadian national exit examination for all specialties is based on the CanMEDS framework: the professional role is assessed directly by questions and indirectly by observation of multiple professional attributes and behaviors. For instance, in internal medicine, there are specific professionalism questions on the written multiple-choice examination, often related to the principles of bioethics. As well, the final oral examination includes professionalism objective structured clinical exam (OSCE) stations addressing issues such as disclosure of adverse events and errors, application of bioethical principles to end-of-life decisions, consent, competency, and standards of accountability. As well, on all OSCE stations, the candidates are assessed for professional behaviors such as compassion. There is also a national licensure examination that includes knowledge questions about professionalism items such as codes of ethics, confidentiality, consent, doctor-patient relationship, self-regulation, and interprofessional issues.

Faculty Development

One cannot expect residents to learn to be professional without faculty knowledgeable in the concepts and practice, and skilled in the teaching and role modeling of professional behaviors and values.[5,15] At our institution, faculty development programs open to all faculty members have been given on teaching and evaluating professionalism, as well as on specific learning methods such as reflection and role modeling. The former have been described in detail.[10] The program included the development of an institutional approach to teaching and evaluation of professionalism, contribution to a definition that is understood by faculty members and for which there is buy-in by teachers, and dissemination with workshops. The attendees usually teach at both the medical student and the postgraduate level, so a coherent "message" is given across the continuum of medical education.

In the half-day workshops on role modeling and reflection, clinical teachers use group discussion, video vignettes, and a guided reflection of their own role modeling to address issues of professionalism that arise during clinical practice, and to learn how to encourage reflection in a safe environment.

We have also developed a faculty development program specifically for residency program directors – a full day on how to develop curricula and use teaching methods for the core competencies, including the professional role, and another full day the following year on developing evaluation methods for the competencies. During these sessions, the program directors reviewed and discussed different methods of teaching or evaluating core competencies, defined measurable behaviors within their specialty that reflect the competencies, identified ways of promoting faculty and resident buy-in, and started to develop specialty-specific evaluation forms.

Focused faculty development activities, some of which are described in Chapter 9, are aimed at Osler Fellows, the teachers for the undergraduate Physician Apprenticeship program. Most of these role model clinicians also teach residents, so the content and skills learned have been translated into the postgraduate level, and the same message is transmitted across the continuum of education.

The Royal College of Physicians and Surgeons of Canada, a national accreditation and standards organization, is developing faculty development on a national scale. They are creating a module for the CanMEDS Professional role. This module will form the backbone for a two-day "train-the-trainer" session for individual "champions" from each university, who will develop expertise in content and teaching and evaluation strategies, and take home resources to disseminate among all residency programs.

LESSONS LEARNED

- Teaching professionalism to residents is not done solely at this level: learning must be sequential and progressive throughout the continuum of medical education. As an institution, our medical school supported the teaching of professionalism at all levels: undergraduate, residency, and in practice. This changed the institutional culture and allowed similar resources to be used across the years, with increasing sophistication and complexity as learners progress through residency. The best level to teach the cognitive base of professionalism may be within the early years, but it must be reinforced, expanded upon, and experiential learning must occur throughout residency. Explicit teaching about professionalism and a congruent message must be integrated at all levels.

- For many, the cognitive base of professionalism contains new concepts and a new vocabulary, which must be explicitly addressed. Formal instruction of this cognitive base must occur for teachers and learners alike. Faculty teachers must be comfortable with the concepts and need to be able to apply and discuss them in the clinical context. Residents must learn and use the same vocabulary and framework as their mentors.

- In our faculty, there were only a few experts in medical professionalism. We found that providing the cognitive base to large groups of residents allowed effective use of this expertise. Over time, other faculty members have become more expert in this content area, and the faculty-wide sessions have been supplemented by program-specific activities.

- Our faculty-wide program has been effective as it has been able to address a critical mass of residents, providing varied perspectives, and efficient use of limited expertise and resources, with sharing and adapting across programs. As well, we have been able to coordinate programs for the residents with the faculty development activities.

- Teaching this topic in a multispecialty environment has been effective: it has allowed us to use teachers in one discipline to teach learners in others. The ability to see that concepts of professionalism, and solutions to professionalism problems, can be generalized has been helpful to residents. In contrast, there are also advantages to having some activities at a program or specialty level: the residents usually know each other and have formed as groups, so that their comfort level in discussions is higher. As well, cases or vignettes can be made specialty specific, and the timing of interventions can be chosen to fit in with other curricular requirements.

- Attitude development and behavior change demand different learning strategies: teachers must be comfortable with, among other strategies, explicit debriefing on role modeling and encouraging reflection as teaching methods is essential. Despite faculty development we still have difficulty providing regular real-world opportunities for residents to internalize the values of professionalism.

- Other authors have described a number of learning strategies to present "professionalism situations" and allow for discussion and guided reflection: a "readers' theatre," a ranking and discussion of challenging situations, role playing, small-group discussion of "relative values,"[5] mentoring programs,[6,15] panel discussions, and multimedia presentations.[20] These descriptions can provide useful ideas and resources to our program directors.

- Residency program directors need specific faculty development to address their needs. They need to know the cognitive base of professionalism and to have a choice of learning and assessment methods. They also need help in leading the culture change needed in their own department and in encouraging buy-in of their colleagues.

- Culture change, and changing the hidden curriculum, is a slow process. External forces to include medical professionalism in a formal curriculum at the resident level started over ten years ago. It has taken this time to develop curricular content and teaching methods, and to engage the residency program directors and general faculty members in this endeavor.

SUMMARY

When planning a program to teach professionalism at the resident level, the program director must recognize that there is a body of knowledge about professionalism that must be learned. More importantly there is a need to apply this knowledge in the residents' context, to allow residents to develop professional attitudes and demonstrate professional behaviors. The means for facilitating this include role modeling, reflection, and experiential learning. To motivate resident buy-in, professional behaviors should be measured so that trainees can be effectively evaluated and progress seen. This remains a challenge. William Osler's comment of a century ago still pertains to our current state of education about professionalism: Give a student "good methods and a proper point of view, and all other things will be added, as his experience grows."[21] This is an admirable goal.

REFERENCES

1. Snell, L, Brazeau, M, Brownell, K, Leonard, P, Magwood, B, Pauls, M, Pope, W, Penner, M, Puddester, D, Robertson A. Report of the CanMEDS Professional Working Group. In Frank, JR. ed. *Report of the CanMEDS Phase IV Working Groups*. Ottawa: Royal College of Physicians and Surgeons of Canada, March 2005, pp. 52–59.
2. Accreditation Council for Graduate Medical Education. ACGME Outcomes Project. Accessed at www.acgme.org/outcome/comp/compFull.asp on January 17, 2007.
3. General Medical Council. *Good Medical Practice*. London: GMC, 1996.
4. ABIM Foundation, ACP-ASIM Foundation, European Federation of Internal Medicine. Medical professionalism in the new millennium: a physician charter. *Ann Intern Med.* 2002 February 5; 136(3):243–246.
5. Klein, J, Jackson, JC, Kratz, L, Marcuse, EK, McPhillips, HA, Shugerman, RP, Watkins, S, Stapleton FB. Teaching professionalism to residents. *Acad Med.* 2003 January; 78(1):26–34.
6. Larkin, G. Mapping, modeling and mentoring: charting a course for professionalism in graduate medical education. *Cambridge Quarterly of Health Care Ethics* 2003; 12:167–177.
7. Ryder, E. Competency 6: professionalism. In Ryder, E, Nawotniak, R, Smith, G, eds. *A Practical Guide to Teaching and Assessing the ACGME Core Competencies*. Marblehead, MA: HCPro, 2007.
8. Cruess, R, Cruess, S. Teaching professionalism: general principles. *Med Teach.* 2006; 28(3):205–208.
9. Stern, DT (ed.). *Measuring Medical Professionalism*. New York, Oxford University Press, 2005.
10. Steinert, Y, Cruess, S, Cruess, R, Snell, L. Faculty development for teaching and evaluating professionalism: from programme design to curriculum change. *Med Educ.* 2005; 39(1):127–136.

11. Hatem, C. Teaching approaches that reflect and promote professionalism. *Acad Med.* 2003 July; 78(7):709–713.

12. Branch, W, Kern, D, Haidet, P, Weissmann, P, Gracey, CF, Mitchell, G, Inui, T. Teaching the human dimensions of care in clinical settings. *JAMA* 2001 September 5; 286(9):1067–1074.

13. Cruess, R, Cruess, S. Role modelling—making the most of a powerful teaching strategy *BMJ* 2008;336:718–721 (29 March),

14. Kenny, N, Mann, KV, MacLeod, H. Role modeling in physicians' professional formation: reconsidering an essential but untapped educational strategy. *Acad Med.* 2003; 78(12):1203–1210.

15. Markakis, K, Beckman, HB, Suchman, AL, Frankel, RM. The path to professionalism: cultivating humanistic values and attitudes in residency training. *Acad Med.* 2000 February; 75(2):141–149.

16. Ludmerer, K, Johns, M. Reforming graduate medical education. *JAMA* 2005 September 7; 294(9):1083–1087.

17. Joyner, B, Vemalakonda, V. Improving professionalism: making the implicit more explicit. *J Urolo.* 2007 June; 177:2287–2291.

18. Cruess, R, McIlroy, JH, Cruess, S, Ginsburg, S, Steinert, Y. The professionalism mini-evaluation exercise: a preliminary investigation. *Acad Med.* 2006 October; 81 (10 Suppl.):S74–S78.

19. West, C, Huntington, JL, Huschka, MM, Novotny, PJ, Sloan, JA, Kolars, JC, Habermann, TM, Shanafelt TD. A prospective study of the relationship between medical knowledge and professionalism among internal medicine residents. *Acad Med.* 2007 June; 82(6):587–592.

20. Marco, C. Ethics seminars: Teaching professionalism to "problem" residents. *Acad Emerg Med.* 2002; 9:1001–1006.

21. Osler, W. On the need for a radical reform in our methods of teaching senior students. *Med News* (New York) 1903; 82: 49–53.

15 Continuing Professional Development: A Focus on Professionalism

Dave Davis, M.D.

INTRODUCTION

The Case for Continuing Professional Development in Professionalism

There are many "gaps" in clinical practice. The Institute of Medicine reports,[1] and those from the Rand Corporation,[2] provide a clear picture of the clinical practice gap: the failure to meet best evidence performance at the time of care. This phenomenon is complex and multicausal, the product of incomplete information, poor information transfer to and retention by the practitioner, poor patient compliance and understanding, and a host of other environmental or setting-specific issues.

This is not the only care gap however: gaps also exist in clinician conduct between what we would normally call professional behavior and those that occur in the real word of clinical practice. These gaps occur when physicians and others fail to follow the tenets of the "Charter on Medical Professionalism,"[3] that is, demonstrate adherence to the principles of the primacy of patient welfare, patient autonomy, and social justice. These two elements, elsewhere described as the science and the art of medicine, contribute to patient's frustrations with health care systems virtually world wide.

The following are examples of the latter problem. They may be illustrative; they are certainly familiar:

- "Turfing": this word denotes a patient transfer or triage from one physician to another when the care of that patient feels more troublesome than it is worth. A widespread phenomenon in medical training

The author is grateful to Laure Perrier, MLIS, of the office of Continuing Education and Professional Development, and the Knowledge Translation Program, Faculty of Medicine, University of Toronto, for her help in providing referencing services.

programs, turfing appears to allocate patient care to meet physicians' rather than patients' needs.[4]

- Commercial influence: many examples exist in which professional educational products and physicians' practices themselves, including clinical practice guidelines and publications, have been biased by the involvement of commercial influences such as those in the pharmaceutical industry. Specialty societies, individual physicians, and continuing education providers have become increasingly dependent on such sources, often – if subtly – to the detriment of professional responsibilities.[5]

- Maintaining humanistic practice in an organizational environment: eighteen family physicians in Seattle participating in focus groups on the subject of professionalism described tensions in balancing organizational expectations and individual physician or patient values. These physicians articulated and weighed their own values with competing values of their patients, the organizations for which many work, and stated values of their profession.[6]

- Personal safety and duty of care: during the Toronto SARS epdieminc, fourteen attending physicians highlighted several themes about values inherent to medical professionalism that arose during this crisis. These include the balance between care of patients and accepted personal risk, confidentiality, appropriate interactions between physicians and patients, ethical research conduct, and role modeling of professionalism for junior doctors. Despite these risks to professionalism, participants in this study amply demonstrated the necessary qualities during the recent health care crisis; however, there were several examples of strained professional behavior witnessed by the participants.[7]

- Self assessment: the literature is replete with examples in which physicians appear unable to judge their past or future performance, or current learning needs and competence, at least to some extent, and without accurate profiles of their practices. In one recent systematic review, this phenomenon is apparent in roughly one quarter of instances, and – of more concern – appears to be most noticeable in situations in which the physician has performed in less-then-optimum fashion yet judges him/ herself to be above average.[8]

Finally, Wofford et al.[9] reviewed formal, unsolicited patient complaints collected routinely at the Wake Forest University Baptist Medical Center in the United States and categorized them in the following manner. The most commonly identified issue was disrespect (36 percent), followed by disagreement about expectations of care (23 percent), inadequate information (20 percent), distrust (18 percent), perceived unavailability (15 percent), interdisciplinary miscommunication (4 percent), and misinformation (4 percent). Multiple categories were identified in (19 percent) complaints.

What can we do in these situations? While significant efforts are exerted in the areas of knowledge translation and putting best clinical evidence into action, similar efforts to include professionalism in the practices of continuing professional development (CPD) providers (and thus physicians) appear minimal or at least lacking. This chapter attempts to address questions related to physicians' professionalism through the lens of the continuing medical education (CME) or CPD provider. For simplicity, we use the term "CPD" throughout this chapter.

Addressing the Gap

What can the medical profession, especially that portion of it dedicated to CPD, do to close those gaps related to deficits in professionalism? This chapter offers some insights into the delivery of continuing education in general, with particular reference to professionalism where the literature permits.

Consider this scenario:

You are the chief of a local emergency department. You have been concerned about the number of prescriptions written in your Emergency Department for oxycodone, a highly potent and addictive pain medication. This is often prescribed in large quantities, frequently for relatively minor injuries such as sprained ankles or acute low back pain, and often against the backdrop of high patient volumes, high demand, and expectations. It also comes on the heels of a meeting with your hospital's public relations officer in which she states that the number of patient complaints – about staff members dealing with certain cultural groups, not communicating with patients, prescribing inappropriate medications to "get rid of" certain patient types such as the homeless, among other issues – seem to be on the rise.

All of this bothers you enormously and you wish to address the problem. It occurs to you you might employ your department's grand rounds, held monthly and attracting almost full attendance by your staff (though attendance has been dropping off recently). You turn to your local CPD director and ask the question, "How can I make these rounds more interesting and informative? How can I get them to look at their behavior and change it? How can I address other complaints of a professional nature in my department?"

This is not an uncommon scenario, either clinically or educationally; many physician-teachers and course organizers are confronted with the dilemma of organizing CPD activities, and/or presenting to or preparing educational sessions and activities for colleagues, other health professional audiences, and the public. As in the case of the emergency chief described above, or in fact where there is any element of reflection or a sense of quality improvement, there is frequently a strong desire to improve the CPD product, to make it more effective.

This scenario is different than undergraduate teaching or residency training, marked by the "captive audience" nature of those audiences, and with built-in measures and methods of feedback to such learners. On the positive side of the ledger, CPD, like the work of clinicians themselves, using effective educational interventions, can effect practice change and even health care outcomes[10] – on a more immediate and possibly rewarding basis than undergrad teaching and residency training. On the challenging (if not exactly negative) side of the ledger, CPD activities rarely require mandatory participation, or demonstrations of competence, or performance. In this scenario, one is engaged in a process of communication with peers – colleagues with their own practice needs, learning styles, and requirements, and – moreover – their own areas of expertise.

This chapter outlines a three-step process to make CPD more effective. They are captured here as steps in decision making: 1) deciding who comprises the audience, and what they need or want to know about professional behavior; 2) deciding what and how to convey this to the audience; and 3) deciding on the outcome. The steps, simple-sounding enough, are in fact fairly complex and iterative. They are made only more so by the topic of professionalism, a subject not always "top of mind" when speaking to physicians about their CPD needs.

GETTING TO KNOW THE LEARNERS, WHAT THEY NEED AND WANT TO KNOW

The Audience and Their Clinical World

It is a truism in CPD that one needs to know one's learners or students; here, "Who's the target audience?" is a favorite planning phrase. The answer is not so simple.

In the scenario above, there are many considerations. First, methods of payment affect clinician-learners' abilities to maintain or deliver practice competencies and to perform at their best relative to professional behaviors. We know, for example, that declining rounds attendance may imply a stricter fee-for-service environment, a frequent occurrence in the North American setting, in which time away from practice settings is not reimbursed. In other settings, physicians may be incented for attending CPD activities. For example, practices enrolled in the Practice Incentives Program in Australia may receive payment for participating in Quality Prescribing Initiative activities (i.e., clinical audits, case studies, practice visits).[11] Second, little explanation needs to be undertaken to describe the environment of virtually every emergency department in most busy centers – long wait times, less-than-adequate numbers and mix of staff members, numerous problems related to social and not medical pathology, even dangerous and risky patient encounters. In many ways, this pressure on service delivery and a tightly constrained environment can describe virtually every clinical practice setting.

Fortunately, there are countervailing forces in the form of local and national professional and regulatory guidelines that compel physicians to participate in CPD. These guidelines suggest a minimum number of hours of formal continuing education for a wide variety of physician groups. It is useful to know what these are in each jurisdiction, and where possible, to tailor presentations to meet them. For example, in the case of the Royal College of Physicians and Surgeons of Canada, additional CPD "points" may be gained by asking physicians to perform pre-workshop charts audits, post lecture structured reading and reflection exercises, or personal learning projects resulting from participation in a CPD activity.[12] There are also of course strong internal motivators and a desire to maintain high levels of professional practice.

There are further practice distinctions as well. As increasing emphasis is placed on interprofessional practice, and as recognition grows about the importance of the team, the audience may comprise teams of clinicians – professionals engaged in burn care, for example (plastic surgeons, physiatrists, nurses, physical therapists, and psychiatrists).

The Adult Learner

While it is useful to view the target of CPD activity from the perspective of the clinician, it is also important to see him or her as a learner.

Although there are many theories of adult education, the work of Fox et al.[13] is possibly the most helpful here. This study asked these questions, "What did you change last in your practice? What caused that change?" – of over 300 North American physicians. There were three clusters of responses, important to us in understanding how to incorporate professionalism in CPD. First, physicians undertaking any change disclosed that they had an image of what that change was going to look like – the surgeon taking up a laparoscopic technique, the physician wanting to take on a nursing home practice imagined himself more comfortable and competent with geriatric patients. Second, the forces for change were widespread – while some drew from traditional educational and CPD experiences, many more were intra-personal (e.g., a recent personal experience), or from changing demographics (e.g., aging or changing populations and patient demands). Third, the changes varied from smaller "adjustments" or accommodations (e.g., adding a new drug to a regimen within a class of drugs already known and pre-scribed) to much larger changes characterized as "redirections," for exam-ple, adopting an entirely new way or method of practice. Here, more minor changes might be accomplished with a brief CPD presentation, even a didac-tic lecture. Clearly, however, larger changes require a much richer CPD experience – perhaps encompassing a lecture, a highly interactive session such as a hands-on workshop, and possibly refresher or practical experience in the work setting. There are many lessons here for those planning CPD in professionalism: the image of the professional physician, the forces for change (internal or external to the physician), the degree of change required, and the agents to help promote it.

There are also other theories and models of adult learning of which Knowles' work may be the most widely known.[14] He describes the adult leaner as needing educational experiences that are relevant to practice set-tings and needs, conducive to learning styles, nonthreatening, and support-ive. Some authors, such as Schön[15] and Kolb,[16] describe the internal process of learning. Schön, for example, describes the pervasive force of "reflection," suggesting that a potent learning mechanism is secondary to self-appraisal and awareness built from clinical experiences, leading to a building of a new and expanded competency or "zone of mastery."[15] Similarly, Kolb uses the notion of experience, suggesting that learners move from the concrete (a case for example) to the more abstract (such as understanding more about the pathophysiology of a disease) and back again.[16] Geertsma suggests that clini-cians move through three phases being primed about a particular problem or gap in knowledge by some clinical experience, focusing on the exact extent and nature of their learning gap, and following up with an appropriate learn-ing plan such as reading or speaking with a colleague.[17] Finally, among this not exhaustive list, Bandura places all learning in a social and environmental context, indicating that learning and its application takes place in the clinical setting, requiring us to focus in this area.[18] Similar to Fox's theories of change, there are lessons here for professionalism and CPD.[13]

What Do Learners Need or Want?

Like the word, "location" in considering real estate values, the words "needs assessment" assume major importance in CPD – they are the sine qua non of planning. A variety of needs assessment techniques are available to identify subjective needs (defined as those expressed by learners), and objective needs (defined as needs observed by others, identified through group comparison, or defined by experts). Each needs assessment strategy enables the collection of different types of information, and each has a body of literature on methods and effectiveness; a multifaceted approach provides a more comprehensive understanding of the situation.[19] We provide here a short listing of these techniques, with a special emphasis on those tools or methods that might inform the topic of professionalism.

Subjective Needs Assessment

Subjective needs assessment may seem a relatively simple task, along the lines of asking the question, "What do you want to learn about?" Adequate self-assessment however has proven more difficult than anticipated,[20] and a rigorous application of methods may be needed to obtain high-quality data.[21–23] There are several examples of subjective needs assessment techniques that may be of special use in eliciting physicians' reflections on "professionalism" and their own needs in this area.

They include, but are not limited to:

- Questionnaires: among the many positive attributes of a questionnaire are its flexibility (quantitative and qualitative surveys are both commonplace) and its confidentiality. Web-based surveys have become more prominent, allowing for rapid deployment and collection of answers in a collective, anonymized fashion. Further, such surveys lend themselves to the use of Likert or global rating scales, which can determine attitudes by asking respondents to indicate their agreement or disagreement, on a several-point scale, to such statements as, "I believe that physicians should maintain perfect patient confidentiality."
- Focus groups: these are small groups, chosen at random or purposefully, and led most often by a neutral party, often unrelated to the topic at hand, or the setting from which the participants are drawn. Such groups often elicit deeply felt beliefs and practices, learning needs, practice patterns, and other issues at stake in a discussion about professional behavior.
- Reflection methods: there are many tools such as diaries or log books that permit the clinician-learner to record details of a practice day, difficult encounters, patient and system problems, and other data. In an interview situation, these can be used to prompt a discussion of educational needs in professionalism, while in an educational setting, outlined below, they may be useful in generating ideas, teachable moments, case material, and other points for discussion.

Objective Needs Assessment

Objective needs assessment strategies include chart audits, peer review (whereby doctors assess each others practice), standardized patients to rate task performance, observation of physician practices, and reports of practice patterns such as regional prescribing practices. Examples of gaps representing the last phenomenon domain are not difficult to find: in congestive heart failure, for example, nearly one third of patients do not receive adequate treatment posthospitalization.[24,25] There are countless other examples, each instructive to the CPD provider, that may be drawn from different data sources – one's own referral practice, recent government publications, health services reports, the literature and so forth. It is interesting – and perhaps educationally useful – to think about the degree to which improving professional behaviors (increasing communication and listening skills, for example) would help to close this gap.

In the domain of professionalism, data sources eliciting direct, helpful, and objective measures are somewhat less available. It is likely that peer assessments or opinions gained from any number of colleagues (nurses and other coworkers, for example) such as 360 degree assessments would be of benefit. Further, the use of patient surveys regarding professional issues may also be helpful, providing measures for feedback to physicians.

DECIDING ON THE CONTENT AND FORMAT: INCORPORATING PROFESSIONALISM INTO CPD

In planning the content of any CPD intervention – rounds, workshops, conferences, small-group learning experiences, audit and feedback, opinion leader-mediated activities, and others – one needs to consider the objectives of the activity. More globally, it is useful to think of what knowledge, skills, and attitudes the activity is intended to impart or change. In considering professionalism, it is unlikely that knowledge alone accounts for any deficits; most physicians know about issues of patient confidentiality, respect for other team members, punctuality, use of language, and other matters. Instead, it is more apt to be the case that attitudes have been modified by practice realities or experiences, by the physician's own internal drivers or the culture of a team or organization; or that physicians' skills or performance have been modified over time.

Thus, the creation of an effective CPD intervention in this area presents – rather than a simple and straightforward process of communicating facts or information – an opportunity to create a truly engaging and far-reaching strategy. To optimize adoption of different attitudes, improve retention of new skills, and to effect practice change, the effective CPD provider must weave a path through many contexts – that of the individual and his/her training and setting, that of his/her learning style and experience, and finally that of the more objective picture of practice and performance gaps. Weaving each of these into the goals of the presentation of CPD activity – the desired knowledge, skill, attitude, or practice change desired by the intervention itself. There are many tools or methods to help in this process; these are explored below.

Choosing the Format

It is constructive to think of the format or method in CPD less as a grand rounds session, lecture, or presentation and more as an intervention. In this manner, one broadens the scope of the educational encounter and makes the provider/teacher think more creatively about ways in which he/she can effect performance change in the learner and improve practice outcomes. Green's PRECEED model,[26] which incorporates elements that are characterized as predisposing, enabling, and reinforcing, helps with this conceptualization of the intervention. This section will deal with two key concepts: making the presentation (rounds, lecture, refresher program, update, or other conference) as effective as possible and enabling the transfer of information back into the practice setting.

Enabling Learning: The CPD Intervention

Four decades ago, Miller described the classical learning experience as "Rows of lecture desks, laden with pitchers of water," a speaker at the front, communicating in a one-directional manner.[27] Though research regarding formal CPD methods[28] has moved us ahead somewhat, there are still many gaps in the practice of effective CPD. While there are many elements to making CPD more effective and more closely adherent to the principles of adult education,[14] two stand out as key to the provision of CPD – increasing the relevance to the practice setting or needs of the learner and enhancing engagement in the learning experience. These two key concepts overlap somewhat but are useful descriptors of effective formal CME and CPD activities.

Increasing Relevance: The Clinical Scenario

There are many ways in which the relevance of CPD activity may be enhanced by the addition of patient scenarios or vignettes. They reflect actual clinical cases, frequently modified to protect patient privacy and to exemplify details of history, diagnosis or management – and in this case, issues of professional behavior. They promote reflection and interaction, increasing the relevance of the presentation. Several are explored here in some detail.

- Standardized patients: Trained patients or actors are useful adjuncts to any educational session. They are relatively less commonly employed in the CPD setting, but may be useful here[29–31] to present, display, or test issues of patient confidentiality, sensitive communication skills, and other measures.
- Videotaped encounters: Such videotapes may use simulated or real doctor-patient encounters or patient accounts of their experiences. Often used as "trigger tapes," these methods are useful in promoting reflection within learners, and discussion between and among them.
- Feedback: Employing data or information received from patients, peers, team members, and others about perceived behaviors frequently provides grounds for reflection on one's own assessment of behaviors compared to external observation. This is particularly useful when considering the relatively low correlations between clinicians' self-perceptions and those of others. The use of 360 degree measurements appears to be growing and is generally reasonably well accepted.
- The written case: Paper- or computer-presented cases are simple, easily constructed, and inexpensive. They may be given out during or before a lecture/presentation to stimulate discussion and problem solving.

Increasing Engagement

Derived from the work of Steinert and Snell,[32] and built on the concept of reflection on action as a key element in learning,[15] the effective lecture or presentation presents several ways to increase interactivity. Lectures, for example, may include a suggestion to think about a problematic case, such as the one described above. This process may be made a little more powerful by providing time in the lecture to do so, suggesting that participants write down a problem, or three questions they have, before the presentation. Similarly, the lecturer might provide a Likert-like scale, multiple choice, or similar quiz to be completed before, after, or during a lecture.

The most obvious, frequently used and easiest way in which to improve interactivity with the lecturer – and thus with the topic of professionalism – is to increase the traditional question and answer (Q&A) session. At the University of Toronto, "Saturday at the University" planners found that a large, two-hour block of lecture time could be effectively broken up into sequential ten-minute periods of lecture and Q&A.[19] Other Q&A methods include the audience response system either computerized[20] or one using participant-held colored cards. Other methods may include debates, panelists, written questions, and mandatory question periods.

Advocated for decades by our adult education colleagues, and the goal of much faculty development activity,[33] the notion of increasing interactivity between learners speaks to the principles of Knowles and others about the intelligence and experience of the audience.[13,14] Based on a relatively large literature,[32,34,35] these methods include buzz groups, "think-pair-share" methods, and "stand up and be counted."

Other Options in Creating CPD Interventions

There is a wide varied array of interventions, loosely categorized as "non-traditional" methods, guideline implementation strategies, or knowledge translation tools.[36] These include such measures as reminders at the point of care, academic detailing, decision support systems, protocols and guidelines, newsletters, emails, learning portfolios, care maps, quality improvement techniques, checklists, and other tools. For the most part, they are beyond the scope of this chapter, although they may prove useful in future considerations of professionalism and CPD.

One of these in particular, however, deserves mention: the educational opinion leader. Over two decades ago, Stross[37] described the selection of one or more peers by clinicians. Once nominated, these individuals were trained to better understand best practices in a variety of clinical areas, and to act as change agents within their own communities. Randomized controlled trials of these agents have proven fairly to moderately successful, changing performance and/or health care outcome measures in atleast some of the anticipated outcomes. It seems likely that in the area of professionalism, where so much is culturally grounded in the setting, such interventions may be helpful adjuncts to the more traditional and programmatic intervenient outlined above.

Faculty Development

Itself a subset of CPD, faculty development is the subject of a sizable literature and increasing importance. Relative to the topic of professionalism in CPD, it may be useful to think of each step outlined above as the building blocks in raising awareness about educational techniques and their application: in this way they may form a "curriculum" for faculty members, enabling them to be more effective presenters and CPD planners – especially in the area of professionalism. In the case of our emergency room chief, for example, she may begin her engagement in this process by recruiting two or three colleagues in her department or elsewhere, invite them to a session that includes the discussion of educational issues described in this chapter, and thus begin their training.

ASSESSING THE OUTCOME

There are many reasons and methods by which to know the outcome of CPD activities. They follow the outline provided by Dixon's several-level outline of the evaluation of CPD activities.[38] The levels include perception of the educational activity, competency (knowledge, skill, or attitude), performance change, and finally health care outcomes. These are outlined below, with special emphasis on professionalism. Other models of change (Miller, for example) may be equally useful.[27]

Perception of the Learning Event

From the narrow perspective of our scenario, measures of perception offer more than that conveyed by the classical "happiness index." Beyond the confines of overall ratings of quality of presentations, postcourse questionnaires may be enlarged to incorporate a number of features such as match with learning objectives, appropriate use of audiovisual materials, the degree to which interactivity was achieved, relevance, and other topics.[31] Also from the perspective of professionalism, a postintervention questionnaire might ask, "Has the course (or rounds, seminar, newsletter, etc.) made any difference to how you view your interactions with patients?"

Competence

For the purpose of this chapter at least, a consideration of competence includes knowledge, skills, and attitudes relative to professionalism, the classic triumvirate of this dimension of impact on the learner. Tests for each of these are widely available and may include[32,33,34,39,40]:

- Knowledge: multiple choice examinations, true-false tests
- Skills: performance simulators (e.g., ACLS or anesthesia mannequins), interviews with standardized patients
- Attitudes: global rating scores

Arnold's recent review of the professionalism literature offers some useful insights about themes or novel approaches in measurement instruments, and describes pragmatic or theoretical approaches to assessing professionalism.[41] She found that a circumscribed concept of professionalism is available to serve as a foundation for next steps in assessing professional behavior. While the current array of assessment tools is rich, their measurement properties require increased robustness. She suggests that future research should explore rigorous qualitative techniques; refine quantitative assessments of competence, for example, through objective structured clinical examinations; and evaluate separate elements of professionalism.[42–46]

Performance Change and Health Care Outcome

While it may be difficult to demonstrate performance or health care change as the result of a lecture or presentation, many CPD interventions and health care environments allow an opportunity to demonstrate such outcomes. Patient or 360 degree questionnaires may assess observations of physicians' and others' professional behavior. Such measures are often best considered as iterative – that is, they may be used to help in the ongoing planning of CPD interventions, as a needs assessment tool.

CONCLUSIONS

This brief chapter has outlined several steps in making the CPD experience more effective – from both the perspective of the individual CPD teacher and the broader viewpoint of the provider/organizer of such experiences. Captured as brief, take-home points, they include the following four principles with a special emphasis on professionalism. First, know the audience – its composition, background, practice milieu, needs, and experiences. Second, know the objectives and goals of the intervention, choosing from a broad and wide range of interactive and relevant methods, adding postintervention enabling and reinforcing materials and methods where necessary. And third finally, know and plan for the outcome – and wherever possible, measure it. This last step then becomes – in an attempt to make all such CPD experiences iterative – integral to further planning, involving the first two steps.

REFERENCES

1. Institute of Medicine (U.S.). Committee on Quality of Health Care in America. Crossing the quality chasm: a new health system for the 21st century/Committee on Quality Health Care in America, Institute of Medicine. Washington, DC: National Academy Press, 2001.

2. Chinman, M, Imm, P, Wandersman, A. *Getting to Outcomes 2004 Promoting Accountability through Methods and Tools for Planning, Implementation, and Evaluation.* January 2004. Sponsored by the Centers for Disease Control and Prevention. Rand Corporation. Available at: http://www.rand.org/pubs/technical_reports/2004/RAND_TR101.pdf. Accessed September 14, 2007.

3. ABIM Foundation. American Board of Internal Medicine; ACP-ASIM Foundation. American College of Physicians-American Society of Internal Medicine;

European Federation of Internal Medicine. Medical professionalism in the new millennium: a physician charter. *Ann Intern Med.* 2002 February 5;136:243–246.

4. Caldicott, CV. Sweeping up after the parade: professional, ethical, and patient care implications of "turfing". *Perspect Biol Med.* 2007;50:136–149.

5. Kassirer, JP. Professional societies and industry support: what is the quid pro quo? *Perspect Biol Med.* 2007 Winter;50:7–17.

6. Ellsbury, KE, Carline, JD, Wenrich, MD. Competing professionalism values among community-based family physicians. *Acad Med.* 2006;81(10 Suppl.):S25–29.

7. Straus, SE, Wilson, K, Rambaldini, G, Rath, D, Lin, Y, Gold, WL, Kapral, MK. Severe acute respiratory syndrome and its impact on professionalism: qualitative study of physicians' behaviour during an emerging healthcare crisis. *BMJ.* 2004;329:83.

8. Davis, DA, Mazmanian, PE, Fordis, M, Van Harrison, R, Thorpe, KE, Perrier, L. Accuracy of physician self-assessment compared with observed measures of competence: a systematic review. *JAMA.* 2006;296:1094–1102.

9. Wofford, MM, Wofford, JL, Bothra, J, Kendrick, SB, Smith, A, Lichstein, PR. Patient complaints about physician behaviors: a qualitative study. *Acad Med.* 2004 February;79:134–138.

10. Davis, DA, Thomson, MA, Oxman, AD, Haynes, RB. Changing physician performance. A systematic review of the effect of continuing medical education strategies. *JAMA.* 1995;274:700–705.

11. Australia. Health Insurance Commission. *Practice Incentives Program.* Available at: http://www.medicareaustralia.gov.au/providers/incentives_allowances/pip.shtml. Accessed September 14, 2007.

12. Royal College of Physicians and Surgeons of Canada. *CPD Program Guide.* 2006. Available at: http://rcpsc.medical.org/opd/cpd/prog-guide_e.pdf. Accessed September 14, 2007.

13. Fox, RD, Mazmanian, PE, Putnam, RW. *Changing and Learning in the Lives of Physicians.* New York: Praeger Publications, 1989.

14. Knowles, MS, Holton, EF, Swanson, RA, Holton, E. *The Adult Learner: The Definitive Classic in Adult Education and Human Resource Development.* Houston, TX: Gulf Publishing Company, 1998.

15. Schön, DA. *Educating the Reflective Practitioner: Toward a New Design for Teaching and Learning in the Professions.* San Francisco, CA: Jossey-Bass Publishers, 1990.

16. Kolb, D. *Experiential Learning: Experience as the Source of Learning and Development.* Englewood Cliffs, NJ: Prentice Hall, 1984.

17. Geertsma, R, Parker, RC, Whitbourne, SK. How physicians view the process of change in their practice behavior. *J Med Ed.* 1982;57:752–761.

18. Bandura, A. *Social Foundations of Thought and Action: A Social Cognitive Theory.* Englewood Cliffs, NJ: Prentice-Hall, 1986.

19. Grant, J. Learning needs assessment: assessing the need. *BMJ.* 2002; 324(7330): 156–159.

20. Norman, GR, Shannon, SI, Marrin, ML. The need for needs assessment in continuing medical education. *BMJ.* 2004;328:999–1001.

21. Boynton, PM, Greenhalgh, T. Hands-on guide to questionnaire research: selecting, designing, and developing your questionnaire. *BMJ*. 2004;328: 1312–1315.

22. Boynton, PM. Hands-on guide to questionnaire research: administering, analysing, and reporting your questionnaire. *BMJ*. 2004;328: 1372–1375.

23. Boynton, PM, Wood, GW, Greenhalgh, T. Reaching beyond the white middle classes. *BMJ*. 2004;328:1433–1436.

24. Antonelli Incalzi, R, Pedone, C, Pahor, M, Onder, G, Carbonin, PU; Gruppo Italiano di Farmacovigilanza nell'Anziano. Trends in prescribing ACE-inhibitors for congestive heart failure in elderly people. *Aging Clin Exp Res*. 2002;14:516–521.

25. Weil, E, Tu, JV. Quality of congestive heart failure treatment at a Canadian teaching hospital. *CMAJ*. 2001;165:284–287.

26. Green, LW, Kreuter, M, Deeds, S, Partridge, K. *Health Education Planning: A Diagnostic Approach*. Palo Alto, CA: Mayfield Press, 1980.

27. Miller, GE. Continuing medical education for what? *Med Educ*. 1967; 42: 320–326.

28. Davis, D, O'Brien, MA, Freemantle, N, Wolf, FM, Mazmanian, P, Taylor-Vaisey, A. Impact of formal continuing medical education: do conferences, workshops, rounds, and other traditional continuing education activities change physician behavior or health care outcomes? *JAMA*. 1999;282:867–874.

29. Davis, P, Russell, AS, Skeith, KJ. The use of standardized patients in the performance of a needs assessment and development of a CME intervention in rheumatology for primary care physicians. *J Rheumatol*. 1997;24:1995–1999.

30. Craig, JL. The OSCME (Opportunity for Self-Assessment CME). *J Contin Educ Health Prof*. 1991;11:87–94.

31. Kantrowitz, MP. Problem-based learning in continuing medical education: some critical issues. *J Contin Educ Health Prof*. 1991; 11:11–18.

32. Steinert, Y, Snell, LS. Interactive lecturing: strategies for increasing participation in large group presentations. *Med Teach*. 1999; 21:37–42.

33. Hewson, MG. A theory-based faculty development program for clinician-educators. *Acad Med*. 2000;75:498–501.

34. Silver, I, Rath, D. Making the formal lecture more interactive. *Intercom*. 2002 October; 15:6–8.

35. Thomson O'Brien, MA, Freemantle, N, Oxman, AD, Wolf, F, Davis, DA, Herrin, J. Continuing education meetings and workshops: effects on professional practice and health care outcomes (Cochrane Review). In *The Cochrane Library*, Issue 2. Chichester, UK: John Wiley & Sons, Ltd. 2004

36. Davis, D, Evans, M, Jadad, A, Perrier, L, Rath, D, Ryan, D, Sibbald, G, Straus, S, Rappolt, S, Wowk, M, Zwarenstein, M. The case for knowledge translation: shortening the journey from evidence to effect. *BMJ*. 2003;327:33–35.

37. Stross, JK. The educationally influential physician. *J Contin Educ Health Prof*. 1996;16:167–172.

38. Dixon, J. Evaluation criteria in studies of continuing education in the health professions: a critical review and a suggested strategy. *Eval Health Prof*. 1978;1:47–65.

39. De Buda, Y, Woolf, CR. Saturday at the university: a format for success. *J Contin Educ Health Prof.* 1990; 10:279–284.

40. Miller, RG, Ashar, BH, Getz, KJ. Evaluation of an audience response system for the continuing education of health professionals. *J Contin Educ Health Prof.* 2003;23:109–115.

41. Arnold, L, Shue, CK, Kalishman, S, Prislin, M, Pohl, C, Pohl, H, Stern, DT. Can there be a single system for peer assessment of professionalism among medical students? A multi-institutional study. *Acad Med.* 2007 June;82:578–586

42. Hays, RB, Davies, HA, Beard, JD, Caldon, LJ, Farmer, EA, Finucane, PM, McCrorie, P, Newble, DI, Schuwirth, LW, Sibbald, GR. Selecting performance assessment methods for experienced physicians. *Med Educ.* 2002 October; 36:910–917.

43. Southgate, L, Hays, RB, Norcini, J, Mulholland, H, Ayers, B, Woolliscroft, J, Cusimano, M, McAvoy, P, Ainsworth, M, Haist, S, Campbell, M. Setting performance standards for medical practice: a theoretical framework. *Med Educ.* 2001 May;35:474–481.

44. Scoles, PV, Hawkins, RE, LaDuca, A. Assessment of clinical skills in medical practice. *J Contin Educ Health Prof.* 2003;23:182–190.

45. Schuwirth, LW, van der Vleuten, CP. The use of clinical simulations in assessment. *Med Educ.* 2003;37(Suppl. 1):65–71.

46. Shaw, ME, Wright, JM. *Scales for the Measurement of Attitudes.* New York: McGraw Hill, 1967.

Definitions of Professionalism

DICTIONARY DEFINITIONS

Oxford English Dictionary, 2nd Edition, Oxford, UK, Clarendon Press, 1989.
The occupation which one professes to be skilled in and to follow. a. a vocation in which a professed knowledge of some department of learning or science is used in its application to the affairs of others or in the practice of an art founded upon it. b. in a wider sense, any calling or occupation by which a person habitually earns his living.

Webster's 3rd International Dictionary of the English Language, Springfield, Massachusetts, Merriam Webster, 1981.
A calling requiring specialized knowledge and often long and intensive preparation including instruction in skills and methods as well as in the scientific, historical, or scholarly principles underlying such skills and methods; maintaining by force of organization or concerted opinion high standards of achievement and conduct, and committing its members to continued study and to a kind of work which has for its prime purpose the rendering of a public service.

SOCIAL SCIENCES LITERATURE

Paul Starr, The Social Transformation of American Medicine. New York, Basic Books, 1984, p. 15.
Professional authority can be defined, in part, by a distinctive type of dependency condition – the dependence on the professional's superior competence. Dependence also arises at times from the emotional needs of clients and the administrative functions of the professions, created especially by the welfare state. And as I have indicated, the legitimating of professional authority involves three distinctive claims: first that the knowledge and competence of the professional have been validated by a community of his or her peers; second that this consensually validated knowledge and competence rests on rational, scientific grounds; and third, that the professional's judgment and advice are oriented toward a set of substantive values such as health. These aspects of legitimacy correspond to the kinds of attributes – collegial, cognitive, and moral – usually cited in definitions of the term profession. A profession, sociologists have suggested, is an occupation that regulates itself through systematic,

required training and collegial discipline, that has a base in technical specialized knowledge, and that has a service rather than a profit orientation, enshrined in its code of ethics.

William Sullivan, Work and Integrity: The Crisis and Promise of Professionalism in North America. New York, Harper Collins, 1995, p. 2.

Professionalism is a very loosely defined term. Originally, of course, it referred to the classic honorific occupations of medicine, the bar, and the clergy. These occupations certainly enjoy high status. When asked to rank the most desirable jobs, Americans have consistently placed medical doctors just below Supreme Court justices, the top ranked job. Lawyers, clergy, dentists, college professors, and architects always appear among the top twenty ranks. Professions are typically described as occupations characterized by three features: specialized training in a field of codified knowledge usually acquired by formal education and apprenticeship, public recognition of a certain autonomy on the part of the community of practitioners to regulate their own standards of practice, and a commitment to provide service to the public which goes beyond the economic welfare of the practitioners.

Elliot Freidson, Professional Dominance: The Social Structure of Medical Care. Chicago, Illinois, Aldine, 1970, p. xvii.

It is useful to think of a profession as an occupation which has assumed a dominant position in a division of labor, so that it gains control over the determination of the substance of its own works. Unlike most occupations, it is autonomous or self-directing. The occupation sustains this special status by its persuasive profession of the extraordinary trustworthiness of its members. The trustworthiness it professes naturally includes ethicality, and also knowledgeable skill. In fact, the profession claims to be the most reliable authority on the nature of the reality it deals with. *Note*: Freidson in his 1994 book *Professionalism Reborn* (p. 16) suggested that he believed it extremely difficult to define professionalism. "In all, then, it would seem that in the present state of the art of theorizing about professions, recent comments on the issue of definition missed the mark. The definitional problem that has plagued the field for over half a century is not one created by squabbling peasants to be solved eschewing definition entirely . . . . The problem I suggest lies much deeper than that, it is created by attempting to treat profession as if it were a generic rather than a changing historic concept with particular roots in an industrial nation strongly influenced by Anglo-American institutions."

Hafferty F.W. Definitions of professionalism: a search for meaning and identity. Clin Orthop Relat Res. 2006; 449: 193–204, 200.

My preferred medical definition of professionalism is built around the tripartite framework of (1) core knowledge and skills, (2) ethical principles, and (3) a selflessness and/or service orientation. The key here is to differentiate between ethics and service versus altruism. My preferred core sociological definition is grounded in Sullivan's tripartite of (1) expert knowledge, (2) self-regulation, and (3) a fiduciary responsibility to altruism. Finally, with its emphasis on civic engagement, is Wynia et al.'s (1) devotion to service, (2) a profession of values, and (3) negotiation with society (to balance medical values with other societal values).

SELECTED DEFINITIONS FROM THE MEDICAL LITERATURE

Swick H.M. Towards a normative definition of professionalism.
Acad Med. 2000; 75: 612–616.
The following are the categories listed by Swick. In his article, each is followed by an explanatory narrative.

> Medical professionalism, then, comprises the following set of behaviors:
> Physicians subordinate their own interests to the interests of others.
> Physicians adhere to high ethical and moral standards.
> Physicians respond to societal needs, and their behaviors reflect a social contract with the communities served.
> Physicians evince core humanistic values, including honesty and integrity, caring and compassion, altruism and empathy, respect for others, and trustworthiness.
> Physicians exercise accountability for themselves and for their colleagues.
> Physicians demonstrate a continuing commitment to excellence.
> Physicians exhibit a commitment to scholarship and to advancing their field.
> Physicians deal with high levels of complexity and uncertainty.
> Physicians reflect upon their actions and decisions.

Wynia M.K., Latham S.R., Kao A.C., Berg J.W., Emanuel L. NEJM. 1999; 341: 612–616.
Three core elements of professionalism, each different in nature, are necessary for it to work properly. First, professionalism requires a moral commitment to the ethic of medical service which we will call devotion to medical service and its values. This devotion leads naturally to a public, normative act: public profession of this ethic. Public profession of the ethic serves both to maintain professional's devotion to medical service and to assert its values in societal discussions. These discussions lead naturally to engagement in a political process of negotiation, in which professionals advocate for health care values in the context of other important competing societal values.

Cruess S.R, Johnston S., Cruess R.L. 'Profession': a working definition for medical educators. Teach Learn Med. 2004; 16: 90–92.
Profession: An occupation whose core element is work based upon the mastery of a complex body of knowledge and skills. It is a vocation in which knowledge of some department of science or learning or the practice of an art founded upon it is used in the service of others. Its members are governed by codes of ethics and profess a commitment to competence, integrity and morality, altruism, and the promotion of the public good within their domain. These commitments form the basis of a social contract between a profession and society, which in return grants the profession a monopoly over the use of its knowledge base, the right to considerable autonomy in practice and the privilege of self-regulation. Professions and their members are accountable to those served, to the profession, and to society.

Stern D.T. (ed.). Measuring Medical Professionalism. New York,
Oxford University Press, 2005, p. 19.
Professionalism is demonstrated through a foundation of clinical competence, communication skills, and ethical and legal understanding, upon which is built the

aspiration to and wise application of the principles of professionalism: excellence, humanism, accountability, and altruism.

MEDICAL ORGANIZATIONS

American Board of Internal Medicine. Project Professionalism, 1999 (revised).
Professionalism in medicine requires the physician to serve the interests of the patient above his or her self-interest. Professionalism aspires to altruism, accountability, excellence, duty, service, honor, integrity, and respect for others. The elements of professionalism required of candidates seeking certification and recertification from the ABIM encompass commitment to the highest standards of excellence in the practice of medicine and in the generation and dissemination of knowledge, a commitment to sustain the interests and welfare of patients, a commitment to be responsive to the health needs of society. These elements are further defined as follows:

Altruism is the essence of professionalism. The best interest of the patients, not self-interest, is the rule.

Accountability is required at many levels – individual patients, society, and the profession. Physicians are accountable to their patients for fulfilling the implied contract governing the patient/physician relationship. They are also accountable to society for addressing the health needs of the public and their profession for adhering to medicine's time-honored ethical precepts.

Excellence entails a conscientious effort to exceed ordinary expectations and to make a commitment to lifelong learning. Commitment to excellence is an acknowledged goal for all physicians.

Duty is the free acceptance of a commitment to service as commitment entails being available and responsive when "on call," accepting inconvenience to meet the needs of one's patients, enduring unavoidable risks to one's self when a patient's welfare is at stake, advocating the best possible care regardless of the ability to pay, seeking active roles in professional organizations, and volunteering one's skills and expertise for the welfare of the community.

Honor and integrity are the consistent regard for the highest standards of behavior and the refusal to violate one's personal and professional codes. Honor and integrity imply being fair, being truthful, keeping one's word, meeting commitments, and being straightforward. They also require recognition of the possibility of conflict of interest and avoidance of relationships that allow personal gain to supersede the best interests of the patient.

Respect for others (patients and their families, other physicians and professional colleagues such as nurses, medical students, residents, subspecialty fellows, and self) is the essence of humanism and humanism is both central to professionalism and fundamental to enhancing collegiality amongst physicians.

Royal College of Physicians of London. Doctors in Society: Medical Professionalism in a Changing World. London, Royal College of Physicians of London, 2005, p. 14–15.
Medical professionalism signifies a set of values, behaviors, and relationships that underpins the trust the public has in doctors.

The values, behaviors, and relationships are as follows:

Medicine is a vocation in which a doctor's knowledge, clinical skills, and judgment are put in the service of protecting and restoring human well-being. This purpose is realized through a partnership between patient and doctor, one based on mutual respect, individual responsibility, and appropriate accountability.

In their day-to-day practice, doctors are committed to integrity, compassion, altruism, continuous improvement, excellence, working in partnership with members of the wider health care team.

These values, which underpin the science and practice of medicine, form the basis for a moral contract between the medical profession and society. Each party has a duty to work to strengthen the system of health care on which our collective human dignity depends.

Royal College of Physicians and Surgeons of Canada

"Professional Role Document": The professional is a person who belongs to a group (a profession) which possesses specialized knowledge, skills, and attitudes which have been obtained after a long period of study and which are used to benefit other members of society. The term professionalism is used to describe those skills, attitudes, and behaviors which we have come to expect from individuals during the practice of their profession and includes such concepts as maintenance of competence, ethical behavior, integrity, honesty, altruism, service to others, adherence to professional codes, justice, respect for others, self-regulation, etc.

American Board of Internal Medicine Foundation. American College of Physicians Foundation. European Federation of Internal Medicine. A Physician Charter. Brennan T. and 17 co-authors. Medical professionalism in the new millennium: a physician charter. Lancet. 2002; 359: 520–522 and Ann Int Med. 2002; 136: 243–246.

The charter outlines three fundamental principles and ten professional responsibilities which are listed below. In the published version, an explanatory paragraph follows each of the categories.

Fundamental principles:

- Principle of primacy of patient welfare
- Principle of patient autonomy
- Principle of social justice.

Professional responsibilities:

- Commitment to professional competence
- Commitment to honesty with patients
- Commitment to patient confidentiality
- Commitment to maintaining appropriate relations with patients
- Commitment to improving quality of care
- Commitment to improving access to care
- Commitment to a just distribution of finite resources
- Commitment to scientific knowledge
- Commitment to maintaining trust by managing conflicts of interest
- Commitment to professional responsibilities.

Association of American Medical Colleges.
The AAMC uses Swick's list of attributes as its working definition.

Accreditation Council for Graduate Medical Education
Residents must demonstrate a commitment to carrying out professional responsibilities and an adherence to ethical principles. Residents are expected to demonstrate:
- compassion, integrity, and respect for others;
- responsiveness to patient needs that supersedes self-interest;
- respect for patient privacy and autonomy;
- accountability to patients, society and the profession; and,
- sensitivity and responsiveness to a diverse patient population, including but not limited to diversity in gender, age, culture, race, religion, disabilities, and sexual orientation.

Revised Version. February, 2007

Core Attributes of Professionalism

ATTRIBUTES OF THE HEALER

Caring and compassion: a sympathetic consciousness of another's distress together with a desire to alleviate it.

Insight: self-awareness; the ability to recognize and understand one's actions, motivations, and emotions.

Openness: willingness to hear, accept, and deal with the views of others without reserve or pretense.

Respect for the healing function: the ability to recognize, elicit, and foster the power to heal inherent in each patient.

Respect for patient dignity and autonomy: the commitment to respect and ensure subjective well-being and sense of worth in others and recognize the patient's personal freedom of choice and right to participate fully in his/her care.

Presence: to be fully present for a patient without distraction and to fully support and accompany the patient throughout care.

ATTRIBUTES OF BOTH THE HEALER AND THE PROFESSIONAL

Competence: to master and keep current the knowledge and skills relevant to medical practice.

Commitment: being obligated or emotionally impelled to act in the best interest of the patient; a pledge given by way of the Hippocratic Oath or its modern equivalent.

Confidentiality: to not divulge patient information without just cause.

Autonomy: the physician's freedom to make independent decisions in the best interest of the patients and for the good of society.

Altruism: the unselfish regard for, or devotion to, the welfare of others; placing the needs of the patient before one's self-interest.

From: McGill University Faculty of Medicine Undergraduate Program on "Physicianship".

Integrity and honesty: firm adherence to a code of moral values; incorruptibility.

Morality and ethical conduct: to act for the public good; conformity to the ideals of right human conduct in dealings with patients, colleagues, and society.

Trustworthiness: worthy of trust, reliable.

ATTRIBUTES OF THE PROFESSIONAL

Responsibility to the profession: the commitment to maintain the integrity of the moral and collegial nature of the profession and to be accountable for one's conduct to the profession.

Self-regulation: the privilege of setting standards; being accountable for one's actions and conduct in medical practice and for the conduct of one's colleagues.

Responsibility to society: the obligation to use one's expertise for, and to be accountable to, society for those actions, both personal and of the profession, which relate to the public good.

Teamwork: the ability to recognize and respect the expertise of others and work with them in the patient's best interest.

The Teaching of Professionalism

Vignettes for Discussion

FOR UNDERGRADUATE PRE-CLINICAL MEDICAL STUDENTS

First identify the elements, characteristics, or attributes of professionalism raised by each of the following cases. You may then discuss solutions to the problem.

Case #1

You notice a colleague reading the chart of a patient who is a personal friend of the colleague. He has not been involved in the patient's care. You know that the chart has some sensitive personal information in it.

Case #2

The medical school assigns families to first-year students for early clinical experience. You are on an elevator and hear a student discussing his assigned family, including the names of the family, in derogatory terms.

Case #3

A drug company representative gives you a stethoscope with the name of an expensive cardiac medicine prominently displayed on it.

Case #4

A student observes an exemplary student during the end of semester final using a textbook during a major closed book examination.

Case #5

A patient and family that you have been assigned to follow gives you information that may influence care and asks that you do not tell anyone, including the patient's doctor.

FOR UNDERGRADUATE CLINICAL MEDICAL STUDENTS

First identify the elements, characteristics, or attributes of professionalism raised by each of the following cases. You may then discuss solutions to the problem.

From: McGill University Faculty of Medicine Undergraduate and Postgraduate Teaching Programs.

Case #1

A final-year medical student believes the attending surgeon is inebriated while performing an operation.

Case #2

A senior resident asks a medical student to put in an arterial line. The student has never seen or performed this procedure before. The resident explains the technique, then tells the student to proceed and leaves.

Case #3

A physician on an overseas flight diagnoses a probable myocardial infarction in a foreign visitor. The patient is upset at the prospect of entering a strange health care system and requests that the physician accompany him in the ambulance to the hospital. The physician, who has other commitments, agrees.

Case #4

You are a student in general surgery. When on call, a woman arrives in the ER with acute appendicitis. The woman is operated on by the chief resident, with you assisting and the attending surgeon supervising. During the case, the chief resident injures the cecum and has to perform a partial cecectomy along with an appendectomy. The next morning on rounds, he tells the patient that "everything went perfectly."

Case #5

You see a patient with severe cellulitis in the ER with a senior resident. The patient reports that she has been treating herself with intermittent washing with alcohol and salt water and then applying corn syrup to the area. When presenting the patient to the attending, the resident starts with "This must be the dumbest lady alive ..."

Case #6

You receive a call from the nephew of a patient of yours asking for information about his health. His uncle, who is your patient, suffers from coronary artery disease and diabetes that is poorly controlled.

FOR RESIDENTS AND CONTINUING PROFESSIONAL DEVELOPMENT

First identify the elements, characteristics, or attributes of professionalism raised by each of the following cases. You may then discuss solutions to the problem.

Case #1

Your daughter is scheduled to graduate from high school this afternoon. As you are preparing to sign out to a colleague, one of your long-time patients presents in the ER with chest pain. You enter the ER and a partner in your group practice is already there to evaluate the situation. As you know that he is competent and conscientious, you go to reassure your patient. He pleads with you to stay.

Case #2

A general hospital has asked all attending staff to work one weekend day and one night per month in the ER. A full-time attending refuses to work nights or weekends.

Case #3

An emergency room physician, seeing increased young people involved in car accidents due to alcohol, organizes a series of visits to high schools in the community to present the problem and the effects of alcohol on students.

Case #4

You have become close friends with one of your colleagues and notice that at social events he frequently drinks excessively and he admits that he binges on weekends. You are on call with him and you notice alcohol on his breath.

Case #5

A long-time patient of yours requests a note from you documenting a nonexistent illness in order to recover cancellation penalties from the airlines on a nonrefundable ticket.

Case #6

Doctor Dell practices in a rural community. He has no training or experience in clinical trial methodology. A drug company offers him $100.00 for each patient he recruits from his practice to evaluate a medication in postmarketing surveillance.

FOR BASIC SCIENCE FACULTY

First identify the elements, characteristics, or attributes of professionalism raised by each of the following cases. You may then discuss solutions to the problem.

Case #1

A student in a master's program in epidemiology decides to leave after one year without fully completing his research. He wishes to go to medical school and asks his supervisor for a recommendation. The student has been told his work is good and he has published several papers. His supervisor wishes him to finish his research. The supervisor sends the recommendation well past the deadline.

Case #2

A professor of physiology observes an honors student using a crib sheet during a major examination.

Case #3

During an anatomy laboratory, a professor of anatomy observes two students throwing a human heart back and forth in a playful fashion.

Case #4

A professor of pharmacology has an appointment with a student to go over his evaluation. He has discussed the student's performance with colleagues and all agree that it is unsatisfactory. He is concerned that if the evaluation is unsatisfactory, he may expose himself to time-consuming appeals and confrontation. He tells the student his performance is below average, but will grade it satisfactory overall.

Case #5

The medical school assigns a family to first-year students for early clinical experience. A professor of biochemistry is on an elevator and hears a student discussing his assigned family, including the names of the family, in derogatory terms.

APPENDIX D

A Matrix for "Matching" Teaching Methods to Attributes

Attributes of Professionalism	Educational Methodologies							
	Formal Lectures	Small Group Discussions	Case Discussions/ Clinical Vignettes	Experiential / Independent Learning	Role Modeling	Role Plays / Videotape Reviews	Independent Learning	Other
Caring and Compassion								
Insight								
Openness								
Respect for the Healing Function								
Respect for Patient Dignity and Autonomy								
Presence								
Competence								
Commitment								
Confidentiality								
Autonomy								
Altruism								
Integrity and Honesty								
Morality and Ethical Conduct								
Trustworthiness								
Responsibility to the Profession								
Self-regulation								
Responsibility to Society								
Teamwork								

Glossary of Educational Methodologies:
Formal Lectures.......................: traditional lectures, grand rounds, large group presentations
Small Group Discussions.........: interactive discussions in non-lecture, non-clinical settings (e.g., workshops, journal clubs, sit-down rounds)
Case Discussions/Vignettes.......: presentation and discussion of clinical cases in a variety of settings
Experiential Learning...............: learning while participating in patient care (e.g., managing ambulatory patients, hospital work, community service)
Role Modeling...........................: the acquisition of attitudes or skills by observing and patterning the behaviour of others
Role Plays/Videotape ....: the use of videotapes and role plays for learning
Independent Learning ....: the independent use of educational resources (e.g., books, journals, film, internet) in the pursuit of learning
Portfolios..................................: a collection of papers and other forms of evidence that demonstrate that learning has taken place
Narratives ....: written accounts of personal experiences

Sample Grid for Use with Discussion of Vignettes

This grid is used in conjunction with the professionalism vignettes found in Appendix C. The learner is asked to read the vignettes and identify the elements of professionalism raised in each case, and using this information, discuss their approach to the issue.

		Case #1	Case #2	Case #3	Case #4	Case #5
Caring and Compassion	A sympathetic consciousness of another's distress together with a desire to alleviate it.					
Insight	Self-awareness; the ability to recognize and understand one's actions, motivations and emotions.					
Openness	Willingness to hear, accept, and deal with the views of others without reserve or pretense.					
Respect for the Healing Function	The ability to recognize, elicit and foster the power to heal inherent in each patient.					
Respect Patient Dignity & Autonomy	The commitment to respect and ensure subjective well being and sense of worth in others and recognizes the patient's personal freedom of choice and right to participate fully in his/her care.					
Presence	To be fully present for a patient without distraction and to fully support and accompany the patient throughout care.					
Competence	To master and keep current the knowledge and skills relevant to medical practice.					
Commitment	Being obligated or emotionally impelled to act in the best interest of the patient; a pledge given by way of the Hippocratic oath or its modern equivalent.					
Confidentiality	To not divulge patient information without just cause.					
Autonomy	The physician's freedom to make independent decisions in the best interest of the patient and for the good of society.					

Altruism	The unselfish regard for, or devotion to, the welfare of others; placing the needs of the patient before one's self interest.							
Integrity and Honesty	Firm adherence to a code of moral values; incorruptibility.							
Morality and Ethical Conduct	To act for the public good; conformity to the ideals of right human conduct in dealings with patients, colleagues, and society.							
Trustworthiness	Worthy of trust, reliable.							
Responsibility to the Profession	The commitment to maintain the integrity of the moral and collegial nature of the profession and to be accountable for one's conduct to the profession.							
Self-Regulation	The privilege of setting the standards; being accountable for one's actions and conduct in medical practice and for the conduct of ones colleagues.							
Responsibility to Society	The obligation to use one's expertise for, and to be accountable to, society for those actions, both personal and of the profession, which relate to the public good.							
Teamwork	The ability to recognize the expertise of others and to work with them in the patient's best interest.							

From: McGill University Faculty of Medicine Postgraduate Core Competencies Program: The Resident as Professional, 2007.

Sample Questions to Guide Discussion about the Social Contract

Small-Group Leaders' Guide with Suggested Responses

"There are rights, statutes, privileges, and obligations of the profession".

1. **What does the concept of the social contract mean to you?**
   - That there are obligations/expectations of physicians
   - That society has obligations toward the profession. Those obligations must be fulfilled to maintain the trust needed for negotiations.

2. **Who are the parties in this contract?**
   - Physicians and their collective profession
   - Patients and their collective (public)
   - Government

3. **Who negotiates the social contract?**
   - Many, with both direct and indirect influences
   - Physicians, health professionals, patients, patient advisory groups, health establishments, pharmaceutical and medical supply companies, the public, governments, the media, etc.

4. **What happens when expectations of the contract are not met?**
   - Professional lapse—loss of trust and a shift in the privileges accorded to the profession, that is, self-regulation, respect, status
   - Societal lapse—loss of trust and a tendency of MDs to regard work as an "occupation." Loss of commitment and altruism.

5. **Give concrete examples of some of the expectations of the social contract, as it applies to your setting now or in the future.**
   - That is, in self-regulation – "squealing" vs. obligation
   - Altruism/lifestyle
   - Relationship to society, in an underfunded system with too few health care professionals
   - How to promote change as individual/through organizations
   - Relationships to fellow professionals.

From: McGill University Faculty of Medicine Postgraduate Core Competencies Program: The Resident as Professional, 2007.

Professionalism Program for Residents: Suggested Outline for Small Group Facilitators

A faculty member will lead each small group, with a senior resident as co-leader.

The goal of the small-group discussion is to let the residents apply the material from the plenary and promote discussion in an interdisciplinary, cross-specialty format.

1. **Introduction of session and participants (ten minutes)**
   - Ask residents to introduce themselves, say what discipline they are in, and state their expectations for the afternoon.
   - Group leader(s) will briefly review the small-group activities and goals ("to apply core concepts in residents' clinical and professional practice").
   - Mention that many participants will have done some of this before as medical students, but it is now reframed for the resident's context, and for the updated version of the social contract.
   - Choose a scribe (or the co-leader can do it).

2. **Identifying issues and related values using vignettes (fifty to sixty minutes)**
   - Ask the residents to read chosen vignettes and identify the elements/attributes of professionalism raised by each (the residents will have the cases but not the "elements"; responses can be scribed on a flip chart or on the "grid" each resident has).
   - Then, ask the residents how they would handle each situation. What would they do? What professional values would they use?
   - There is no need to complete all vignettes if things are going well and discussion is valuable.

Take a stretch and snack break here.

3. **Discussion of the social contract (forty to sixty minutes)**
   - This is a group discussion, the goal of which is to ensure the residents understand the basic concepts of the social contract and can apply them in their own setting.

From: McGill University Faculty of Medicine Postgraduate Core Competencies Program: The Resident as Professional, 2007.

- The questions will be used to trigger discussion. The group leaders have "suggested answers." There are no "right" answers. The residents should be encouraged to think of concrete clinical examples that apply in their setting.

4. **Wrap-up and evaluation (fifteen minutes)**

- Ask residents what important key point or concept they will take away, and how they will apply it. Summarize on a flip chart. Group leaders please bring copies of flip chart notes to organizers at end of session (with your name on it).
- Evaluations to be completed and handed to you before residents leave.

Sample Evaluation Form for Residents' Half-Day Program on Professionalism

Please rate the following statements by circling the number that most reflects you opinion	Strongly disagree	Disagree	Neutral	Agree	Strongly agree
The overall program					
The program addressed my needs	1	2	3	4	5
The program enabled me to learn about professionalism	1	2	3	4	5
The time allocated was adequate	1	2	3	4	5
The program was well run	1	2	3	4	5
I would recommend a similar program to my colleagues	1	2	3	4	5
The plenary session					
The information was clearly presented	1	2	3	4	5
The information was pertinent and relevant	1	2	3	4	5
The time allocated was adequate	1	2	3	4	5
The small-group session					
The session allowed me to apply plenary concepts	1	2	3	4	5
There was opportunity for interaction	1	2	3	4	5
The small-group leaders were excellent facilitators	1	2	3	4	5
I enjoyed meeting with residents from other disciplines	1	2	3	4	5

From: McGill University Faculty of Medicine Postgraduate Core Competencies Program: The Resident as Professional, 2007.

For each of the following statements please identify the extent of your knowledge or skill on a scale of 1–5 (1 = not at all, 5 = to a large extent), *before* and *after* you attended the resident half-day on professionalism

My ability to …	Before workshop					After workshop				
	Not at all			To a large extent		Not at all			To a large extent	
Define professionalism	1	2	3	4	5	1	2	3	4	5
Identify the attributes of professionalism	1	2	3	4	5	1	2	3	4	5
Integrate concepts of professionalism in my clinical setting	1	2	3	4	5	1	2	3	4	5
Describe the social contract between physician and society	1	2	3	4	5	1	2	3	4	5
Discuss how the social contract applies to my setting	1	2	3	4	5	1	2	3	4	5

What did you like most about this workshop?
What could be improved?
What key point(s) or concept(s) will you take away?
Give an example of how will you apply what you have learned.
General comments about the session?
Residency Level: R2___   Other (specify)_____ Discipline _____

Thank-you. Please return this evaluation to your group leader before leaving.

Index